Living with
Restenosis
2-in-1 book

Includes:
Surviving a Successful Heart Attack
-and-
Chronic Total Occlusion:
After the Heart Attack, the Statins and
Restenosis

Mike Stone

Living with Restenosis: 2-in-1 book is intended solely for informational purposes and is not intended as personal medical advice. Personal medical advice should be obtained from your own doctor or other qualified medical authority.

http://www.heartrecovery.net

While every precaution has been taken in the preparation of this book, the publisher assumes no responsibilities for errors or omissions, or for damages resulting from the use of information contained herein.

Heart Recovery Publishing
2028 Sawmill Rd.
River Ridge, La 70123

ISBN: 1452836167
EAN-13: 9781452836164.
Cover design by the author

To Esty and the kids-
Naamah, Sagi, Rakefet and Tuval

Special thanks to Professor A. Teddy Weiss, Hadassdah Hospital
Mount Scopus, for getting me through that certain weekend,

and to

Dr. Hisham Nassar, Hadassah Hospital Ein Kerem who
performed the angiogram, angioplasty and inserted the stent,

and to

the very dedicated staff at both hospitals.

Preface
Living with Restenosis

Living with Restenosis is a 2-in-1 book including *Surviving a Successful Heart Attack* and *Chronic Total Occlusion: After the Heart Attack, the Statins and Restenosis*. Why a 2-in-1 book? Aren't they both independent entities? On the one hand, they are. They can be purchased separately. On the other hand, each one is incomplete. They compliment each other; they convey the whole story.

Surviving a Successful Heart Attack (SASHA), first published in 2004, covers a more naive period of my life. Good health was something to be taken for granted, heart attacks were only for fat people or smokers, cholesterol was that bogey substance to be minimized at all costs, and terms such as 'stent' and 'statins' were not part of my vocabulary.

Heart attacks happen to other people, not to non-smoking normal weight people as myself, until reality strikes -- HEART ATTACK! And then the real reality; the physical recovery from the heart attack was nothing when compared to the recovery from the statins, which so disrupted my professional and personal life.

SASHA also covers the period of my life when cholesterol transformed from foe to ... not foe. It covers the period of discovering that my first 50 years of personal dietary guidelines were based on mass-media advertising, huge corporations, and worst of all, bad science. It ends with me standing on both feet, after recuperating from both the physical heart attack and the statin-induced side effects; however, what next – to what direction?

Chronic Total Occlusion (previously published in 2007 as *The Next 20,000*), is that new direction. To the casual reader, the lifestyle changes I have made may be construed as radical, eccentric. That is what makes *CTO* incomplete. Without experiencing the emotional scars described in SASHA that have remained following those two statin-induced side effect years, the reader of 'CTO' will not be able to appreciate a lifestyle I now accept as totally normal.

Table of Contents

Surviving a *Successful* Heart Attack

Mike Stone

Published by LULU Press
3131 RDU Center, Suite 210
Morrisville, NC 27560

First Edition: July, 2004
Second Edition: August, 2005
ISBN 978-1-4116-0834-4
Cover design by the author
          Photograph on back cover: Yogev (Yogli) Yehuda

Author's note

Not being an avid reader, I never thought that one day I would author a book let alone one relating to the medical field. Initially I had envisioned a short essay and/or a pamphlet regarding the positive role that bicycle riding played in my post heart attack life. At the time I contemplated releasing it as an eBook – the wonder of the internet. I could have uploaded it and it would be immediately available world wide.

As I compiled more and more information, my pamphlet expanded into a 200 page work and I developed an itch to have it published hard copy, rather than see it as a virtual internet file. This meant contacting a publisher, preferably through a literary agent. The feedback from the agents was similar. "Why is my book different and better than competitive works on the market?" An interesting question indeed. I never had any intention of writing a 'better book' nor competing with any other existing book relating to heart attacks.

As the book was nearing completion, I decided to explore the avenue of self publishing and stumbled upon a recent technological development known as POD – Print on Demand.

This was the ultimate solution for me. While I do hope to reach a maximum number of people, even without a single sale, I have already profited. Obviously I cannot turn back the clock and prevent the heart attack I had three years ago, however, the vast amount of knowledge that I acquired while researching this book, will do much to prevent my next heart attack that may have been on the way. This book may now be finished, however my learning process continues.

I would like to acknowledge several individuals whose valuable contributions made it possible for me to finalize this project.

First and foremost, my wife Esty who *stood by* me during my two dark years and *put up* with me while I spent an endless amount of hours assembling data.

I am also grateful to Ziona Ben–Hamo for proof reading and to Al Brandler and Rich Stone for their comments regarding the preliminary manuscript.

I am indebted to Garry Borsi for his constant source of inspiration.

Thanks to Tony Wiseman and Orit Josefi of the Outlook Organization, for doing what they do.........

And finally, to 'Dad' for his comments regarding the final manuscript.

Mike Stone
July, 2004

Preface

I am neither a doctor nor a nurse. Once upon a time I did earn a Boy Scout merit badge in first aid but that was about forty years ago. What then gives me the authority to write a 'Health' type book?

Three years ago, at the age of 51, I found myself on the way to the Emergency Ward while undergoing a heart attack. In retrospect, I can say that I was most fortunate in seeking immediate medical help at the time of the attack, however I later discovered that there was a considerable amount of information not covered in the Rehab Program regarding the ***real recovery*** from a heart attack. Understandably, no two people emerge from this type of experience at the same level of health, and no two people react exactly in the same manner to medication that becomes a daily necessity. Not everything written in this book will apply to everyone who has had a heart attack. There definitely is life after a heart attack; however it is different not only from the obvious physical standpoint, but also from the mental and/or emotional standpoint as well.

This is not a typical *how to* book. I will leave the writing of the "Heart Attack Guide for Dummies" to someone else, assuming it has not already been written. This is the story of an average non-smoker, non-overweight, ordinary guy who surprised everyone with his heart attack; that is everyone except my wife Esty who constantly warned me that a heart attack was on its way, and the unpleasant surprises along the way to mental/emotional recovery and self-acceptance.

Who is this book for? First and foremost it is for the heart attack victim. Should he/she react in a similar fashion to my experience to the medications, the results should not come as a total surprise. Secondly, to his/her spouse and immediate family – an understanding and comprehension of *what's going on* may prevent a potentially tense situation from exploding into a relationship strained unnecessarily.   And to the general public that is concerned about a potential heart attack in the future, you may decide to give up the cigarettes, get rid of some of the excess baggage and begin an exercise regimen compatible with your age and general health, preferably after consulting with a physician.

I have deviated a bit from my initial thoughts regarding *for whom this book is for* because of the events in the three year post heart attack period I personally encountered and what I have learned. It is now my hope that the medical establishment that deals with cardiology will become more attuned to the potential upheaval in the *quality of life* that post heart attack patients may experience and certainly no less important, to re-examine the real reason that caused the heart attack in the first place.

What originally started out as a layman's book of answers for other heart patients has evolved into more of a book of questions.........

1

4788.3

10:09

March 15, 2003

51.0

26.50

4788.3

2

The Before Years

That first chapter was great, was it not? I promise that it will be clear by the end of the book. Theoretically, this is the first real chapter. I mentioned in the Preface that I'm just an average non-smoker, non-overweight, ordinary guy. I should also mention that for years I swam two - three times a week. Friends and business associates saw me as being in great physical condition for a man of my age.

Why then the heart attack? Were the causes linked to my genetics, my environment or to my personal habits or was it a combination of all three factors?

Most doctors would probably answer that it was a combination of all three factors. This analysis would technically be correct. It does sound logical that an individual reacts to one's own environment and to some degree on his/her genetic makeup and natural stamina. The doctor's report that I received upon discharge from the hospital revealed my condition prior to entering the hospital. It was determined one of the contributing factors for my heart attack was the existence of heart disease in the family. Three years before my heart attack, my mother at age 75 had a heart attack and underwent a quadruple bypass operation. Conventional medical wisdom dictated that I inherited the *bad genes* and the potential to have a heart attack from her.

But as a layman without the benefit of years of medical school training, my own observations and twenty-twenty hindsight had told me that the heredity argument in my case was a bit overdone. My heart attack resulted more from my personal choices, habits and interaction with my immediate environment.

♥ ♥ ♥

Let us start with the early years. What was so awful about my environment?

Actually it was not awful. It was typical! I was born in Brooklyn, N.Y. in 1950 and moved with my family to Baltimore at the ripe old age of two and I remained a Baltimorean throughout my college days. Ahhhh, those early days. Things were much simpler then. A Ford was a Ford, and a Chevy was a Chevy. One was able to distinguish a '55 Chevy from a '56 Chevy from *the* '57 Chevy.

We were the first TV generation. Picture tubes were only black and white. You did however have a choice of several different screen sizes depending on the size of your wallet. There were not many confusing buttons and you had a choice of only three channels: #2, #11 or #13.

The next blockbuster to hit the market and the living room resulted from Swanson's innovative solution to dispose of (market) 270 tons of leftover Thanksgiving turkey. What was that solution? A three-compartment aluminum tray, containing a portion of turkey, corn bread dressing and gravy, and buttered peas and sweet potatoes packaged to look like a small television -- the original TV dinner!

Many a preteen was weaned on a TV dinner balanced on his/her lap while being hypnotized staring at the small TV screen. It was great from the standpoint of Mom -- from the freezer to the oven and then to the TV all in twenty minutes.

And from the standpoint of us kids, the TV dinners were a real treat. Nobody gave too much thought to nutritional values in those days beyond the four basic food groups.[1]

Do you remember those real home made dinners when just about everything was fried in Crisco? It was truly the miracle age of convenience cooking. Terms such as saturated fat, hydrogenated and partially hydrogenated fat were a generation away from our every day vocabulary. Veggies? Forget it, unless it came out of a can or was part of a TV dinner, which somehow made them tasty. Now don't forget dessert. Our favorite was what my Dad called *idiot cookies.*

What's an *idiot cookie*? In its raw state, it was found in the refrigerator section of the supermarket, packaged to look something like an extremely fat hot dog.

Preparation was quite simple. First cut them into slices about an inch long and then cut each slice into 4 quarters. Place them on a baking pan in a 350°F oven for about fifteen minutes and then like magic they would melt down to form real cookies. They were great! Healthy? I kind of doubt it but we ate tons of them. Why the name *idiot cookie*? I assume that when my Dad's mother made cookies the old fashion way, it took much longer to prepare and the finished product undoubtedly was a whole lot healthier too.

The homemade dinners were something else; however as kids, we usually enjoyed lunch much more. There were two kinds of lunches. One was the *indoor* lunch and the other was the *outdoor* type. The *indoor* lunch could be subdivided into two categories. This would best be described as the *stay at home* kind and the other as the *school* kind. In reality, they were quite similar as they were both sandwiches. When it came to sandwiches, I differed a bit from the other kids as to my preferences. The overwhelming choice at school was peanut butter and jelly. Skippy, Peter Pan or Jif were the staples -- smooth or crunchy, every kid to his own. The type of jelly was generally irrelevant.

The Before Years

Quite frankly, I was not into the typical sandwich. I was known throughout my elementary school career as the Cream Cheese Kid. Needless to say, it was a full fat cream cheese. In my opinion the ultimate sandwich was a Philadelphia brand cream cheese spread lavishly between two slices of white bread. A typical lunch would consist of two or three of these concoctions. In fact, one could say that I had become addicted to cream cheese. At snack time, I would forgo the bread and just dig in with a spoon. I also had my own special way of eating a cream cheese sandwich. My initial assault on the sandwich would start with peeling off the not too tasty brown crust of the bread and consume that first, and then savored the best part for last. I would then squish the remaining part of the sandwich together which for some unknown reason seemed to make it taste even better.

I was more creative at home and consequently tried cream cheese on toast. Big Mistake! Instead of toasting the bread first, I made the sandwich and slipped it into a slot in the toaster. The first sign that something was amiss occurred when the toaster partially popped back up and my sandwich appeared to be firmly cemented in the toaster slot. I did the only logical thing in this situation and that was to insert a fork into the slot to pry out the remnants of the sandwich. That was Big Mistake #2 which understandably dwarfed Big Mistake #1. Wooooooo! I lived to tell the story but I never did that again.

My taste buds gradually expanded to new horizons and as I approached adulthood, I acquired a taste for peanut butter. Did I mention the term *hydrogenated* before? It was not yet a part of my vocabulary.

Now we have the second kind of kids' lunches. Let us call this the *outdoor* type. This too can be subdivided into two types: the outdoor type *with parents* and the outdoor type *without parents*. The *with parents* type meant going to a real restaurant and choosing food from a menu. Although this was a novelty which usually meant getting dressed up in an itchy shirt and tie, it did not occur too frequently and therefore had only a negligible effect on my dietary makeup. The outdoor type *without parents* meant eating outside with friends and/or eating alone. This generally meant Gino's fast food which was very popular during school vacation time and during the long summer break. Years before I first set eyes on the Golden Arches, our place was at Gino's. Why the name Gino's? If you have been paying attention up until now, you will remember that I grew up in Baltimore.

I was a crazy Baltimore Orioles fan but there was that *other* sport in the city and that was called football. Do you remember the Baltimore Colts? Way back then, their legendary quarterback Johnny Unitas is still remembered as the best quarterback to ever grace a football field. The only other teammate that I can remember from those Colts days is Gino Marchetti. Gino played in the NFL in the late fifties and early sixties. He was not only an All-Pro defensive end but was voted by sportswriters in 1969 as the best defensive end in NFL's first 50 year history.

I do not recall if the restaurant that bears Gino Marchetti's name was actually owned by him, if it was franchised or just someone paying to use his name. I must admit that eating at Gino's started my long lasting love affair with fast food. A hamburger back then cost 15¢, French Fries 12¢, a Coke 5¢ and only 32¢ for a meal fit for a king. That 32¢ ceiling was shattered when I added the second burger. In time, the industry advanced to doubles and to quarter pound slabs of beef.

As a teenager, I would mow the yards of neighbors for $1.75 to $2.25 a pop and the proceeds of my labor enabled me to dine at Gino's and similar fine establishments quite frequently. Later in life I could have given Homer Simpson a run for the money in a doughnut consumption competition. I was addicted to Dunkin Donuts and was known to have eaten more than my share of Oreo Cookies and Three Musketeers.

I also remember that at this stage in my life and throughout my college days, I was always one of the skinniest kids in the class. In Junior High School (what they now call Middle School), I remember a gym teacher looking me over and his sarcastic comment: "Don't they feed you at home?"

My love of eating and taste for the 'fine foods' lasted for years. The dining hall at the University of Maryland was always closed Sunday evenings, which prompted my roommate and me to stroll down to Route #1 where we would each finish off a family sized pizza with a Coke. He too had a good appetite. (That's right, College Park. I remember the Terps playing at Cole Hall under Lefty Driesal, who promised to make the U of M the UCLA of the east. It did happen, only 30 years later, and not under his reign.)

Several years after I graduated from college I moved to Israel, and as a permanent resident was drafted into the regular army. I was considered a bit unusual as I was the same age as my Battalion Commander. I received my Corporal stripes while he was already a Lieutenant Colonel. Most of the other soldiers did not know my real name but they came up with a nickname for me and I was known as *The Dahsan*. The English translation is *compactor* as in garbage compactor.

Looking back at the straw that broke the camel's back which brought about my heart attack cannot be blamed solely on my former eating habits. This will be discussed later, however I feel certain that they had a significant contributing effect, which is why I provided this background information

3

Health Conscious

How many times have you heard someone ask "Where were you when you heard that President John Kennedy was assassinated?" I remember exactly. I was in Miss Twilley's eighth grade social studies class when the announcement came over the loud speaker.

I also remember exactly where I was when I heard that Prime Minister Yitshak Rabin had been assassinated. I was in 'beautiful downtown' Bethlehem on reserve duty. It was Saturday night, November 4, 1995.

It was the day before, on November 3rd, that I made my transition from the 'eat anything' attitude to a health oriented eating conception. I have made several transitions since then according to different eating doctrines. However this transition stands out as significant because it represents a complete break from all the eating habits I had enjoyed since birth for the previous 45 years. And ironically, it all happened by mistake!

That morning I arrived home on leave supposedly for the weekend. I received a package from Uncle Al that contained three books. Two of the books were on computers which was my field for the past twenty years. The third book was something about nutrition or whatever but definitely not my kind of book.

Later that afternoon I received a phone call from my commanding officer informing me that he had forgotten to mention that I was the standby ambulance driver for the weekend. I was to return immediately to Bethlehem as the regular ambulance driver had already left for the weekend. It was suggested that I bring some reading material to negate the anticipated boredom on this assignment

Needless to say, that phone call pushed my panic button and I started running around the house gathering odds and ends that I would need for the weekend as well as for the upcoming week. I needed to pack my clean undies, socks, snacks and whatever goodies I could quickly lay my hands on. Then I headed for the computer room and latched onto the newly arrived package from Uncle Al. Somehow I just assumed that the book I laid my hands on was one of the two computer books that I just received. Unfortunately I was wrong!

You can imagine the hurry I was in to get out of the house. Unfortunately I didn't take the time to verify if I had one of the two computer books. Keep in mind that this was after the 1993 Oslo Accords[*], and before the present Intifada[**]. Things were generally quiet and only a minimum number of soldiers were left on duty for the weekend.

Upon returning to Bethlehem and settling in for the weekend with absolutely nothing to do except to wait for an emergency call, I decided to find a comfortable position to plant my rear end and to see what's new in the computer world. I opened my knap sack, felt my way through the undies, socks and goodies until I reached the book, pulled it out and Surprise! Surprise! I found it difficult to believe that I had two whole days with nothing to do (hopefully) except to read in order to

---

[*] Agreement between Israel and the Palestinian Authority - first stage – the P.A. would combat terrorism and Israel would withdraw from Palestinian population centers

[**] Palestinian armed uprising

occupy myself only to discover that both of the computer books were still at home. I had inadvertently packed the health book. I tossed the health book back into the knap sack and was really disgusted with myself because of my slip-up.

The monotony of doing nothing hour after hour and waiting for an emergency call had a silver lining. My hectic schedule leaves me with very little free time which I could call my own. Despite the fact that I didn't have access to the computer books while I was on this assignment, I decided to cut my losses and focus my attention on this health book. The book was "Dr. Dean Ornish's Program for Reversing Heart Disease."[2] As soon as I started reading it, I realized that it had become difficult to put the book down. This book had opened up a new world for me regarding taking personal responsibility for my overall wellness. For the past forty-five years I had eaten whatever came to mind and as much as I pleased. During my entire life, I had blocked out all thoughts regarding the health aspects of every day eating. From the last chapter, I was the 'Dahsan', remember?

If I had to summarize the Ornish system in a few words, it would be a high complex carbohydrate, low fat vegetarian and fruit diet. The book is not a diet book as the name implies. Basically it is an all encompassing program for reversing heart disease. The diet portion of the book is only one of three main topics. In addition to eating habits, the other two topics cover exercise for the body and meditation for the soul.

Meditation was never a part of my makeup. My impression of meditation had always been something reserved for people with too much free time on their hands with no ambition to perform anything useful. I was always much too busy for that! I didn't need some guru telling me how to find my inner peace.

Exercise was a sort of outlet for me. In the past decade, I had gone swimming about three times a week early in the morning before going to work. The routine was to leave the house in the morning carrying my work clothes and swimming gear, getting in a quick thirty or so laps in the pool, quick shower, getting dressed and continue on to work.

It was the eating habits in the book that impressed me the most. The eating theory of Dr. Ornish is basically to eat fewer calories and at the same time burn off more calories through exercise. His scientific theory is based on the fact that protein and carbohydrates contain four calories/gm while fat has nine calories/gm. According to his logic, if you decrease the amount of fat in the diet, you will consume fewer calories while not necessarily eating less food. If the amount of food is not drastically reduced then the metabolism rate will not decrease significantly. This he claims is the reason many diet plans plateau after several weeks, making additional weight loss more problematic. And certainly no less important, Dr. Ornish touts that his low fat routine is significantly more heart healthy. The Ornish regimen is high on carbohydrates and fiber.

Carbohydrates are divided into two main categories. The good category is known as complex carbohydrates and these include whole wheat, brown rice, fruits and vegetables. These carbohydrates are high in fiber and are not absorbed rapidly. They do not cause a rapid rise in blood sugar which can cause an immediate increase in the insulin response. High fiber food gives one the feeling of being 'filled up'. Dr. Ornish highly recommends copious amounts of food that contain these complex carbohydrates. The bad category is known as simple carbohydrates and these include sugar, bleached white flour and white rice (refined starch). Calories from this category do not fill you up and are quickly absorbed into the blood stream causing your blood sugar to increase rapidly.

Fiber is also divided into two categories: water soluble and non soluble. Foods high in soluble fiber are very healthy for various body functions. It delays glucose absorption, and is believed to lower cholesterol. Fruits, vegetables and oats are good examples of food containing soluble fibers.

The book also recommends eating non soluble fibers which promote regular bowel movement, prevent constipation, and remove toxic waste through colon in less time. Wheat bran, whole wheat products, and fruit and vegetable skins are examples containing non soluble fibers.

When I arrived home from my assignment in Bethlehem, Esty could not believe how my short stint there could have possibly changed my eating habits so dramatically in such a short period of time. I do not recall if I reached Dr. Ornish's target of ten percent level for fat intake, however my fat intake had dropped significantly. Low fat dairy products became the rule in the Stone household. A three percent fat milk gave way to one percent fat content; fat content in cheese dropped from the traditional nine and/or five percent to one-half percent.

Ironically, I don't recall having seen skim milk on the local supermarket shelves. Perhaps that was because it was never on my shopping list. I also reduced my meat intake substantially. Whole wheat bread replaced the bleached white flour varieties. I would now bring my lunch to work from home instead of eating out. My standard lunch consisted of several low fat cheeses on whole wheat bread. This was in addition to a fruit or vegetable such as a carrot, apple or banana.

At my place of work, a graphic designer's desk was located directly behind my desk. I returned to my desk one day after a short break to find a whole wheat sandwich cutout on colored paper pasted to the edge of the screen of my computer. Graphic designers apparently have a sense of humor. Several days later and again after a short work break, I found a picture of a carrot taped to my computer screen. In time, an apple, cucumber and a banana joined the parade. Despite the fact that

I have changed jobs several times, the graphics have accompanied me from job to job and from computer screen to computer screen.

I do not remember the number of years that I was a Dr. Ornish groupie nor do I remember when we started to part company. Undeniably, his book made me cognizant of my poor eating habits prior to my exposure to his book. As a result of my Ornish period, I began looking at food labels for content and eliminated fried and (until recently) high fat foods from my daily diet. This is not to say that I would not eat junk food occasionally but I became aware of what foods to generally avoid.

♥ ♥ ♥

Dr. Ornish's high carbohydrate, low fat diet has attracted a significant amount of controversy. Another best seller to hit the market was The Atkins Diet authored by Dr. Robert Atkins[3] who advocates a regimen of high fat and protein but no carbohydrates.

Dr. Atkins' theory is a 180 degree turnaround from the Dr. Ornish perspective which advocated lots of complex carbohydrates. Dr. Atkin's contention is that the overeating of carbohydrates causes blood sugar levels to rise which in turn causes increased insulin production to break down the sugar. It is this increase in insulin that causes the physical craving for additional carbohydrates. This then becomes a never ending cycle of eating that leads to weight gain and a variety of related health problems.

If you are now confused about proper nutrition, let me assure you that both Doctors Ornish and Atkins are accredited physicians. However their analysis of the cause and the possible remedy of overweight people and disease are contradictory to say the least. Dr. Ornish's theory claimed that excess weight and the resulting health problems were caused by an excess of fat consumption. Dr. Atkin's revolutionary approach advocated eating as much fat as the dieter craved while eliminating the carbohydrates.

The non-carbohydrate theory is based on a phenomenon called ketosis. Conventional medical theory states that it is the carbohydrates that are converted by the body into sugar which is considered to be the gasoline that runs the body. Ketosis is the system in which the dieter eliminates practically all carbohydrates from the diet including complex carbohydrates. This in turn forces the body to start burning the stored fat reserves as body fuel. This in turn results in weight loss. Since the consumption of carbohydrates is substantially reduced, the body does not produce an excess of insulin.

High carbs and low fats
- or -
low carbs and high fats

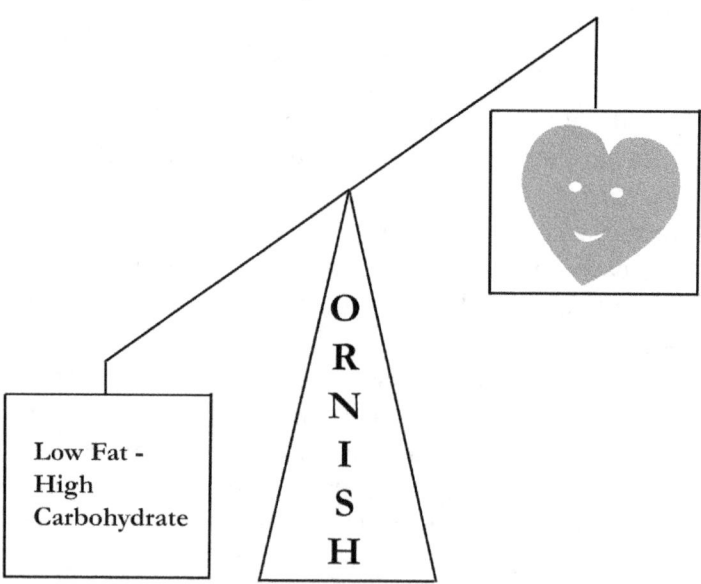

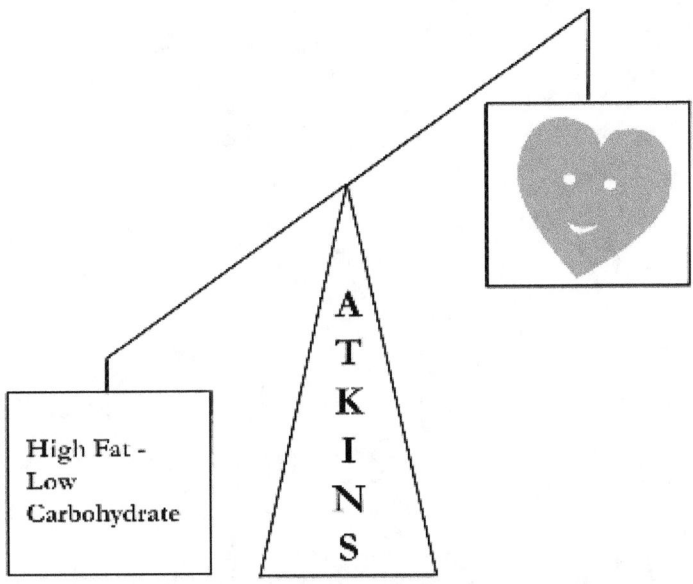

Both claim their doctrines promote health, not to mention weight loss/control. Both systems claim that the other causes damage to health. Two doctors from two different worlds! Apparently medical science is not the exact science that I grew up believing it to be.

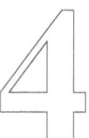

Mom

Genetic heart disease in my immediate family was never considered to be a problem. This line of thought took an immediate turn in March-April of 1998. My oldest son Sagi who had turned thirteen years of age celebrated his Bar Mitzvah on April 2nd and the festivities were celebrated with a sizeable in-house party on April 4th. My parents were the guests of honor who made the very l-o-n-g trip to Israel from New Orleans. It is not an easy trip -- especially for septuagenarians. Between pre-boarding time in New Orleans plus approximately five hour connecting time at JFK airport in New York and actual flight time add up to a twenty-four hour trip. That equates to twenty-four hours of irregular eating and sleeping time in addition to many hours of cramped quarters during flight time. Recuperating from jet lag on a trip of this magnitude usually takes a few days for younger folks and possibly a bit more time for the aging population

The following day, March 29th, I returned to work. I was relatively certain that the folks would be sleeping most of the day bouncing back both mentally and physically from the long trip. Unfortunately there was a mix-up with my Mom's suitcase at the airport upon arrival and her suitcase containing her clothes for the festivities was accidentally switched with another suitcase.

That morning my mother had still not fully recouped from the trip. After not sleeping well the first night in Israel, she was quite concerned about her missing wardrobe and the need to start replacing missing clothes for the upcoming events. Early that morning Esty contacted the airport. We had tried to contact them the night before but were not successful. Fortunately the missing luggage was located and my folks and Esty departed on the one and a half hour trip back to the airport to reclaim her suitcase. Despite the good news in retrieving her suitcase, Mom was still not feeling much better. Esty thought it advisable to have a doctor examine her.

After checking with our health clinic, it came to Esty's attention that as tourists my parents could not be examined by our family doctor at the clinic. She then made an appointment for an examination that evening at a private clinic. I had already returned from work by early evening and my parents and I headed off to the private clinic. We were expecting the obvious that it was going to be simply exhaustion from the long trip and in another day or two she would be back to normal.

The doctor decided to perform an electrocardiography; the procedure measures the electrical impulses that are discharged every time the heart beats. The apparatus prints out the results during the entire procedure. After the electrocardiography (a.k.a. EKG or ECG), he informed me that Mom was going thru a heart event. I do not recall if he actually used the term *attack* but she had to get to the emergency ward immediately at the nearest hospital. The doctor suggested that we not wait for the ambulance as time was critical and we would make better time if we drove there ourselves rather than wait for an ambulance.

At the emergency ward, the doctors confirmed immediately that she was going thru a heart attack. Mom simply could not believe it. Although she was not feeling that well, she was not feeling that terrible either. After all, having a heart attack is serious business and it would seem that someone experiencing an attack would certainly have no doubts that he/she is going thru an actual heart attack.

Considering that she was in the midst of a heart attack process, Mom was in exceptionally good spirits -- and why not? It was because she was going thru it at.......Hadassah Hospital in Jerusalem! She remembered as a young girl all the fund raising events sponsored to raise funds for Hadassah Hospital, which was then a source of great pride for the Diaspora. During her first visit to Israel in 1982 (when Esty and I were married), one of the *must things* to do on her sightseeing list was to see the Marc Chagall stained glass windows at Hadassah Hospital. Now she was getting the grand tour of the hospital from the inside -- being taken care of by Hadassah doctors, being fussed over by Hadassah nurses – *wait until the gals back at home hear about this*!!

♥ ♥ ♥

This was the first time I had ever experienced someone close to me going thru a heart attack. According to conventional medicine, heart attacks are caused by atherosclerosis, a chronic disease characterized by normal thickening and hardening of the arterial walls resulting in a loss of elasticity. There are three main coronary arteries that convey oxygen rich blood to the heart. What then causes arteries to become narrowed or blocked? In addition to aging, do you remember when we discussed junk foods, especially fried foods? According to Dr. Ornish's theory, it all comes down to fat. It is not that fat is inherently bad for you and as Dr. Ornish claims, the body needs fourteen grams of fat per day in order to function properly. However, the problem is what happens to the excess fat that the body does not need, especially saturated fat which the body will convert to cholesterol.

Cholesterol is also manufactured in the liver. As per Dr. Ornish, the body does not have the mechanism to get rid of excess cholesterol either by urinating or thru bowel movements. It gets absorbed into the blood system and over a period of time, it starts to accumulate on the walls of the arteries. It is this plaque that contributes to the narrowing of the arteries which ultimately will cause blockage and in turn this blockage will impede the blood flow in the arteries.

Dr. Atkins downplays the connection between heart disease and fat consumption. He contends that there are four deadly consequences all linked together by a single metabolic occurrence that contributes to heart disease. The consequences: upper body obesity, glucose intolerance, high triglyceride levels and hypertension. If you have not already guessed, the common cause for all -- excessive insulin production caused by eating carbohydrates.

As I mentioned earlier, I am not a doctor and therefore I will not offer a hint to which school of thought explains the cause of heart disease. The point is that heart disease is real, widespread and is a silent killer.

♥ ♥ ♥

For those of you that are not familiar with a Bar Mitzvah, the ultimate absolute **last** thing that you would want to happen during Bar-Mitzvah week is to have an out of town (out of country!) guest (parent!) have a heart attack! (Actually I can think of something worse, but I prefer not to specifically mention it.........).

Her condition became stabilized after feeding her intravenously with blood thinners, clot dissolvers, and artery expanders. She started to feel better until they reduced some of her medication. This was the day of the planned festivities, Thursday, April 2nd and the guests started to arrive in droves. We did celebrate on schedule without Dad who remained at Mom's bedside

Actually, there was an unexpected family member present at Thursday's events. The day after Mom was admitted to the hospital, my sister Carol called up and asked Esty if she would like her to fly over (as I previously mentioned, Bar-

Mitzvah week has its own rules of being busy/coordinating/going nuts without any other extraordinary events also going on simultaneously). Esty did not give it a second thought if the offer was just a rhetorically polite empty offer or a real sincere offer to come, which I think was the actual case. However Esty immediately responded with big "yes" and the next day Carol was here.

Meanwhile, starting from April 3rd, Mom was feeling well again, and she was scheduled to have an angiogram performed on April 8th.

An angiogram is a medical procedure in which a flexible tube called a catheter is inserted into a coronary artery in the groin area and is guided manually via the coronary artery into the heart. Some surgeons prefer entrance to the artery thru the hand. A special dye is then injected thru the catheter into the bloodstream and is viewed on an x-ray screen. The cardiologist can then see the path and flow of the dye and can determine whether he/she will perform an immediate angioplasty to open up any clogged arteries.

Angioplasty is a medical procedure that has been in use since the late 1970's. It is officially known as PCTA or Percutaneous Transluminal Coronary Angioplasty. A second balloon tipped catheter is placed within the original catheter and is guided to the blocked area. It is then inflated and deflated several times until the narrowed area has been enlarged to permit a satisfactory blood flow. A big advantage of using angioplasty when applicable is that the patient can be back on his/her feet within a day or two after the procedure as compared with bypass surgery which requires weeks if not months of serious recuperation time.

We were all overly optimistic that the findings of the angiogram would result in a relatively simple ballooning of Mom's clogged artery and that she would be back on her feet in short order and getting on with the rest of her life. Up to this point, Mom was hospitalized at the Mt. Scopus branch of Hadassah hospital in Jerusalem. Most major operations including heart procedures are done at a sister branch of Hadassah hospital about a half hour drive across Jerusalem -- the Ein Kerem Branch of Hadassah Hospital.

It was no problem getting her over there. She was wheeled down to a transit vehicle, the type which is used to pick up shift workers. It was being used now as a shuttle to transport workers and patients up and back between the two hospitals. After exiting the hospital, she got off the wheel chair, climbed onto the vehicle and sat in the first available seat. Dad traveled with her in the van and Carol and I went by car.

The angiogram was performed smoothly by the cardiology professor at the Ein Kerem branch. When he gathered all of us together to give us his findings, we were all of the opinion that the
worst was all behind us.

What a shock! Angioplasty cannot be performed in Mom's case and he and his staff recommended a quadruple bypass as soon as possible and strongly recommended that the operation be performed immediately in Israel. He and his staff felt that it would be too risky to fly Mom back to the U.S. for the operation.

Both Carol and I agreed to the cardiologist's suggestion and we called brother Rich in the States to fill him in. He too agreed that the operation be performed in Israel. It was unanimous among us three kids. Dad was not all that excited about having the operation in Israel but there are times when a parent's veto is not enough to overrule a major decision. The date of the operation was set for April 14th.

After recuperating from the angiogram, Mom was transferred back to Hadassah Mt. Scopus again in an old van. There was nothing unusual about the return trip and she resumed her blood thinning medication while awaiting the upcoming operation.

Between the angiogram and the upcoming scheduling for the bypass operation, two noteworthy events occurred. Rich preferred to be with   Mom at the Hadassah Hospital rather than to receive updated briefings from half a world away. He quickly finalized his flight plans and he was on his way to Jerusalem. On the brighter side, this turned out to be an unexpected family reunion but our hidden anxiety regarding Mom's condition was well contained especially in Mom's presence.

On the afternoon of Rich's arrival, Dad, Carol and I were at Mom's bedside which had become our daily routine. I decided to go home, shower, have a quick lunch and catch up with some much needed sleep before heading to the airport to pick up Rich. I had been home a few minutes when the phone rang. It was Carol. She informed me that Dad was now being worked on in the emergency room! Apparently the physical exhaustion and anxiety had finally caught up with him. His chest pains were enough to have him admitted to the hospital.

A change in plans was in order! Carol was now in the emergency room with Dad and requested that I return to the hospital to be with him. She wanted to be with Mom who was on another floor. Rich was quite surprised to find that it was Esty and not me waiting at the airport to greet him. They drove directly to the hospital and by the time he arrived, he was well briefed regarding the rapidly changing situation.

The day before the bypass operation, Mom was again transported back to the Ein Kerem branch of Hadassah Hospital. Again, it was an old van with no seat belts. She felt quite insecure on the trip. It was not the thought of the pending surgery that bothered her; it was the unbuckled bumpy ride.

The next morning, Dad was left to fend for himself at the Mt. Scopus branch of Hadassah. Rich, Carol and I were at Ein Kerem to be with Mom for her operation. It's a strange feeling saying "good luck" and "see you later" to someone so close to you being wheeled away from the preparation room to the actual operating theatre wondering if there will actually be a 'later'. The operation seemed to drag on indefinitely.

Mom

When the surgeon f-i-n-a-l-l-y appeared, he informed us that everything went off as planned and that there were no unexpected surprises. We would be able to see her the next morning when she awoke. Carol had a return ticket the following day and because of the extenuating circumstances, we received special permission to enter the post operating room very early next morning. With nothing else to do in Ein Kerem, the three of us returned to Mt. Scopus to report the good news to Dad. Needless to say, he was overjoyed when we broke the news to him.

Early the next morning, the three of us, Carol, Rich and I were off to see Mom. Dad was still at Mt. Scopus at the time. We dressed in sterile white gowns over our clothes before entering the post operational room to visit with Mom. She was awake at the time but was still very groggy. She thought that a scenic picture hanging on the wall across from her bed was her chest X-ray. The first thing she said was "Carol, what are you still doing here?" Carol had originally planned to be in Israel for a week and wound up staying two weeks. Mom knew that Carol was to leave Israel the morning following her operation. Mom thought that she was out of it for several days and that Carol had again postponed her trip back to the U.S. because things were not going too well.

It took a while to persuade Mom that it was really the very next morning after her operation and that we arrived at the hospital very early specifically for Carol to say good-bye before her trip back to the U.S. We were all somewhat relieved that Mom had recognized us despite her groggy condition and that she was well aware what was happening around her. We also called up Dad to give him an update, who by this time was also feeling much better, as the couple days of being stuck in a hospital bed gave him the time to catch up on some much needed rest.

Within a day or so, Dad was released with a clean bill of health. He had arranged for sleeping quarters at Ein Kerem for the next several days until Mom's release. With the emergency over, Rich was on his way back to New Orleans. Mom was released on April 20th. The hospital staff assumed that Mom could make her way downstairs on her own from her room on an upper floor to her waiting vehicle at the entrance to the hospital. Fortunately we were able to scrounge up a beat up wheel chair which was in worse shape than Mom, and Mom was on her way to the nearest elevator, the first leg on the way home.

What started out as a two week Bar Mitzvah trip turned out to be a two month change of venue. There is always a bright side to every story. First of all, the kids were able to see their Grandma and Grandpa for a longer period of time than originally planned especially since they were staying with us. Secondly, Mom's heart attack was not caused by her trip to Israel. The heart attack was on its way long before this trip and it could have caught up with her at a local supermarket, while driving alone or any other time and place and the results could have been catastrophic. On May 28th the trip was finally over and the folks departed Israel for the trip back to New Orleans.

About six months after Mom's operation, Carol had her son's Bar Mitzvah in Baltimore. It was hard for me to believe that only a short six months ago his Grandma had undergone a quadruple bypass operation and was now dancing the night away

5

The Attack

With Mom's attack already considered an historic event, life continued. We returned to our daily routines-- getting up in the morning, coming home from work and possibly some shopping, schlepping the kids on the way home from work, dropping into bed exhausted. Slight variations to the daily rituals included a dip in the pool several times a week, preferably in the morning. After all, one has to keep in shape! On weekends, we liked to get away from the house. This included but was not limited to visiting out of town relatives, outdoor camping, etc.

Spring 2001 was a particular stressful time at work. Both Esty and I desperately needed a vacation away from the daily grind. We set our sights on Paris since neither one of us have been there before. We just had to get away from everything for a week. It was to be an escape from her work, my work, and the daily chores that come with being a parent.

The flight to Paris was uneventful but pleasant. We filled up our days to the fullest with a great deal of sight seeing, French cheese, dry red wine and of course, *beaucoup* sex. Back home our daily exhausting routine, lack of time and energy had its way of putting a damper on our amorous activity.

That's what vacations from time to time without children are all about. As far as sex is concerned, if you average out the huge *over doing* done on vacations, especially in the settings of a foreign country, with the *under doing* during normal daily routine, the overall average comes out to be about........ average!

We arrived in Paris in the wee hours of the morning on Friday, April 27th. Our return flight was scheduled for Thursday, May 3rd. The following Wednesday, our last full day in Paris, after a quiet evening munching on delicious French bread, cheese that only the French know how to make, vin rouge - that's red wine for you uncultured and uncouth individuals, and of course, another rump in the sack, I was taking a leisurely shower as Esty wanted several more minutes of unstressed, unhurried lay-in-bed time before getting up. The program for the day was to take the train to Versailles and spend most of the day at the magnificent Versailles Gardens.

While in the shower, I started to experience strange sensations. All of a sudden I started to feel an overall weakness. The weakness spread to my left shoulder, arm and hand and I also started to have shortness of breath. I felt as though my left hand was unable to hold or grasp anything. Yet, I did not feel severe pain at all. It was more like moderate discomfort. Despite the fact that I was not feeling well, I believe I smiled and was thinking "Are these the symptoms of too much sex in too short a period of time"? After all, I was fifty-one years old at the time, some thirty – thirty-five years after my biological peak performance period.

I was relatively certain that this could not possibly be a heart attack as I had already heard first hand what going thru a severe 'heart attack' feels like. While visiting our good friend and neighbor Itsik in a hospital two and a half years earlier, I had run into a colleague from my previous place of employment. He was the same age as me and I inquired as to why he was wandering around the intensive care ward in the hospital blue/green pajamas. His answer shocked me. He said that he was in the midst of moving to a new apartment a week earlier and while conversing with the moving people who had just arrived to start loading, and BOOM, he had suffered a 'heart attack'! After my expected reaction of WOW, he explained to me what it felt like to have cardiac arrest. He felt that someone had lodged an axe directly into his heart. The pain was excruciating. Although he was now feeling much better, his eyes were wild with excitement as he unfolded his 'attack'.

I remembered that night at the hospital vividly. It was not only the briefing describing my colleague's 'heart attack' but my friend Itsik who was hospitalized the day before of complications that developed from his bout with the flu which had put him in the intensive care unit. After talking with Itsik for several minutes, Esty and I told his wife Rina that we would pop in to see them the following morning in the hospital which was on our way to work. We left the hospital and went directly home. Upon arriving home a half hour later, we were horrified to find a message waiting for us. Itzik had passed away minutes after we had left them.

As I remembered that last night with Itsik, and my colleague's description of something I was definitely not experiencing, I quickly washed off the soap in the shower, and returned to bed to lie down and rest for a while until the feeling of discomfort and weakness passed.

After getting back into bed, the discomfort and weakness in my left shoulder and hand did not seem to improve immediately. Esty kept her composure (she later admitted that on the inside she was shaking like a leaf) and at the time did not externally exhibit any particular concern regarding my temporary bout with:

1. indigestion from last night, or

2. exhaustion from all the intimate episodes the
    past week, or

3. a combination of both.

I wonder if there was ever a study made of the human female species to determine if they feel a personal achievement regarding their ability to physically exhaust their mate!

Meanwhile Esty started looking thru the papers and booklets we had brought along in the event of a medical emergency. After a short rest period, the restlessness and discomfort passed as quickly as it had come. I decided to stay a bit longer in bed to recuperate but within several minutes the same discomfort returned. Esty managed to locate several doctors and now the question was 'do we or don't we phone a doctor?' Again, my discomfort left me and I remained in bed another fifteen minutes. I felt fine, got dressed and resumed normalcy as if the previous half hour never occurred. I was back on my feet. Esty showered, we had breakfast and then headed out to Versailles.

An additional treat awaited us in Versailles. It was the only day since we arrived in France that was not raining or foggy. The sun was shining and after a tour thru the magnificent palaces, we walked down to the beautiful lake. We rented a small row boat and rowed around the entire lake until it was time to return the boat. I felt terrific! The next day was Thursday, our air departure date. Early morning and afternoon was reserved for more sightseeing and in late afternoon, we headed for the airport for the trip home.

Bright and early Friday morning I visited my health clinic and informed them as to what had happened to me several days earlier. My regular doctor had not been working for several months and I requested a substitute doctor to give me an EKG. According to the 'Rules', since I was currently feeling OK and because this was Friday and the country was already partially shut down for the weekend, I was scheduled for an EKG on Sunday at the clinic's associated Coronary Institute. This upset me since I did not want to wait the whole weekend not knowing whether or not I had a serious problem. I went to see the head doctor on duty and he instructed the nurse on duty to perform the EKG immediately.

Both the head doctor and my substitute doctor looked over the resulting EKG print-out and said that presently everything seemed fine. If it indeed was a minor attack in Paris, it had passed and everything now checked out. However, if the same symptoms reappear in the future, I should **immediately** go to the emergency room of the nearest hospital.

For the time being, life went back to normal -- going to work every morning, occasionally hitting the swimming pool in the morning, shopping, kids schlepping...and even the intimacy part was back to 'pre vacation normal'. To be more explicit, adjusting to the daily variables such as both Esty and I being home at the same time; I did not doze off early on the living room couch; she did not doze off early; I am in the mood; she is in the mood; she has the energy for it; I have the energy for it; she is not too busy with kids; I'm not to busy with the kids. Shall I go on?

♥ ♥ ♥

The next several months were extremely stressful at work. Looking back, I believe the real problem was my mishandling of the stress at work. It controlled me rather than I control it!

On Wednesday, July 11, 2001, I left work at a normal hour. Esty had picked me up and we drove off to visit Rakefet who was at a young counselor's training summer camp for the week. It was parents/family visiting night. Her camp was located about a half hour drive from Jerusalem. After a several hour visit with her, we continued westward to the old city of Jaffa. There our good friend Hanna was giving a surprise fiftieth birthday party for her ex- husband Boris. The party was held at an upscale restaurant in Jaffa. We arrived too late for the main course but just in time for dessert.

Boris and I are very good friends. I met him in 1977 when be both did our basic boot training together. We have been in contact ever since that time. If you are curious as to why an ex-wife would arrange a surprise party for an ex-husband, it is because that they still have two children in common to care for and both extended families still feel the family ties despite the fact that they have been divorced for ten years. At the end of the long full day, we finally arrived home and crawled on all fours into bed .

The following day (Thursday), I had a horrendous day at work. Esty had again picked me up from work and was not too pleased with my current state of affairs. That evening we were off on a much longer trip up north to visit with Tuval who was at camp for the week. It was also parents/family visiting night in his neck of the woods. On the way up north we stopped off at a McDonalds' for a quick dinner. It was only occasionally that I would still eat junk food. Perhaps it was the lasting effects from my Ornish days. That night I had an urge for something really tasty, like a Big Mac with French fries and a diet coke (as if the diet coke somehow makes the whole meal 'healthy'). We continued up north and finally arrived at our destination. We waited patiently thru the ultra long show that the counselors and kids put on annually. Every year the theme changes but the monotony of the event never changes. Fireworks were next on the agenda and f i n a l l y we got to meet with Tuval for a little while. We arrived home quite late that night again on all fours. The only thing left on our agenda was to go to sleep and as soon as possible.

Friday July 13th, 2001: I'll remember this day probably until my last. I woke up really tired. And why not? I had a rough week at work -- two very late nights -- and now finally, the week-end. How I would wait for the week-end! And as usual on Fridays, first stop was going to the pool.

What's nice about Friday swims is that I know that I'm not in a hurry to finish as soon as possible and hurry off to something else. This is in contrast to the couple of times I swim in the middle of the week before work, to finish the thirty or so laps as fast as possible and then hurry off to a shower, get dressed then on to the job. Fridays are my time. I do not have to limit the laps, and usually on Fridays would do between forty – fifty laps. Going back and forth would make me feel more energized, as I would always feel both really refreshed and pooped after long Friday swims; a healthy sort of 'pooped' feeling as compared to the depressing fatigued feeling after a long day at work.

That particular Friday, however, was different. Instead of picking up a second wind after several laps, I felt that the laps were getting harder and harder. After finishing only sixteen laps, I decided that I had had enough; I was just too overtired.

I showered, dressed and left the pool to start some local errands. I bought dairy products and other perishables for the week-end, stopped off at the pharmacy for some odds and ends, and returned home to perform other Friday rituals at home. First of course, was to cut the grass. After that, I cut Rina's (Itsik's widow) grass. Then there was fix this, fix that, at home. Close to three-fifteen p.m., Esty who at the time worked every other Friday, arrived home from work.

About a half hour after I finished the chores for the day, I again started to feel the same symptoms I felt in Paris several months ago. This time both Esty and I knew exactly what it meant. We knew it was time to go immediately to the hospital.

The question was should we wait for an ambulance or have Esty drive me directly to the nearest hospital which was the Mount Scopus branch of Hadassah Hospital in Jerusalem. Since we live way out in the boondocks we thought it prudent to leave immediately for the hospital's emergency room. It was

Friday afternoon and most everyone was back at home from work for the Sabbath which meant that there would be very light traffic. The trip to the hospital was extremely uncomfortable despite the fact that I was not in great pain. I found it difficult to sit quietly and I thought the ride to the hospital would never end. As we approached the hospital, we encountered a red traffic signal. I glanced around for oncoming traffic and since I could not see any, I told Esty to drive thru the red light. It was at that point that Esty realized how serious the situation had become.

Within thirty – forty minutes from the time I started to feel quite badly, I was in the emergency room hooked up to an EKG. The doctor on duty asked me to rate on a scale of 1 – 10 the severity of the pain. My thoughts went back to my friend with 'an axe thrust into his chest' which rated a solid category 10. I rated my pain situation as a number 3. The EKG confirmed that I was indeed having a heart attack and I was quickly hooked up to intravenous feeding delivering clot dissolvers, blood thinners and artery expanders. A more professional lingo interpretation as follows:

Clot

- **Thrombolysis** is the medical term for the breaking up of blood clots, which also leads us to several more similar sounding words that are a must to learn for impressing your guests at your next cocktail party.

- **Thrombosis** is the formation or presence of a blood clot inside a blood vessel or cavity of the heart.

- A **thrombus** is a blood clot that forms inside a blood vessel or cavity of the heart.

- An **embolus** is a blood clot that moves through the bloodstream until it lodges in a narrowed vessel and blocks circulation.

Or as Palladin (TV late fifties) would say 'Have thrombus, will travel', which would now be an embolus.

- **TPA** (Tissue Plasminogen Activator) - Blood Clot Dissolver

Artery Expanders:
- Nitrocine (Glyceryl Trinitrate) is commonly used. It increases the size of blood vessels of the body allowing the heart not to work so hard to circulate the blood therefore decreasing the amount of oxygen needed for the heart to operate efficiently.

Most heart attacks are caused by a clot that blocks one of the coronary arteries. The clot usually forms in the coronary artery that had been narrowed/ hardened due to atherosclerosis. The internal layer of the arterial wall now covers a buildup called plaque which can rupture causing a piece or pieces to separate from the artery. The clot is actually the separated pieces of plaque.

Within a sort period of time the pain and discomfort receded and I was feeling normal again. Upon being stabilized, I was taken to the coronary intensive care section for observation. I remember thinking to myself "just my luck, I wait all week for the weekend, the weekend has barely started, and I have this happen.

Why couldn't this have happened on Sunday morning, the start of the work week in Israel? Now they will probably keep me here until Saturday night and I will be back to work on Sunday -- some fun week end!" Considering that I was feeling well and it was Friday evening, I sent Esty home to be with the kids for what is usually a nice Friday night dinner with everyone at the table.

Later that evening when one of the male nurses happened to walk by, I started to get that heavy, dead feeling in my left shoulder and hand in addition to shortness of breath. Despite my monitors being hooked to a master control board which was constantly being monitored by other staff members, I called the nurse to my bedside and informed him that I was having considerably more intense pains than my previous discomfort. He quickly went to the other side of my bed for a better view of my heart monitor screen.

Most of the hospital staff on duty that evening in the intensive care unit was of Russian origin including the male nurse at my bedside. I do not remember if his next words were in Russian or Hebrew but he said something to the effect 'Hey fellows, look what's going on with this guy'! The nearby staff came to goggle at my monitor and their gibberish chatter gave me the impression they were watching an instant replay in slow motion of a major sporting event.

They immediately added Integrilin, a clot blocking blood thinning drug, to my intravenous feeding. Again within a reasonably short period of time, the pain and discomfort dissipated. Several hours later, the same thing reoccurred. The pain and discomfort was not as severe as the previous session but enough for the staff to further increase the dosage of Integrilin. The cardiologist on duty informed me that I have what they call 'a clot that's playing with me'. Apparently it had not yet dissolved despite the increased dosage I received and it was still large enough to get caught up in an area where the passageway had become abnormally narrow.

The next morning, Esty came by with the kids and was happy to see that I was feeling fine, but was a bit shocked to hear that since she left to go home the previous evening, I had gone thru two additional attacks. Later that day my two sisters-in-law with their husbands also made the long trek from Beer-Sheva to visit me.

I was now feeling quite well and had no idea why the staff would not let me get off the bed and why they were getting so upset with me for not laying still enough in bed. As far as I was concerned, what happened the previous twenty-four hours was now history. Whatever I previously had, has been corrected and I now was wondering what I was still doing in the hospital. I was relatively certain that the angiogram that was scheduled for the next morning was just 'going to be for the record' and within a few days I would be back to my normal schedule.

Esty and the kids were the last visitors with me that evening. They all returned home to get organized for the upcoming week. Esty planned to drop by the following morning before I was to be taken to the Ein Kerem branch of Hadassah Hospital for my angiogram. Later that evening, the head nurse brought me a small bowl of water, wash cloth and towel to freshen up. I was still not allowed to get off the bed. Everything was progressing as expected.

Early the following morning, Esty arrived just prior to my trip to Ein Kerem. She had intended to follow me by car primarily to establish a return route for the trip back home that evening. I was still not allowed to get off the bed and I assumed that they would arrange for a wheel chair for my short trip to the transit vehicle as was the case with my Mom three years earlier at this same facility.

The first of four surprises was about to take place. The staff that had been taking care of me that morning had up until then seemed very calm and professional. They entered my room and informed me that in another couple of minutes I would be on my way to Ein Kerem.

However, there was something in the air that had changed; it was subtle, but noticeable just the same. The professional *calm* that the staff had been exhibiting had suddenly changed to *tension*, which seemed strange at the time, and it was not until much later on that we found out why.

The second surprise was on the heels of the first surprise. Instead of bringing me a wheel chair to take me to the transit vehicle as in the case with Mom, an intensive care ambulance staff consisting of doctor and driver entered the room with a portable bed from their ambulance. As I was being transferred over from the hospital bed to the ambulance bed, the local staff was busy transferring all of my intravenous connections. They also unplugged my hospital oxygen line and hooked me up to a portable oxygen tank.

And a third surprise (which I was not aware of at the time): Esty had just said good-bye to me and that we would meet at Ein Kerem. She left my room and was in the hallway walking out when she encountered the shift head-nurse. Esty also said bye to her and that she was on her way to the car, to which the nurse in shock and disbelief answered back "What! Aren't you riding with him in the ambulance?!?" Esty had no idea at the time why the nurse responded to her in that manner.

I was lifted onto the fancy intensive care ambulance and off we went. I was expecting a nice leisurely, somewhat slow ride to Ein Kerem which is located on the opposite end of the city. After all, Mom's trip back and forth on a transit vehicle going over the identical route was slow but not very comfortable. Just as soon as we left the hospital grounds, the ambulance's lights started flashing and the siren started to scream. In another five minutes we would be entering a long stretch of road which is always backed up for miles during rush hour and this was rush hour. I was curious to see just how a screaming, blinking ambulance would work its way thru it. The road was clogged with traffic and just as the Red Sea opened up for Moses, so did the two lanes ahead of us. The right lane of traffic moved slightly to the right and the left side of traffic moved slightly over to the left and we went right on thru.

The doctor that was in the ambulance with me was constantly asking me questions. "How was I feeling? Did I feel a little better or somewhat worse? How did I feel during the actual attack?" As we were slicing thru traffic, I raised my head slightly to look out the rear window to monitor our progress thru the crowded streets. The doctor did not seem to comprehend how it was that I was so enjoying myself on the ride -- especially in the 'condition that I was in'.

When we arrived at the hospital in Ein Kerem, I was wheeled from the ambulance directly to the angiogram room bypassing the patients in the waiting area who were waiting for their prescheduled angiograms.

Once inside the hospital and on the table, I encountered my fourth surprise of the day. It involved the radiologist who was preparing me for the angiogram. I had never seen anyone in the health industry profession move so quickly and methodically in preparing me for the angiogram. It was though he was alerted that a VIP was arriving and was told to pull out all of the stops. I remember thinking that if this chap keeps up this pace patient after patient, then he is liable to wind up with a heart attack just like me!

Dr. Nassar, the Senior Interventional Cardiologist at Hadassah, took over within minutes after preparations were completed. He lowered a portion of the huge machine very close to my body and administered a local anesthesia in the upper right groin area. He then proceeded to perform the angiogram. This was not a pleasant procedure but not as uncomfortable as the actual heart attack

During the angiogram procedure, the cardiologist pinpointed my problem. He located a ninety percent blockage within my LAD artery and he then performed an angioplasty. In order to keep the narrowed area open and/or preventing it from collapsing, he then inserted a stent into the problem area.

A stent is a spring like wire mesh metal tube that is placed in the artery to keep it open following the angioplasty procedure. The wire mesh is collapsed and is put over the balloon catheter. After it is moved into place, the balloon is inflated; the spring expands and permanently locks in position. This supported area can close in time and should this occur, the failed outcome is called restenosis. Recent technological advancements led to the development of special coatings to the stents resulting in a decrease in this occurrence.

The entire angiogram/angioplasty/stent procedures took several hours. I was then wheeled into a recovery area just outside the angiogram room. I was feeling fine. My blood had become so thin following the increases in medication due to the additional two heart attacks that it was unable to coagulate properly. I continued to bleed from the entrance area in my groin. A number of weights were placed over the groin area to keep the wound closed. As my condition continued to improve, I was taken to a lesser degree recovery room in order to be under observation until the following morning at which time I would be returned to the Mount Scopus branch.

I was again hooked up to blood thinners to make certain that nothing was caught up in my new stent. My groin incision started to bleed again. The night before my heart attack, I slightly scraped my head on the car door while it was opened. It was a very small scratch and was hardly visible. My blood had continued to thin and caused that slight scratch on my forehead just above my eye to start bleeding again. This was now bandaged and unfortunately there was some bleeding under the skin which turned the whole area around my eye a pretty shade of black and blue. It appeared as someone had clobbered me in that area. The doctors decided to stop the intravenous blood thinners. In lieu of weights on the groin incision, they closed the incision tightly with a large clamp that resembled a type of clamp used to hold glued sheets of plywood together. The clamp stopped the bleeding in no time at all. There was a slight side effect to this procedure as my leg turned an unhealthy yellow color. The discoloring did not bother me; however it did upset several of my friends that visited me later that afternoon. The clamp was removed that evening and the incision remained closed. Normal coloring also returned to my leg.

The next morning started with a change of venue. I was now allowed solid foods which had been stopped the evening before my angiogram. I was now able to get out of bed for the first time since Friday afternoon. For those of you that have lost track, we are at Monday morning. Now, after three days of staying practically motionless in bed, I was sitting up, resting for a few minutes, putting one foot down, waiting, and putting the second foot down, resting for a few minutes and then very slowly standing up on my own volition. I automatically set my sights on the 'John' in my room. Very slowly, step by step I walked to the bathroom. It was a great feeling. It was not because hospital bathrooms are such an aesthetic place to urinate. In my case, this outhouse was like a dream come true. It was a fantastic improvement over the damn bed pans I had been using the past three days.

Noontime rolled around and I was wheelchair bound to a dinky transit vehicle, a sure sign that I was on the road to recovery. We arrived at the transit vehicle and since I was given the OK to walk, I climbed out of the wheelchair and into the van. The ride back to Mount Scopus was uneventful which suited me just fine. Upon arrival at Mount Scopus, I was put into another wheelchair and was taken to a standard internal ward as a regular patient. I had officially graduated from the intensive care category. The staff encouraged me to start walking slowly around the corridors, which I was happy to do.

The rest of the week was basically uneventful. I was given an Echo procedure to determine the extent of the permanent damage that my heart had sustained in the attack(s). The following statement is probably the most important in this entire book:

For anyone who thinks that he/she is going thru some type of cardiac related problem (I purposely do not want to use the term heart attack, because most people do not believe that this is actually happening to them) it is critical for this individual to seek correct medical attention as soon

as possible. In the event that he/she is having a heart attack, the extent of the permanent damage to the heart is directly related to the actual start of the attack and the time that proper first aid relief is administered.

The pains and discomfort felt in the chest/shoulder/arm/hand areas are a result of the heart not receiving enough oxygen rich blood resulting from a blockage along the way. After a period of time, the heart cells in the blood depleted areas start dying. The longer the time lapse, the more areas in the heart will cease to function. **This damage is irreversible.**

An Echo Test, also known as Echocardiography or Cardiac Ultrasonography, is a test utilizing ultrasound to evaluate cardiac chamber size, wall thickness, wall motion, valve configuration and motion. It also displays the overall visual functioning of the heart. This technique is similar to ultrasound which is used to check the fetus of the unborn child. The test is performed externally and is painless. The results of my echocardiograph indicated that the permanent damage to my heart was minimal. Again, I cannot emphasize enough the importance of receiving essential first aid as soon as possible in the event of a heart attack.

I was released to go home on July 20th -- a total of eight days in the hospital.

Going Home and Hospital Rehab

Before I was released from the Mount Scopus branch of Hadassah Hospital, I, like most other patients, was visited 4 times a day by a nurse wheeling a cart of medicines -- early in the morning upon wakening (sometimes the *upon wakening* part was externally caused….), in the afternoon shortly after lunch, in the evening after supper, and at bedtime. The daily recuperating routine at the hospital changed dramatically when I was discharged. The onus was now on me to remember to take my medication in a timely manner.

- Plavix (for three weeks only)
- Aspirin
- Lopresor/Neo Block (twice a day)
- Tritace
- Lipidal

Plavex

A complication that can arise from having an angioplasty procedure performed with a stent implant is that a residual buildup of blood could remain inside the stent which in time can cause another blockage. During the weeks following the stent insertion, a thin film of cells will grow over the framework of the stent and eventually coating it as if it was part of the artery wall. The purpose of the Plavix (Clopidogrel) medication is to prevent the blood from sticking to the metal stent framework during this critical first month post stent insertion. A later generation of stent technology that involves chemically coating the stent, substantially reduces the chance of blood adhering to the stent.

Aspirin

Aspirin acts as a blood thinner which makes it less likely for the blood to clot. A daily regimen of Aspirin plus Plavix significantly contributes to the free flowing of blood thru the stent as well as thru the arteries.

Lopresor/Neo Bloc

Lopresor / Neo Bloc are types of medication known as **Beta Blockers** (Beta – Adrenergic Blockers). They relieve stress to the heart by lowering the rate of the heart beat. This results in lower blood pressure and reduces the heart's demand for oxygen. They also have a positive effect in improving the survivor rate for heart attack victims and are accredited to having reduced sudden cardiac arrest by twenty – thirty percent.

Tritace/Ramipril

Tritace / Ramipril are types of medication known as **Ace Inhibitors** (Angiotensin Converting Enzyme Inhibitors). As the term 'inhibitor' implies, these medicines inhibit/block a specific enzyme in the body that is responsible for causing the blood vessels to narrow. If the blood vessels are not abnormally narrowed, they will allow for a normal oxygen rich blood flow to reach the heart. Consequently, the heart will not have to labor as much which in turn may reduce the risk of further damage to the heart due to cardiac arrest. Ace Inhibitors help control the volume of blood in the body. Less blood to pump makes it easier for the heart to function satisfactorily. Like the Beta Blockers, ACE Inhibitors are also accredited with reducing the risk of death by twenty – forty percent.

Lipidal/Pravastatin (Pravachol)

Pravastatin is a cholesterol-lowering drug, and is a member of a group of medications called **statins**. Pravastatin blocks a key step in the body's production of cholesterol and is used to lower cholesterol levels in people with high cholesterol. The 'charts' recommend patients to keep their LHL, the bad cholesterol level, at less than 100. This figure is based on U.S. health guidelines. This medication is usually taken late in the evening preferably before bedtime. Most cholesterol synthesis in the body occurs between midnight and three a.m.

You are now approaching the end of my Medication Course 101. Upon discharge from the hospital, I was given a report summarizing my condition upon arrival and the events of the week:

ACUTE ST ANTERIOR WALL MI –
THROMBOLYTIC RX
PTCA + STENT TO LAD
HYPERTENSION
HYPERCHOLOSTEROLEMIA

And for the translation:

ACUTE (abrupt) MI (Myocardial Infarction –Heart Attack)
ANTERIOR WALL (Front side) ST (Wave – EKG reading)

THROMBOLYTIC RX (Clot medication)
PTCA (Angioplasty) STENT (insertion of the 'spring')
LAD (location: Left Anterior Descending coronary artery)
HYPERTENSION (High blood pressure)
HYPERCHOLOSTEROLEMIA (High cholesterol)

Friends and family who came to visit me that Friday when I returned home could not believe that they were visiting someone who had just started a recuperation period after suffering a *heart attack*. Other than my black and blue eye, there were no physical signs that I had gone thru critical surgery. I felt great, wide awake, refreshed and I was in very good spirits. I could not understand why the Professor of Cardiology at Hadassah Hospital said that I would have to remain at home for a month or two (I had no problem with that). Also, following my recuperation period, my work day would be limited to a four hour per day schedule for the following two months. I have to admit that it was only several years after my stent implant while researching this book, that I discovered the reason why I was taking Plavix and why it was so important not to push myself too fast or too hard during the first month of recuperation.

I also had no problems with the advice to start an exercise program ASAP. The very first morning after coming home from the hospital, I was out walking in my neighborhood at a rather slow pace. It wasn't because of aches or pains, I just wanted to play it safe. Every day I walked a bit further and in a short period of time I increased the tempo to my normal pace.

The following week I began my rehabilitation course at Mount Scopus. Sessions were twice weekly for a period of six weeks. These were two hour sessions. The first hour was a lecture period and the second hour was the exercise portion of the program.

The lecture series ran the gamut of topics that contribute to heart disease, i.e. lack of exercise, poor eating habits, the heredity factor, etc. Emphasis was placed on good eating habits that included keeping foods with saturated fats down to an absolute minimum and to avoid red meats and keep a lid on the eggs. These foods have a tendency to raise our LDL cholesterol, which is the *bad* cholesterol. We learned that fish and chicken are excellent substitutes for red meats. Olive oil is not a saturated fat and is high in monounsaturated fat which is at the top of the list for 'healthy' oils. Olive oil is relatively expensive, and we learned that the ultimate alternative is canola oil, which like olive oil, is high in monounsaturated fat and low in saturated fat.

Each participant had his/her current situation explained by the head of the rehab program, exactly what was performed, the permanent damage that was sustained and what the significance was regarding recovery and ultimately how it would affect daily life once getting back to a normal routine. We also learned about conditions that contribute to heart disease and how big a role stress plays in the overall picture. We became acquainted with new words in our vocabulary for fixing the many facets of heart disease such as angiogram, angioplasty, bypass surgery, etc.

At the beginning and end of each exercise session, our blood pressure was taken and recorded. We were then hooked up to portable EKG monitors that registered our heart rates. Next on the agenda was a series of stretch exercises that made us aware of some muscles we didn't know existed. We were also put thru the paces on a stationary bicycle, a walking machine and a bicycle type workout machine that strengthened the upper body parts including the arms.

All the participants in this Rehab Program had a small electronic device strapped around his/her waist which was connected to the signal forwarding receptacles. The results were submitted real time to a large monitor hanging from the ceiling. The Physiotherapists and nurses were then able to constantly monitor each of our pulse rates and EKG readouts and be able to act accordingly in the event of an emergency. The intensity rate of each machine was gradually ratcheted up every week to increase our stamina.

You may recall that when I was given an angiogram, it was followed by an immediate angioplasty and that a stent was implanted. We were surprised to learn that because of potential complications while undergoing angioplasty and subsequent stent insertion, these procedures are performed only when it is deemed necessary. Arteries that are blocked up to seventy percent are not ballooned. A thirty percent opening in an artery is considered adequate and does not warrant an angioplasty procedure.

The completion of the exercise sessions at the Rehab Center was not meant to be the individual's termination of a body building program. It was only an interim step on the road to recovery. The emphasis was to encourage us to take half hour walks on a daily basis starting at a slow pace and gradually increasing that pace until reaching a level of normality and eventually reaching a good aerobic workout.

As per my cardiologist's advice, I started taking my daily walks a day after I was discharged from the hospital. The walk started at a snail's pace. Despite the fact that I was feeling fine there was still an element of apprehension. How would I know if I was about to take one step too many? As the days went by, I gradually increased the pace of my daily walks and felt comfortable with the progress I was making. Believe it or not, I was really starting to enjoy myself. I would arise early and take my walk in the cool hours of the morning. It was amazing how comfy one could get recuperating at home. Compare this to the hectic normal schedule of pre heart attack days. Crawling out of bed early in the morning, literally flying off to work, and crawling back home on all fours later that evening and at times, very late at night.

It was not too long after I was discharged from the hospital that I noticed by ten a.m. I was starting to feel 'zonked' and I began taking morning naps which felt good. The naps started to become a daily habit. I was not certain whether it was because of the luxurious life of not having to do anything or possibly making up for the sleep I lost during the past several hectic months prior to my heart attack.

About six weeks after my heart attack, the cardiologist professor who had been monitoring me from the time of my initial hospitalization, allowed me to partake in more strenuous activities. I was delighted to hear this as the daily walks were beginning to bore me out of my mind. I was now permitted to swim and to ride a bike. I was very anxious to get back into the pool.

Do you recall the Sagi Bar Mitzvah story? One of the presents Sagi received from us was a twenty-one gear mountain bike. It was not exactly a top of the line model but compared to my thirty year old, ten speed rusted out relic that I had not ridden in years, Sagi's bike felt like a two wheeled Rolls-Royce.

Getting back into the pool after a long absence was an eerie feeling. I could not help thinking about the last time that I was in the pool and the struggle to complete only sixteen laps on the morning of July 13, 2001. The only swimming stroke I learned was the breast stroke. That what happens when one learns to swim at the very young age of thirty-five. On the brighter side, the breast stroke allows for swimming slowly and indeed, the first few laps were *very* slow. The first ride on Sagi's bike was also very slow and did I mention that my neighborhood is quite hilly? I can think of only one place in my neighborhood where there are 150-200 meters (165-220 yards) of flat area. My first bike ride was only about fifteen minutes – back and forth in the small flat area. I again had the same feeling of apprehension as that first walk, and that first lap in the pool. How could I know if I was over exerting myself?

I adapted quite rapidly to the swimming and biking as they were welcome alternatives to walking. As my endurance, strength and self confidence started to improve, the number of laps and pace at the swimming pool started to increase accordingly.

As time went by, it was becoming obvious that despite the morning naps which at times were supplemented with short afternoon snoozes, I was still running out of gas during early evening hours. I could not understand why I was considerably more energetic when I was discharged from the hospital as compared to the end of a several weeks of rehab at home. Something did not add up! I was now constantly tired and had a sluggish feeling during the day. I noticed that my blood pressure was not only much lower than my regular elevated blood pressure but was now constantly lower than the accepted standard of 120/80.

Immediately following one of the rehab periods of twenty minutes on one of the exercise machines, my blood pressure reading was lower than normal. My cardiologist subsequently reduced the dosage of my ACE inhibitor prescription. This prescription adjustment didn't seem to do much for my constant feeling of fatigue but it did adjust my blood pressure to an acceptable level.

After six weeks of a leisurely life at home, I returned to the real world of work. I started working about four hours per day for the first two month period but it was back to the real word just the same. Prior going back to work, I was living the life of a king. The first thing upon awakening in the morning, I had to make a 'big' decision. Would it be the bike this morning or the swimming pool? Hmm! That wasn't too stressful. Next on the agenda was to eat a good leisurely breakfast, read a bit and perhaps watch a little TV and possibly time for another nap. Before I knew it, lunch time snuck up on me. Again some more reading, possibly some TV and another nap if necessary and lo and behold, it was already dinner time.

Up to this point, I did not have to do any serious thinking. The constant sluggish feeling and the 'do not feel like doing anything' feeling did not rock the boat while I was recuperating at home. No earth shattering decisions were made during this period. Going back to work changed all that. My daily routine was now due for a rude awakening!

My morning exercises before leaving for work continued unabated and gave me a sense of accomplishment. The morning nap went by the wayside as there was no way that I was able to plug this into my schedule. I started to run out of gas earlier and earlier every evening. Just as soon as I got home from work, I would head for my comfy living room chair across from our TV set and within minutes I would be fast asleep – totally exhausted. I was now always tired, and I assumed that as time went by, I would recoup my strength and eventually would be able to get back to my pre-attack routine without my recently adopted nap time.

7

What's wrong with me?

O ne day at work I ran into a chap named Dado who was a brother to my good friend Yossi. Yossi and I had lunch together quite frequently and I learned that Dado suffered a heart attack about a year earlier and had a stent implant 'somewhere'. I was very curious to know what medicines he was taking.

After swapping preliminaries, I let him know what I was currently taking. He distinctly remembered the Neo-Bloc that he was given and the side affects that sapped out his energy and alertness. Six months after his heart attack, his doctor had taken him off all of his medication with the exception of aspirin. His lethargic condition dissipated and he is started to feel extremely well.

It was not until a year later while having lunch with Yossi did I learn that Dado had not only been a star soccer player but he was also the team captain of Jerusalem's prestigious Betar Jerusalem Soccer Club. The team had previously won several premier league championships as well as a number of national cups. Dado had been the first team captain that had the honor of raising the National Cup. We will return to Dado later on......

In January 2002, I had my first semi annual checkup at the hospital. That was shortly after my chance meeting with Dado. I took a complete series of blood tests in addition to a stress test on a walking machine. All the test results were quite good especially the computer generated stress test. I informed the head of the cardiology department who was following my case, about my constant fatigue, sluggishness, and my frame of mind of simply 'feeling out of it'. He decided to take me off the Neo-Bloc and closely monitor the results afterwards.

In addition, he was not satisfied with my LDL level of 115 and doubled my dosage of Lipidal. Within a few days, I felt that I could 'breathe again'. I was no longer conking out early in the evening and was able to stay up for longer hours. This was my first positive sign that I was on the way back to recovery and return to my previous life style.

Other problems still remained. Although I no longer felt the need for a nap during the day, the mental sluggishness continued and I was unable to shake it. Other negative changes were also happening with increased frequency. A number of daily routines that had been automatic and accomplished without consciously thinking about them could no longer be taken for granted. I began locking the car while leaving the car keys in the ignition. This was happening more and more frequently. I started unintentionally leaving my cell phone in the car.

A first aid solution to this problem was to make a duplicate key and carry this in my wallet. I was cognizant of these memory lapses and needless to say, it did not sit well. The duplicate key did not eliminate the frustrating feeling of "what's happening to me?" It did however, enabled me to open the car door without too much trouble. I refined my exiting the car routine by taking a mental inventory count of car keys and cell phone before exiting the vehicle. This new strategy only took a second or two and it was probably not noticeable to my non enlightened passengers. This was a big change for me.

What was once a simple chore now had to be executed purposely.

Gone were the days when I would arrive at my office with my car keys automatically in my left front pocket and my cell phone in my right pocket. This force of habit task which had previously been accomplished without ever thinking twice about it now became much more complicated. I added a third item to the list of things I would take to the office. It was a music cassette which I enjoyed while fighting traffic on the way to the office. Now I started to leave the car with only two out of the three items I had intended to bring with me. I discovered that when I removed the cassette from the radio, this seemingly uncomplicated maneuver would erase from my mental 'things to do list', the task of removing the car keys from the ignition.

Gradually I was able to update the car exiting procedure to include the third item. This additional mental concentration overload caused me to lock the car one day with the windows wide open and I did not discover this until one of my co-workers called this to my attention just as I was about to leave the parking lot.

I became aware of another situation that had surfaced which became problematic. I was able to see and hear perfectly well yet I was not able to comprehend video signals and audio sounds that I saw and heard. This was another form of conking out but now I was on my feet and wide awake. This brings to mind the windows I left open in my car when I locked the doors. Somehow the open windows didn't register.

Another similar example occurred when I put a sheet of paper on top of my briefcase one evening with the intention of taking it with me to the office the next day. The following morning my concentration was funneled on getting out of the house and off to work as quickly as possible. I had to see the sheet of paper lying on top of the brief case when I removed it. Instead of inserting the paper into the briefcase, I simply set it aside and left the paper in my house after I had left for work.

What's wrong with me?

The list of seeing things in front of me and not being able to register those things in my mind was beginning to overwhelm me.

My verbal communication also suffered. I recall one of my assistants asking me a question regarding a project that we were working on. I understood every word she said but I was unable to comprehend the question. I got out of this situation by responding "What do you think we should do?" She gave me her answer, and again, I understood every word she said but I could not understand her answer.

And to make matters worse, not seeing was followed by not remembering. I am not referring to some complicated statistic or piece of data. In this instance, it was the name of a co-worker sitting in the next room. I saw him in the hallway adjacent to our rooms. He was talking to someone and I was about to say "Hey…" and I realized that I could not remember his name. As luck would have it, I was able to glance at the door to his office and see his name on the door.

And the fun continued! I started having trouble making daily, routine decisions. When having to make a choice in relatively simple matters such as what to wear, or what to spread on my sandwich for lunch, the answers puzzled me. There was an episode of the Simpsons in which Mr. Burns found himself for the first time in a supermarket. He wanted to purchase some ketchup. In one hand he held a bottle that was labeled ketchup and in the other hand he held a bottle labeled catsup. He kept looking back and forth at the two bottles and saying out loud "catsup…ketchup …catsup…ketchup". He simply could not make up his mind.

I began to notice that my mental concentration and my ability to analyze situations and to plan ahead, had undergone a metamorphose and the change left a lot to be desired. Doing immediate tasks at hand was no problem. I did not feel that I was walking around inebriated or in a stupor. I was able to concentrate on specific tasks providing that I was left undisturbed. The problem was that I lost the connection between the immediate tasks with other parallel tasks that would also require some type of attention. At work I began not to see (notice) things on the computer screen and since I had been in the computer field for twenty years, this also was very disturbing.

On a recent project, I remembered going into my boss's office to inform him that on a particular opening web page on our site, a problem with an application with a link on the page had been solved. The page could now be uploaded to the internet. All my concentration regarding the particular page was focused on that one specific application. When he asked me about some of the icons on the page and clicked them, they were inoperative. I remember standing there dumbfounded thinking to myself "How in the world did I not think of clicking the icons to verify that they also work?" Here I was claiming the page was complete when in reality it was the original problem that I had solved successfully but it never occurred to me to check anything else on the page. In addition, I lost the ability to see clearly some future date and/or event and to coordinate future tasks that gel together as a project.

Another way to look at this problem can be compared to driving our Mitsubishi sedan at night with the bright lights on. Besides being able to see far off in the distance, I can also see quite well in the near distance which encompasses the shoulders of the road (side vision). This is how my mind would work regarding my project responsibility. When working on a project, I would be constantly aware of parallel aspects going on at the same time. I may not have seen all the small details that had to be accomplished to finish the project, but I would definitely stay on top of the coordination and the assembling the major parts for the project's finish.

That is how I previously visualized the way projects would end, months before the actual finish. This is not to say that I lost the beam altogether. My concentration had become like a flashlight beam, very narrow and no side vision which allowed me to see several meters (6½ feet) ahead of me only.

What's wrong with me?

My decision making abilities also changed. I found that I would be making poor decisions based upon short sighted considerations only.

In addition to confusion and forgetting things, I felt that there were changes in my mood and frame of mind. One can almost say a lack of frame of mind. While everyone in my immediate surroundings would be in a positive mood, I would be in a zero mood, not necessarily a bad mood but rather an apathetic mood, which was neither good nor bad. This of course would be preferable to bad moods that I would get into with only the slightest provocation.

I started to sense the world around me differently. I have normal hearing and with eye glasses my vision is twenty-twenty. I had the feeling that I was hearing everything quite well but it was as if I had cotton stuffed in my ears that somewhat delayed the sound from reaching my inner ear in real time. I could see everything perfectly while wearing my glasses, however it was as if the lenses were not only several millimeters thick, but rather a whole foot thick, which also caused a delay in real time before the picture entered my mind (please excuse the use of both the metric and American system of measurement systems, but you get the point).

It was almost as though there was an additional factor separating/filtering my own personal sensors from the outside world. My hands could feel but it was as if I was wearing invisible thick gloves that filtered out the direct touch.

Equally frustrating was being told something which I understood at the time but after a time lapse of only a few minutes, I would not remember it. One day a friend of mine requested that I complete a minyan[*] as it was important for him to say Kaddish[**] in memory of his late father. He spoke to me about twenty minutes ahead of time. I heard, I acknowledged, I

---

[*] the quorum of 10 adult Jews required for communal worship
[**] Jewish prayer recited in the daily ritual of the synagogue and by mourners at public services after the death of a close relative.

understood but within twenty minutes I forgot! It was not until several hours later that I remembered that I promised to attend.

It also follows that the combination of being physically/mentally zonked out and being in a bad/zero mood all of the time just does wonders for one's sex life. I was not sure if it was because of the lack of interest that caused a decline in my physical abilities, or the decline in my physical abilities that caused the lack of interest, or maybe a combination of both. These are well known and documented side effects of some post-heart attack drugs that we have to take, especially the drugs taken to insure that blood pressure does not exceed normal levels.

Although there apparently is still life after a heart attack, but it was turning out to be a different type of life from that which I was accustomed to.

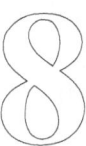

Self Rehabilitation - Physical

I still remember how good I felt after being discharged from the hospital. This was before I developed an adverse reaction to the medications I was taking. At the ripe old age of fifty-one, I was not about to hang it up and start to vegetate. It did not take me too long to realize that I was not cut out to just walk as my prime exercise activity despite the fact that quite a few people do enjoy a brisk walk daily. I was anxious to get back in the pool. Better yet, I yearned to get on a real bike and not the stationary type bike that we used at the rehab center. As I mentioned earlier, six weeks after my heart attack, I was given permission to partake in both swimming and bicycle riding with the stipulation that I start these exercises at a very slow pace.

I enjoyed riding a bike when I was a kid and even thought I was the last one on my block in my age group to learn how to ride a two wheeler. I did not become a proficient bike rider until the ripe old age of eight. Despite sports not being 'my thing' during my entire school years, I did run junior varsity cross country in high school. I was not very fast but I did finish every race in which I participated by running the whole course. It was not unusual for me to pass about half of the other runners who during the race reduced their run to a walk. I attributed my stamina to my wiry frame which was devoid of a single ounce of fat. Some of the chubbier rascals that had to schlep those extra kilos/lbs simply ran out of gas early.

Bikes have really evolved since my old ten speed antique. I remember the two gear levers that were at the bottom bar and in order to change gears, I had to reach down which was rather uncomfortable. After buying Sagi his twenty-one speed mountain bike (levers on the handle bar) three years earlier, the change was quite apparent. I really enjoyed taking his bike out for a ride every now and then.

Yogev, also known as Yogli, is a friend whom I met at work. He had been conducting extensive research on the type of bike he wanted to purchase for himself and for his girl friend. The time and effort he put into this project was comparable to purchasing a new car. Some of the factors under consideration were: new or used; street bike, mountain bike or hybrid; tire size; single gear up to and including close to thirty gears; shock absorbers; disc brakes; price; etc. Cannondale is considered by many to be the top of the line and is often referred to as the Rolls Royce of mountain bicycles. It also can carry a price tag upwards of $5,000. What helped to finalize Yogli's decision to purchase a bike was the input of another co-worker named Guy who was considered the 'bike professional' of the office. His bike, a Trek 4500 was purchased a year earlier for approximately $600. I thought that price tag was extremely expensive which brought back memories when I purchased a ten speed bicycle at TOYS R US back in 1972 for $65.

Sagi's bike in 1998 cost $200 which I thought at the time was quite exorbitant. What can I say? I'm still used to the purple four cent Lincoln stamps and the ten cent phone calls. After much thought, Yogli decided to buy a Trek but something less professional then the Trek 4500. He settled for the Trek

4300 which cost about $400. As you can see, prices in Israel are a 'bit' more than in the States

After riding more and more in my neighborhood, I decided to upgrade my two wheel relic for two reasons. In the event that Sagi and I would want to ride together, two bikes would be better than 1 and a half bikes. On a more serious note, I considered the purchase of a new bicycle not as an adult toy but an important acquisition to be incorporated into my physical rehabilitation program. The $400 that Yogli had paid for his Trek 4300 bicycle was already a discounted price as it included a second bike at the time of purchase for his girl friend Faran, which by the way is now his wife. Faran wound up with a less expensive model Trek 850.

Several weeks later, which happened to be exactly two months after I had my heart attack, was also Esty's birthday, a date I better not forget! We decided to celebrate by eating dinner in Jerusalem and to rendezvous with Yogli later at the bicycle store. After celebrating Esty's birthday at a restaurant we went out to buy 'me' a new bike. This by the way sums up the type of person Esty really personifies. It's her birthday and I get the new bicycle. Isn't life grand?

Since Yogli had put considerable time in selecting his choice for a new bike and since I valued his judgment, I felt there was no need to reinvent the wheel. I purchased the same model Trek 4300. The only difference was my shiny new bike was red and his was a silver gray. I remember how I felt when I rode Sagi's bike for the first time. WOW! It was like a riding a dream compared to the older run down bikes that I previously owned. After my first ride on my new Trek 4300, I experienced WOW #2 which felt like I was in a completely different league compared to Sagi's two wheeler. I simply could not imagine what riding a Cannondale would feel like.

Bike riding was now the first thing on my agenda after rolling out of bed in the morning. I was off and riding usually before breakfast. My endurance had increased to the level that I was able to ride for an hour without stopping. I decided it was about time to do some serious riding. This meant getting out of my immediate neighborhood and seeing other sites. I was a bit apprehensive about leaving the confines of my development for the first time. It was similar to the feeling I had the first time I sat on a bike after my heart attack when I was given an OK by my cardiology professor to take a short ride.

As I was preparing my equipment for the ride, I could not help but think about Abe Weintraub. I might never have of heard about this amazing story if I had not known his son, Bob, who lives in Beer-Sheva. I met Abe and his late wife Ruthie over twenty years ago when they were here visiting Bob. Abe and Ruthie were from Brooklyn, and when they heard that I had a grandmother still living in Brooklyn, they paid her a visit as soon as they got back to the States. Nice folks the Weintraubs.

Ruthie eventually became sick with Alzheimer's disease. When she was confined to a wheel chair, Abe, then approaching the ripe young age of eighty, started pushing his wife of over fifty years all through the city – for hours – every day. After Ruthie passed away, Abe thought to himself "not only was I walking all day, but also pushing Ruthie's weight. There's no reason why I can not start running by myself."

And start running he did. Marathon races! Between the ages of eighty and ninety, he started and completed nine New York Marathons! At age ninety, he finished the New York Marathon in less than seven and a half hours, a world record for the age 90+ runners. If Abe could run like that at age ninety, there is no reason why I could not undertake a somewhat rigorous bicycle riding program at age fifty-one despite my previous heart attack.

Yogli was trying to organize Friday 'fun rides' with other co-workers in the Jerusalem area. The 'group' finally met for the first time and consisted of Yogli and myself. Yogli assumed the position of Commander & Chief Navigator. My responsibility was limited to supplying fresh home made bread for this venture. We have one of those small bread baking machines that does it all. Esty is the chief operator of this gadget. We met for the first 'group' bike ride at Bet-Zait just outside of Jerusalem and rode uphill back to Jerusalem.

There were numerous stops along the way. After all, uphill is uphill and this was my first bike ride of any significance since my house rehab period started. Besides being cognizant of my surroundings, my eyes were constantly glancing at the pulse measuring device that I was wearing and I made certain that my pulse rate did not exceed the high end of the recommended rate range. In effect, I was constantly monitoring my pulse rate for the entire bike ride. The ride up the hill was thru a very scenic part of the Jerusalem forest as was the stop for breakfast. Yogli took out the fruit he was carrying and I came up with the bread. We refilled our water containers from the water we were schlepping strapped to our backs and delved into our peaceful and pleasant breakfast. We continued uphill towards Jerusalem, turned around and rode back down. The uphill part of the trip was a real drag but the downhill run made the entire trip worthwhile.

I rode about 10km (6 miles) that day and was quite pleased with myself regarding my endurance level. In fact, it felt like quite an accomplishment. I cannot recall exactly what I did when I returned home but I assume that I took a nice afternoon nap, probably a nice long one!

That week at work, word was out that there was now an organized group of bicycle riders that started riding on Fridays. It was irrelevant that the group only had two participants. The rides had started. The following week, our 'group' increased by fifty percent. That's right; we now had three able body participants. Elana from the software support department joined us. Yogli, our Commander at the time was 30ish, strong and an officer in an elite Special Forces army unit. He is presently in the reserves and was recently promoted to the rank of Captain. Elana was somewhere in her mid twenties. The three of us met at the same rendezvous point at Bet-Zeit and rode the same route as the previous week.

About ten minutes after starting out, we were riding at a snail's pace up a steep hill. Elana was now walking her bike. We ran across a local resident who was taking his morning walk. He stopped to talk with us and that suited me just fine as I was ready for a break. He thought it so nice that a father was taking his two grown kids out for a bike ride. He was amused to learn that we were co-workers and not a family. Elana was not too thrilled with the route Yogli had chosen but eventually we all made it to the top after stopping along the way for breakfast.

Having Elana with us was good for publicity. We were now a co-ed group. Fridays had now become a fixed event every week and slowly the group started to grow. If I recall correctly, the maximum amount of riders at any one time was only six. For a while we never had less than three - four riders at any one time and these were not always the same riders. I can think of at least thirteen different riders that rode with us at least one time.

At the beginning the route was more or less the same. We would all park our cars at Bet Zeit and then ride in the direction of Bet-Shemesh which is in the opposite direction of our initial rides. We rode until we felt that we reached the half way mark for the distance we wanted to travel that day. The half way mark depended on several factors such as the endurance of the riders that particular day, the heat, the hour, etc.

When we advanced to the stage where we had finished a ride of approximately 30km (18 miles) irrespective of the number of rest stops, we decided to make it a one way trip. Guy, who had not participated with us on earlier rides, wanted to organize a one way trip from Bet Zeit to Bet Shemesh, a distance of approximately 30km. Because of the differences in the altitudes, the overall direction of the trip would be downhill.

Organizing the car arrangements topped the list of things to be done before the next bike ride. Who would leave their cars at the starting point? Who would leave their cars at the finish line? How would the riders and bikes get back to the starting point? These decisions were not too difficult to finalize but it all had to be arranged beforehand. When Friday morning rolled around, four vehicles met at the finish line in Bet Shemesh, two vehicles remained there for the return trip and two vehicles with the six bikes headed off to the starting point and off we went.

Approximately 25km (15 miles) out of the 30km (18 miles) were on unpaved trails and included stretches where only a four wheel drive vehicle could navigate. The route was parallel to the Sorek River. It passed a dam at the Ein Kerem area and continued thru the mountains parallel to the old Tel Aviv / Jerusalem rail line which is now being rebuilt. The view along this route is fabulous. If I had not known that that we were only a ten – fifteen minute drive from Jerusalem, I would have believed that we were on a bike trip thru the Greek island of Crete.

There is something very peaceful and calming riding thru a trail and listening to the current of the stream along side the route and marveling at the wooded mountains all around. We rode at a comfortable pace and took a number of rest stops. The breakfast stop along the way left everyone stuffed. Unfortunately this was not an ideal feeling knowing very well we had to climb aboard our bikes shortly and head back on the trail. We stopped at a shaded area about two thirds the way of our planned trip with only mountains and trees to look at. The birds were chirping and the scent of blooming spring and wild flowers was everywhere.

Everyone brought something which we all shared. I brought my Esty bread, Guy had his herbal tea – yup, he schlepped his small gas burner with him. Hadas's crepes were made that morning and they were consumed in record breaking time. You may recall the potato chip commercial where you could not eat just one, well, the advertisement could have been written for those yummy crepes. After consuming our fill of goodies, our motley group was now more inclined to take a nap rather than get back on our bikes!

Fortunately we were not too far from our long descent down the mountain to the Bet Shemesh region and once again we were on our way. At the bottom of the descent, there were two points where the trail curved around and the Sorek stream crossed the path and covered it with about a foot of flowing water. Going thru the stream kicked up the excitement several notches. We took another 'breakfast break' after the second stream crossing, munched on the remaining goodies, rested awhile and took off again

Several kilometers later I felt that something was not right. It was an eerie feeling and I could not put my finger on it. Here we are in the middle of nature having a nice pleasant ride, when it hit me. **I had forgotten my backpack at the last stop.** I do not know what bothered me more, the possibility that some other nature hiker might find my abandoned backpack and I might lose my drivers license, credit cards, my spare water and other incidentals or that in the middle of nature and with not a care in the world, I had another mental relapse similar to locking keys in the car. I just experienced another supposedly automatic function that turned out to be not automatic.

Guy and Yogli, the two strongest riders of the group rode back to fetch the backpack. Needless to say, I was delighted and relieved to see them return with it. It was only partial compensation for the awful feeling of helplessness that I felt not being able to remember to take the backpack after the break.

Finally we arrived at the parked vehicles we had left early in the morning in Bet Shemesh. The feeling of the group was ecstatic. This was the trip to end all trips! We all sat down in the middle of the parking lot to stretch our aching leg muscles. We really believed that we had just completed the ultimate 30km (18 mile) bike ride. Our route was mostly trail riding through a beautiful wooded area. It just doesn't get much better than that.

♥ ♥ ♥

During the next several months, Fridays were reserved for our bike rides. The regulars were Yogli and me. Eventually the group dwindled down to just the two of us and this caused a problem that we did not anticipate.

We had started taking longer and longer rides, usually a round trip to the same point. Eventually, Yogli proposed that we meet at a prearranged location, leave one car there and both of us would then drive to the starting point of our bicycle ride. We would then bike ride one-way to where we parked the first car and drive back together to pick up the second vehicle

The unanticipated problem developed gradually. When we started to solicit bike riders, all of us had about the same level of endurance. The girls at the office were not too keen on taking long trips and as the distances grew they became more and more disenchanted. They were the first to drop out. As the mileage/km steadily increased, the enthusiasm of the group of riders declined proportionally except for Yogli and me. I always looked forward to these Friday bike rides and was both surprised and pleased how my endurance kept improving.

My daily morning routine of many years had abruptly changed directions. I was now getting up quite early in the morning and going for my bike ride before work. I also discovered that it did not matter if I was first one to start working at seven a.m. or nine a.m. I would still be in the office until six – seven p.m. and very often much later

This 'important' part of my day I started doing first thing in the morning, and not waiting to see if I have the time/energy to ride during the evening or at night. The daily morning bike rides also increased my stamina which made my Friday tours less strenuous.

I purchased a speedometer/odometer about seven months after I bought my bike. I was a bit fascinated and envious when someone in our riding group had one of these gismos and furnished us with statistics regarding the distance, average and maximum speed. I just had to have one of these gismos primarily to monitor my exercise progress and this was a perfect time for it. On April 5th, 2002 my Trek 4300 was sporting a new addition – a new speedomer/odometer.

The advantage of having an odometer makes it convenient to find excuses to continue riding just a bit more. By the time I installed the odometer, I realized that I did not have a problem in riding 10km (6 miles) every morning before going to work. This now became the target reading for my morning rides. Instead of the clock determining a time element for my exercise program, I subsequently switched gears to calibrate mileage/km which more accurately reflected my progress.

Despite the fact that I was unable to ride every morning I was still averaging 70km (42 miles) per week. This tally included the Friday bike rides. That is not too bad for someone recuperating from a heart attack less than a year earlier. I remember vividly those first bicycle rides of fifteen minute periods back and forth around the flat areas of my neighborhood.

Riding by yourself has its merits as it allows you to daydream without infringing on other chores especially in the work arena or possibly at the dinner table while having light conversations with family members. Daydreaming also has its limits and I would not recommend it in heavy traffic for obvious reasons.

As time ticked by, the distance increased and I was now averaging 11km (6½ miles) per day. With just a little more effort I knew that I could round out these figures upwards to 80km (50 miles) / per week. After three months of bike riding I had clocked 1,100 km (682 miles) which is over 12.2km (7½ miles) / per day. That same day I set a personal goal I wanted to achieve. On April 4, 2003 I want to see at least 4,000km (2,480 miles) on my odometer. This seemed to be a realistic goal as I was already on a yearly pace of 4,400km based on my first three month period. I assumed that I would start to swim several times a week and during the hottest part of the summer I would be riding less. I would also be riding less during the cold rainy days of winter. Yup, 4,000km would do just fine!

It was toward the end of summer 2002 that I took a week off from work for a father/son camping trip. This was prior to back to school time for the kids. Tuval, my youngest son was eleven years old and he helped me pack our tent together with all of our camping equipment which included two bikes and a bicycle touring book. We drove to the northern part of the country not far from Kiryat Shemona, practically a stone's throw from the Lebanese border. Our agenda included rising early in the morning for our daily bike rides. We planned to be back well before the temperature hit the high of the day, cool off in the pool and get ready for the evening meal.

Our tent was erected in a very nice camping ground called Horshat Tal. The facility furnished all the comforts of home such as running water, hot showers, clean bathrooms and a very nice lake for swimming. According to the book, a 30km (18½ mile) trip on level trail riding ground seemed apropos for our first riding day.

The next morning we were up before daylight, loaded the bikes back onto the car and headed off to the starting point for the first ride of the tour. The tour books are filled with useful information such as pointing out historic and important landmarks and other places of interest along the way. There is also a downside to the book regarding critical points along the way especially locating trails which were not always accurate.

As per the tour guide, we set the daily odometer reading to zero and we took off. When we were at the half way mark along the route, the tour map indicated a place to make a right hand turn. We spotted this point but the trail was overrun with foliage and appeared as if no one had traveled this route for quite some time. We thought we would give it a try but it didn't take too long to realize the trail had become impassible. We then made a U turn and returned to the location where the overgrown foliage started. There was still some doubt in our minds whether or not we had made a premature turn off the main road or we were at the right place but the dense foliage simply made the trail non navigable. It was already getting quite hot as it usually does at summer time in the Middle East and so we decided to head back by the same route that brought us to this point. Tomorrow is another day and we will try to do it right next time.

We arrived back at Horshat Tal overheated and sweaty. We quickly got into our bathing suits and plunged into the lake with all the other bathers. Thinking back when this occurred, I consider myself to be lucky that I did not have another heart attack when I hit the water. The water was *extremely* cold. The rapid change in external body temperature was quite a shock. The big unanswered question remained how could this peaceful looking lake be so cold on this very hot summer day? The answer was quite simple. The bulk of the lake water emanates from the Hatzbani River in Hatzbaya, Lebanon which is fed by the melting snows in the mountains. After getting somewhat acclimated to the frigid water, it was possible to swim a meager five minutes before we would turn to a pretty shade of blue. I do not remember what we had for dinner that evening. I imagine it was a father and son barbecue.

The following day I decided to go back to our original route which I thought was the correct choice. I assumed that the trail that was half covered by grass and other vegetation and was run down by the lack of foreign and domestic tourists due primarily to the Intifada. The trail was growing back to the way nature had originally planned the area. We attempted to navigate the disappearing trail again, and again we had to return to our original starting point. It was time to return to our campsite.

After covering just about the entire area which was not in accordance with the official printed version of the bicycle route, we were still very satisfied with our bike riding and the outdoor living for the past several days. The last day of our bike riding we were back on the overgrown trail that took us to a partially paved road that linked up to the proper route and we finished the ride. I know exactly where the book let us astray. Just wait till next year!

Despite the fact that we went astray several times, we did manage to get in some good bicycle riding. We returned home at the end of the week with an additional 200km (125 miles) on the odometer. My daily average had now risen to above 12½km (7¾ miles), approaching 88km per week. Remember the rounding up? If I reach an average daily ride of 12.86km, then I'm already at ninety per week.

Bike riding was slowly now becoming an obsession. The beginning of October was my six month halfway point to reach my quest of 4,000km (2,480 miles) by April 4th. I had already passed 2,350km (1,460 miles) which put me at the fantastic rate of 4,700km (2,914 miles) per year. If I would continue to improve at the current rate I could reach 5,000km (3,100 miles) and indeed I revised my personal goal of 4,000km to reach 5,000km by April 4th, 2003.

9

Self Rehabilitation - Mental/Emotional

I realized immediately after my heart attack, that this did not occur primarily from the 'hardware' located in the middle of my chest cavity but was strongly influenced by the 'software' in my head. (As I have mentioned before, I have been in the computer field for the past twenty years.) My physical appearance did not indicate that I was a candidate to fall prey to a heart attack. Basically, I had none of the known indications to suspect a pending heart attack. I was not overweight, a non-smoker, physically active and supposedly in good condition. What pushed me over the line was my failure to control the stress in my daily life. And what exactly is stress? It is any external stimulus that upsets the dynamic balance of our bodies!

Just about everyone encounters some level of stress in their daily lives. Stress takes many forms and everyone handles it differently. It may start at the breakfast table and you could be under pressure to leave the house as early as possible to avoid the morning rush hour traffic, cope with the other drivers with whom you share the road, and up until now, you have yet to arrive at the office. The stress continues unabated at the office from the time you arrive until the time the lights go out.

The phone calls, the deadlines, the unplanned little set backs that cumulatively mess up project schedules, computer crash, the sick employee that does not arrive for work which is another schedule buster, an employee's child is ill and someone has to stay at home with the child, your boss is in a bad mood, your boss's boss is in a bad mood, etc. The list is endless.

Stress over the last several decades has become well documented. As early as 1950, Dr. Hans Selye,[4] a physiologist from the University of Toronto described the general effect of severe stress which is termed the *General Adaptation Syndrome* (GAS.). GAS is comprised of three overlapping stages: alarm, resistance and exhaustion.

Alarm

This is the first response of the body to an external stressful situation. The body recognizes a danger and mobilizes its physical resources to cope with the stress. Pulse and breathing quicken, and the muscles, now 'on alert' become tense. It is not unusual for an individual to feel the first symptoms of stress such as: upset stomach, diarrhea, fever, headaches, shortness of breath, etc.

Resistance

The body's defense systems have stabilized and the physical symptoms of upset stomach, diarrhea, etc. no longer seem to be present. The body appears to have returned to its normal pre-stress appearance. The body pays a high price for this transformation. During this stage, the body has adjusted to cope with the original stress at the cost of a reduction in its ability to resist stress from other sources.

Exhaustion

At this stage and after prolonged resistance of coping with stress, the body's resources become exhausted and the immune system is weakened. Depending on the individual, the weakest organ system is the first to break down.

Factors influencing the severity and potential consequences of stress are its duration, intensity and its imminence.

In my situation, I believe my first forty-five years of 'eat all you want and whenever you want' set the stage for possible complications in later life. On the other hand, had I lived on a deserted tropical island under ideal living conditions (fine food, Pamela Anderson, e-mail…), I may have lived to a peaceful old age without ever knowing that my cardiovascular system was a ticking time bomb. However, in my non medical opinion, it was the prolonged period of several months of extraordinary stress at work that ultimately pushed me over the line.

Another interesting point is why it is that two different people will physically react differently to the same stressful situation. In 1959, two cardiologists, Dr. Meyer Friedman and Dr. Ray Rosenman[5] formalized their theory regarding different personality types in people, and how the type of personality can influence the physical health of the individual.

Type A people can be categorized and described as people that view everything as urgent. This may include but not limited to the following: walking, talking, eating rapidly, move abruptly, feel impatient with the rate of many daily occurrences that take place, have a tendency to interrupt others, are basically achievement oriented, feel guilty when not doing anything productive, can be hostile or aggressive without serious provocation. They can have a tendency to evaluate themselves and others by numbers. Does this remind you of increasing my annual goal of 4,000km (2,480 miles) to

5,000km (3,100 miles)? This more or less describes me yet I never considered myself as the aggressive type. I still feel uncomfortable being stuck behind a slow driver even though I still have time to get to work early. I also do not like waiting in line.

In contrast, the **Type B** person can be categorized as 'cool' and does not get rattled easily. This individual takes life easy and plays for enjoyment. There is no inclination to prove superiority and harbors little or no attribute that mold the Type A character.

The interesting point here is statistically, Type A people were considered for a long time to be almost three times more likely to have heart attacks!![6]

Bike riding and swimming were the prelude to my physical recovery. It was also the time to 'fix the software upstairs'. This is somewhat of a murky area. I was not the first person to undergo a heart attack and I can not say that there is something wrong upstairs with everyone who does have a heart attack. Unknowingly I had become a pressure cooker, however the excess steam valve was stopped up and there was no way for me to blow off the excess pressure until **BOOM**. The inevitable happened, the system started to shut down and in layman's terms, it is called a *heart attack*.

I was never an outgoing individual. On the contrary, I was quite reserved in my mannerism and kept both the good and the bad bottled up inside. I had no problem with that. I was even proud of it because 'that is the way I am'. That outlook still landed me a wife that is quite suitable for me. We worked hard to build a nice home where our four terrific kids grew up. I would venture to say that our standard of living was more than adequate. Simply put, a lot of people would like to have what we have obtained in life.

While I could not be called a party pooper, social activities were not on the top of my agenda. I was not one to pop over to someone's home for a cup of coffee at the end of the day and get involved in small, meaningless talk. I considered this a waste of time and with the little free time I had, I wanted to use it to better advantage.

It has been said that one of the most important assets we possess is time. As the hours tick by, that time slot is irretrievably lost forever. Whether I am at work or at home there always seemed to be a myriad amount of things that have to be accomplished within a given time slot. Inevitably, one or more of the chores could not be squeezed into the given time frame and would have to be reprogrammed in a future 'free' time slot. And to waste time visiting neighbors??? Give me a break! Esty would laugh at me and would say the reason that I do not visit any neighbors is because I do not drink coffee. My pat answer would be "Coffee is just for grown-ups" and this became my punch line whenever I was offered coffee.

Not being a coffee drinker, I did not see the necessity of the 'ceremony' that accompanies the preparation and drinking of coffee and of course the small talk in-between each sip of the freshly brewed drink. Esty had drastically cut her consumption of coffee in the past several years. When she was still 'addicted' to it and at the end of the day, despite being very tired, she just had to visit a girl friend for the 'ceremony' and the small talk.

Several months after my heart attack, two good friends came by and tried to persuade me to participate in a seminar that they had attended. Their enthusiasm in describing the seminar was sincere and they highly recommended the program. I had heard about these types of seminars, for people *to find themselves, to be all they can be, to improve the quality of their lives and for self improvement.*

While I did not have any objections to others attending these programs, I felt that I had very little or nothing to gain in attending one of these sessions. I did not have to *find myself.* I knew exactly where I was and knew which direction I was going. I had no qualms with the quality of life that I built for myself. I was doing just fine, thank you. I worked hard and enjoyed the fruits of my labor without the input of an outsider giving me advice and therapy on how to manage my affairs. I have always considered these friends to have their feet planted firmly on the ground and were not the weirdo type of individuals seeking some alternative voodoo system of life.

Ten years earlier I would not have heard of such an idea -- not even from my best of friends -- not five years earlier, not one year earlier, not even two months earlier. However the rules of the game had radically changed for me the moment I had the heart attack.

Something apparently was not totally right in the way I had been running my life up until then, and even if the source of the attack itself was partially from external sources (i.e. work related stress), ultimately I myself am to blame as I did not properly know how to handle the excess stress and allowed it to physically defeat me.

The stage may have been set with accumulated plaque lining my arteries, but ultimately it was not my boss, or his boss, or the awful aggressive other drivers, or anyone else who can take responsibility for my fall. The problem (even if I did not know it at the time) was mine, and the responsibility was mine to find a solution.

When my friends spoke to me about attending the seminars, I was already feeling the accumulated draining effects from all the medications I had been taking. To be truthful, I believed it would have been a waste of time to attend the seminars sessions that were scheduled over a long weekend and were expected to last until the early hours of the following day. I thought it best to postpone this program to a later date when I would not feel like a wet wash rag just about every night before dinner time. I just could not shake this 'always tired' feeling.

After my January 2002 checkup (Beta Blocker discontinued, cholesterol medication doubled), seeing that I was able to stay awake longer, I decided that I would attend the seminar that they had recommended, the next one being the following month (February).   It was run by the Outlook organization (http://www.outlook.org.il/english) with other branches in England and in Spain.

I had serious doubts about any real benefits to be derived by attending these seminars, yet it was worth a try. Whatever I might gain from these sessions would definitely be a plus. I had nothing to lose except the fee to participate and the time I allocated to participate in the program. Actually, the sponsors of this program advised the participants that if they felt they did not get anything out of the 4 day series, they would be entitled to a full refund. It was actually a win/win situation.

Besides actually not having anything to lose,   I took the whole Outlook weekend one step further. I was going to take a whole weekend vacation by myself. By February, I was already back to working full time (since the first of November) and I planned my weekend as follows:

The first session of the seminar starts at six p.m. on a Wednesday. On that day, I would work a half day, then take the bus to Tel-Aviv (where the seminar was held). I had already prearranged with Esty's nephew to stay at his apartment, about a fifteen minute walk from the seminar location. He was renting the apartment with some friends, however that weekend he was in Beer-Sheva for the entire weekend. I had his room for myself.

On Thursday, the seminar also starts at six p.m.; however I decided that I would be on vacation from *everything* for the weekend. Instead of coming back to Jerusalem to work, I would take the day off entirely and find something to do in Tel-Aviv.

The sessions on Friday and Saturday start at eleven a.m. which does not leave much time for anything else. Should the seminars fall short of anything meaningful, I would still be treating myself to a mini vacation. Household chores would be on hold as well as work at the office. Daily routine regarding family matters, Esty and the kids, were all on hold for a few days. That mini vacation was just for me!

♥ ♥ ♥

The starting day of the Outlook Seminar did arrive of course, and as planned, I worked that morning, and then took off to Tel-Aviv. I first stopped by the apartment (I wanted to look for it in daylight and not starting searching for it late at night) to drop my stuff off, and headed off to the seminar.

Approximately thirty participants signed up for the program. I recognized a few of them that came from my neighborhood. Besides Tony the trainer, there was his assistant trainer Orit, and their entourage of at least twenty supporters. These individuals were graduates from previous seminars and had volunteered their time for the weekend. Their input was quite valuable and contributed significantly to the success of the program. The program was managed with army type precision and all supporting personnel knew exactly what roll they had to perform.

The seminar basically consisted of lectures, group exercises and/or sharing personal experiences with the group of participants. The first session was primarily lectures followed by group exercises. Several participants had an opportunity to share their experiences with others in the program. The initial session lasted quite late and afterwards I took a nice leisurely walk back to the apartment.

The next morning I awakened to a very unusual situation for me. I am always busy, always something that just has to get done that day, always something to do while I'm at work, or something I want to take care of when I'm home. Well here I was, in Tel-Aviv, first thing in the morning, with absolutely nothing that I **had** to do, and I had all day through six p.m. in order not to do it (I'm not sure if this last sentence is correct grammar wise, but I think you get the point).

During my first seven years in Israel, I lived in the southern part of the country called the Negev. From there I moved to the Jerusalem area. I did have a life before I married and frequently went into Tel Aviv for a variety of reasons. The friends that I had there twenty – twenty-five years ago were no longer there. Remember that old saying 'there is a time and place for everything'? I now had the time and this was the place to start a walking tour of the places that I had not seen for many years.

I started walking southbound and arrived at the Main Bus Station. Actually, that was the name when I was there previously. Nowadays it is called the old Main Bus Station. Sunday mornings at the old Main Bus Station used to be a beehive of activity. There were literally tons and tons of soldiers going back to their bases after a weekend at home. I also spent many Sunday mornings there or to close by Yad Eliyahu waiting to catch a bus back to my base in El-Arish in the Sinai peninsular during my days in the army. This particular area was considered to be the inter-urban activity center of Tel Aviv until a much larger inter-city bus station was constructed in a new location. The old Main Bus Station is still in use serving the local area.

I remembered several streets in the area that were lined with shoe stores on both sides of the street. I strolled down one of the streets and the shoe stores were still there. At the end of the block I turned to enter another parallel street expecting to find a slue of additional shoe stores and to my amazement, this street had undergone a complete makeover. The neat row of shoe stores on this street had been transformed to a honky tonk conglomerate of massage parlors, peep shows and the like.

The entire neighborhood had undergone radical changes since I last visited the area. South Tel -Aviv was never known to be an upscale area. It was now inundated with thousands of foreign workers. Most of these laborers came without their families. A good many of these laborers overstayed their allotted time in the country and were now working illegally in Israel. The area was now reflecting the new character of the changing times.

Continuing my walk, I arrived at the intersection of Allenby and Ben Yehuda streets. I passed a parking lot and felt that there was something strange about the immediate surroundings. Then it hit me! There was a movie theatre at this intersection and now it was gone. It was called The Mograbi. Not only did I remember the theatre, but I am sure it was not just from the outside. I was definitely there inside. (I do not remember what movie we saw, her name, or even what she looked like, but I was definitely there inside!)

I continued strolling further north to an area that was called Kikar Atarim. Twenty years ago it was a well kept tourist area. I can still recall a large concrete building being there with its array of windows circling the building that housed both locals and tourists alike. That was then and this is now. The building was now in shambles. No longer did it have the rotunda window like arrangement intact. The windows were gone as were the tourists and local residents. The whole structure looked as though it took a direct hit by a Scud missile. The bare concrete also showed signs of abuse. And so ended my nostalgic tour of Tel–Aviv for the day.

By this time, I had to start heading back towards the location of the seminar. Not far from the seminar I treated myself to something that I usually do not eat very often. It's a platter of ful - which is a deep bowl filled with hummus (a paste of pureed chickpeas/garbanzo beans), tahini (a smooth paste of sesame seeds), and of course ful (fava beans - ful is a typical Middle Eastern dish, Egyptian in origin) and a hard boiled egg in the middle. It is served with a huge salad on the side and all the pita bread you can eat. After stuffing that all in, I waddled to the next seminar session.

A cross section of the group attending the seminar was quite novel. A random sampling of the participants would closely coincide with the ethnic makeup of Israeli society. You would find youngsters that just finished high school, educated attendees along side of individuals who never graduated from grade school, army and police officers, white collar professionals, blue collar laborers and the unemployed. In addition you will find individuals that enjoyed financial success according to any normal social and/or economic yardstick. You will also find individuals that have been 'lost' since childhood and have remained at the bottom of the economic totem pole after reaching adulthood.

A very interesting phenomenon gradually encompassed the attendees. It was the bonding of the participants at the early stages of the seminar. We all came from diversified backgrounds and the reason for attending the seminar was as varied as the participants themselves. Because of our individual needs, each of us took home a 'different package' of benefits that meshed with our perceived problems. One of the underlying principles of the Outlook program is to encourage each participant to realize his and/or her full potential. I later wondered if it was only coincidental that I bought my new bicycle speedometer/ odometer shortly after I attended the Outlook series of seminars.

I remember several exercises where part of the group exited in tears, and I had no idea why? What could be so special about that particular exercise? But then again, in several of the lecture sessions, the trainer brought up points which gave me material to ponder over for a long period of time. No doubt that several of the other participants who had become so emotional during some of the exercises, may have thought that a lecture that I thought to be very significant was to them the most boring lecture in the world.

The point is that everyone had come for his/her own reasons with his/her background and life experience; some people are looking for something to give them a very significant *kick in the tail* total change of direction in their lives, and some (like myself) came for the *fine tuning*. Basically the seminar offered something for everyone, not necessarily the same things for everyone, but something (something different) for each and every participant.

What also makes the seminar special is the opportunity to experience things in the closed sterile seminar environment that are not possible to experience outside in the real world. After the concluding session late that Saturday night, my interest was aroused enough to immediately sign up for the second seminar in the series, which was to be held several weeks later.

♥ ♥ ♥

The seminar is a four day program that shares the same name as the organization itself, 'Outlook'. It offers a new perspective as to how the individual views himself/herself and his/her relationship with the surroundings. A second four day sequel seminar is called Essence. It deals with the very being of an individual. This second seminar is considerably more intensive than the Outlook seminar and is conducted in a manner that one can view him/herself from the outside looking in. This allows the individual to analyze him/herself under extreme conditions and to take a new perspective in coping with the ongoing challenges of the day. It makes the individual aware of his/her potential and to recognize his/her own capabilities.

It was during this seminar that I received the shock of my life! The Essence seminar alerted me to the fact that my emotions had become totally dysfunctional. I was aware that I was being regulated to some extent by my medication but up until now, I had no idea to what extent.

There were a number of things I was able to do physically just by force of habit such as driving, walking, talking, eating, bike riding, etc. I had consummated these functions just by force of habit and realized my emotions played little or no part in these activities but at Essence, my emotions were put to the test.

Although I was always someone who knew how to hide emotions inside and not reveal them, but I **did** have them, and feel them. When my good friend Itsik passed away suddenly two years earlier, I think I cried for an entire week. I felt the loss deep inside. I **felt!** At Essence I discovered that I had become different from all the other participants in the seminar program. Everything going on that was affecting everyone else in an emotional manner was simply not registering with me. I was not able to relate to a number of other participants who were visibly going through some highly emotional upheavals that moved most others in the program.

I returned to my real world after the Essence Seminar. How I felt during the seminar was no longer significant. What is significant is that it made me aware of my actions in the real world and my emotional relations with the people who were very close and dear to me. This was of course my immediate family and in particular Esty.

What had escaped me before Essence was now quite clear. My prescribed medications had turned me into a walking, talking zombie. I had lost the ability to relate emotionally to others in my immediate surroundings. This was not to say that I was unable to lead a quasi-normal life. Waking up in the morning, going for a bike ride, showering, getting dressed, eating breakfast, driving to work, answering my e-mail, returning home from my place of employment, eating dinner, and eventually going to sleep. Despite this charade, Esty knew that Mike was not the same Mike. I realized that I had a problem with my medication. I also knew that I had recently survived a heart attack and the doctors that pulled me thru this ordeal felt the prescribed medication was mandatory if I was to maintain a satisfactory life style.

A month after I had attended each seminar, Esty also attended them. I was unaware at the time that this was the genesis of *our* recovery from *my* heart attack. Why *our* recovery? Without a doubt, it was Esty that had the most difficult time getting back to our normal lifestyle. Her daily chores were significantly compounded following the moment I entered the hospital. Her new daily routine started the week I was hospitalized. It was quite time consuming running back and forth between home and hospital. This now had to be coordinated with her responsibilities at work, at home running the household, grocery shopping, providing taxi service for the kid's extra curricular activities and the list goes on and on. This was only the beginning of her new schedule.

The most difficult and completely unexpected activity was adjusting to the *new* Mike who had developed significant physiological problems in the recuperative period after being discharged from the hospital after a successful heart operation.

As time went by, the increase in side effects of my medications was taking its toll. I felt that I had become much less fun to live with. In addition, I carried over my frustrations to my workplace and was not certain to what extent this *new* Mike was apparent to my co-workers. I thought of the hypothetical pot bellied individual who tries to impress the ladies at the beach. He holds in his stomach, expands his chest and tries to maintain this posture for as long as possible. At some point, the stomach muscles revert to its normal shape and eventually, he lets it all hang out. So it was with me at work. I would make every effort to keep up a normal appearance as usual, despite it being a very conscious effort, and would let it go when getting home in the evening. The only thing that I now looked forward to was my daily bicycle ride before going to work in the morning and waiting for the longer weekend rides. I was just about oblivious to all my other surroundings.

♥ ♥ ♥

Beside introspection which is what the Essence Seminar is all about, each group finishing the seminar initiates, organizes and carries out a volunteer project for the good of the community. You can read about my group's project at: http://www.outlook.org.il/english/0302.html. The project is geared to let each participant experience what it is like to give for the sake of giving without the slightest thought of any type of remuneration.

This was a new and interesting concept for me. Up until now, I had lived by the doctrine of always getting something for doing something. If I received more than I gave, I profited and conversely, if I gave more than I received, I lost. It's a tough world out there but that's the way it is. Let everyone else take care of themselves!

In addition to the group project, each of the participants was asked to come up with a personal project whether big or small that he/she wanted to accomplish. This could be something he/she had previously contemplated or it could also be something new. Typical personal projects mentioned were: lose 10 pounds (6 kilos) within a certain time frame, finish a course that was started, complete a specific repair job at home with a finite cutoff date, etc. The project I had chosen was in a class by itself.

I am one of those fortunate people who knew and remembered all four of my grandparents. My last living grandparent, my maternal grandmother passed away in 1982. Besides making the world's best apple pies, she also played the piano. One of her favorite pieces was an abbreviated two page version of Tchaikovsky's Piano Concerto No. 1 in B-Flat Minor. The last time I saw her alive was in 1978 when I took a trip to the U.S. to participate in my sister's wedding. During this trip I spent several days with her and waited anxiously to taste her oven fresh apple pie and listen to her play her Tchaikovsky piece.

What can I say? Old age has its way of creeping up on everyone. The apple pie that I had longed for came out of the oven half baked and did not contain the same ingredients and/or taste that I had remembered from years earlier. A somewhat similar situation occurred when she played the Tchaikovsky piece for me. It seemed as though she was missing more notes than she was hitting

You are probably wondering how my late grandmother relates to my personal Essence project. The answer is that the project that I had chosen for myself was to learn how to play the piano. I had specifically in mind that specific Tchaikovsky piece. Coincidentally, the written music mysteriously turned up in my house years ago. My intuition advised me that I would need this abbreviated two page copy if I ever intended to play it. I located a used piano and shortly afterwards I was taking weekly piano lessons from an instructor that lived in my neighborhood.

Learning to play the piano was like learning a new language. Best results are obtained in both categories if one starts at an early age and not at the 'young' age of fifty-two. The piano played an important roll in my rehab program and I enjoyed sitting behind the ivory keys. My daily routine would start with a bike ride, then fifteen – twenty minutes of piano homework. That was now the best part of my day despite the slow progress I was making on the piano.   Then came everything else that the day had to offer me, none of which interested me at all.

The feeling of confusion, the inability to make quick decisions and the nagging amnesia continued to haunt me. These *apparently* were all associated with the side effects of the ACE Inhibiters that I was still taking, at least according to some doctors and nurses I had been in contact with -- at the hospital, and also at my health clinic. They all insisted it was necessary to continue taking this medication. After all, they had the statistics to prove this type of medication was beneficial. I was hoping that my system would overcome these horrible side effects and that I would return to the mental state I enjoyed before taking them.

At my work place where I earn my bread and butter, I felt that I had lost control as to what was going on. Perhaps it wasn't noticeable among my colleagues at the office or with my two assistants or perhaps our clients in other departments that we were servicing. It was an eerie feeling. All fields of the computer industry are constantly changing and my brain was unable to absorb any new type of technology that was applicable and beneficial to my type of work. I felt that is was my two assistants that were now 'holding down the fort' and I was going along for the ride.

One of my assistants was on maternity leave during the summer of 2002. The other one was in the midst of her own personal frustrations due to a salary dispute with the management. I could tell that she was becoming increasingly disgusted with all the foot dragging regarding her employment conditions, especially during a period of more than the usual amount of work coming our way.

A good friend and neighbor Miki, who was the architect that designed our home, was planning a trip to Austria for about five – six couples. Esty was eager to get away for awhile. I was facing a dilemma at my office foreseeing a very possible situation where my disgruntled assistant would be overworked doing the job of 3 for almost two weeks, would just throw in the towel, quit and seek work elsewhere.

In my current frame of mind, this would be a catastrophic situation! I felt so out of control regarding what was happening at work that I decided not to take the dream trip. Esty was now off to Austria and I remained in Israel. The next month, if you recall, I partially compensated myself with the week (camping/riding) vacation up north with Tuval.

Although my mental abilities and mood changes had been impaired, I still managed to keep myself fully occupied. Esty and I had agreed that it was time to spruce up our abode which was long overdue. There were some minor repairs to be taken care of as well as an indoor painting project that had to be addressed. And with Esty being 'out of the way' for the next ten days in Austria (who incidentally was not just a spare wheel with the other couples in Austria, she paired off nicely with our good friend Rina - Itsik's widow), this project was now elevated to the number one priority on the house agenda.

The kids and I got to work. Two walls in the living room changed from white to orange which was Esty's preference. A wall in the adjoining kitchen turned reddish/burgundy and the master bedroom acquired a new coat of pale blue. The remaining wall space on the lower level of our home was given a fresh coat of white paint.

After completing the Essence seminars, I did not need any additional proof that my emotional feelings were still 'out of whack'. I can recall on a number of occasions how happy our reunions were after being separated for an extended period of time (overseas trips, weekend breaks in the middle of reserve duty stints, etc). The longer the separation, the more joyous were the reunions. This was quality time and I cherished every moment of it. Esty's trip to Austria was winding down and she expected me to pick her up at the airport. In normal times I would have done this without thinking twice about it.

In our last phone conversation just prior to her departure from Austria, an enthusiastic Esty said that she just could not wait to meet me at Ben Gurion airport upon her arrival. When I heard this, I was thinking "this is really foolish for me to spend one – one-and-a-half hours each way to the airport and back when she could have come back with someone in the group very easily." Just to make matters worse, when I was getting ready to leave the house for the trip to the airport, my thoughts at the time were "too bad her trip was not for a couple of days longer, then I would have had time to paint the entire first floor." These thoughts would have been unimaginable had I been percolating on all four cylinders.

I mentioned earlier that Esty had also attended the two seminars shortly after I had. Something **very very** important that we both received from the seminars, particularly the Essence seminar, was that the communication between us did not only rise to a higher plateau, but to a higher dimension altogether. This is not to say that I discovered 'secrets' that I had not previously known about her, but the level of – let's call it – our ability to connect – was total.

My attitude towards her homecoming from the Austrian trip came up in a discussion/mini argument we had several weeks later. Under normal conditions, a husband telling his wife after a ten day absence from each other "Too bad that the trip could not have lasted several days longer because I could have finished the painting" could have easily pushed a spouse over the brink. What woman can bear hearing that her husband has lost emotional, physical/sexual feelings for her when absence is supposed to make the heart grow fonder?

Because of the impact the seminars had on Esty, she was able to understand that I was struggling with myself in the twilight zone and my actions had nothing to do with her as a woman. Being over-medicated had taken its toll on me and any intimate relations we had was nothing more than going thru the motions.

I was fortunate not to go thru the ultimate test as to how I would react in the event that Esty would have said "That's it, you have had it – you are out of here." My probable response to this dilemma would be that I would experience no emotion and could have easily said "OK, I will move to the den for now until I find something outside."

As long as we are discussing Esty, there is another factor worth mentioning. I am beginning to believe that there is a gene in the male species called the Jack-Ass gene. Most women are familiar with this gene despite the fact that most males are probably unaware of its existence. It is the gene that causes the male species to act obnoxious to his spouse for the slightest (imagined) provocation. This stupid 'chauvinistic right' has been handed down from generation to generation, and who am I to question this policy? Before my heart attack, when I did allow this Jack-Ass gene to dominate me in a situation with Esty, I realized that she was being hurt but I did not show any signs externally, yet it did bother me emotionally. However, in my over medicated, supposedly rehabilitation period, I *knew* I was hurting her, but I felt nothing inside.

The only thing that seemed to cause me any enjoyment was getting on the bike, enjoying the fresh air, the view, the getting away, the **being by myself.**

Something was out of kilter and yet I knew that I was part of this world. My physical actions appeared to be functioning. It was the robot in me that automatically sent me to work in the morning and back home again in the evening. I would do the normal chores around the house that needed to be done - fix this, fix that, painting, maintaining the garden, etc. Somehow, despite these 'accomplishments', there was something missing and I felt that I was not totally in this world. As in the movie Matrix, I was living in my own parallel world. It is difficult to explain this world other than it was not completely congruous with the real world.

My entire system of senses that I relied on to connect me with the real world was no longer functioning properly. I was functioning, however under the continuous influence of a dental Novocain shot – no, a correction – under the influence of two shots; one into the brain that muddled my ability to reason correctly, caused bouts of confusion and minor amnesia, and another one into my heart which paralyzed all my emotions.

It was inevitable that sooner or later there would be a showdown with my boss. I was hoping that this meeting would not come about until I have the results of my next semi annual checkup, which would shed some light on my future with the firm. A reduction in my medication would enable me to see the light at the end of the tunnel. On the other hand, if the dosage of medication was not reduced, I would have no other choice but to initiate the meeting. At some point, my poor performance was bound to surface and if my boss initiated the meeting, it would be quite obvious that he found a problem with my performance. He was aware that I was having some difficulty with my rehabilitation but he was not cognizant of the magnitude of my problem.

Ironically it was circumstances at work that set the stage for our talk which came at my initiative. My small department was about to start on the largest project in my field since the beginning of my employment with the firm. This project would take at least a half year to complete assuming that everything went as planned. It was to utilize a new technology that required an expertise that was entirely new in the field.

My inability to make routine decisions, my forgetfulness and my overall confusion in coordinating anything involving a few tasks would lead to total chaos in this very involved and costly project. It was time for a one on one critique with my boss and to place all the cards on the table.

My boss happens to be one of the most knowledgeable and impressive individuals that I have ever met in this industry. His professionalism and expertise in his field are unrivaled and his peers that do not know him intimately may get the impression that he is one tough cookie. Co-workers in the office feel that he has similar characteristics as the Israeli fruit called the Sabra which has a tough outer shell but is soft on the inside. In this case, soft has the connotation of a big heart. His office is only two doors away from my office and yet it was not easy to get together with him as his calendar is packed with scheduled meetings all over the country. When he is in the office, his time is at a premium.

In the early part of December 2002, I informed him that we would have to have a talk and he promised it would be in a day or two as he would be in the office for the next several days. I already knew all the things I wanted to discuss with him but had no idea where the conversation might lead to nor did I know what would be the consequence of our talk. In the meantime, life continued.

Esty wanted very much to be part of the supporting crew for the next Outlook Seminar and had hoped that we would participate together as supporters. She thought that by hearing everything again not as a participant but part of the staff would be beneficial. I was not overjoyed with the idea as a good deal of time and work would have to be allocated for preparing for the nuts and bolts of the seminar. The demands on the staff and supporters are much more exhausting than for the participants.

The first preparatory meeting for the upcoming Outlook Seminar was held on Wednesday evening. After work that day, Esty and I traveled to Tel Aviv for the first organizational meeting. I knew some of the other supporters and others I met for the first time. The meeting lasted quite late and we returned home after another one and a half hour drive. The following day, Thursday is the last day of our work week. I had yet to have my meeting with my boss. Many firms in Israel work a half day on Friday but our firm is not one of them. Something strange happened that day. Perhaps it can be attributed to the organizational meeting that was held the night before. I was hoping that I would have that talk with my boss and get all this behind me before the weekend but this was not to happen.

Towards the end of the day, it became apparent that the conversation would not be held until the beginning of next week. At the end of the day, my boss poked his head into my room to say good bye for the weekend and I reminded him of the talk that we had not yet held. He answered that he has a couple of minutes now, if that would be enough time. I answered him that it would not be enough time, and I think he then realized that the talk was not about work, but about me, and he responded "First thing Sunday morning". It was then about six p.m. I still had an hour, hour and a half to finish up what I was working on before heading home.

And now we come to the *strange* part I mentioned earlier. For the longest time, Esty had not seen me coming home from work with anything resembling a smile and especially when I arrived home after eight p.m. That Thursday

95

was different. Beside me giving her a big kiss after I got home I was grinning from ear to ear. Esty was now witnessing a strange phenomenon and was probably wondering "Has Mike finally gone nuts altogether?"

To tell you the truth, I am not exactly sure as to what did happen. Perhaps it was a bit of "Outlook energy" that my subconscious mind picked up from the previous night's preparatory meeting for the upcoming seminar. Or perhaps the meeting brought back something I heard when I was participating in the seminar program as a registered participant and for some reason only now registered.

Up until now my thoughts were that I was approaching life with a half empty glass and it bothered me that the present Mike had far less mental features than the pre-2001 Mike. A radical change occurred between the time my boss had left for the weekend and the time that I arrived back home. My half empty glass had been converted to a half full glass. The change did not affect me physically -- my memory was still not the same, neither was my problem solving abilities. My concentration was still not up to par.

Let's face it. I did survive a heart attack and not only did I survive the attack, but I function quite well considering the ordeal I went thru. Quite a few other heart attack victims who traverse the same motions come out of this situation in a vegetative state. My half filled glass stacks up quite well with others who live in a fantasy world and think they are percolating with a full glass. After all, I have my Esty, my fantastic family, my comfortable living quarters and I am gainfully employed. Life can be beautiful!

After a year and a half of mental anguish, I have suddenly accepted the fact that I am not as sharp as I used to be. I have been in the computer/programming field for twenty years but I was not born into the computer industry. Nowhere is it written that I have to remain in this field for the rest of my life.

The next morning was a morning that I will remember for a long time. The weather was awful – not only because it was chilly, but because it was also pouring rain all morning. During the previous months I had entered into an obsession of bike riding. I was going to ride *sooooooo* much that my semi annual hospital examinations (including the stress test) were going to be *sooooooo* good, that my professor of cardiology would have no choice but to start reducing the dosage of medication that I was taking.

Since the previous evening, I was beginning to re-assess my half full glass theory of looking at life. Perhaps it was because of the medications that I am able to continue my life and without this medication, my condition could very well be considerably worse then it is today. I developed a real passion for bike riding but in the past six months I was not riding for personal enjoyment. I was riding solely to impress my cardiologist/professor by getting a good report card at the conclusion of the stress test.

Enough is enough! Today I will ride for myself because I enjoy bike riding and I wasn't about to let insipid weather hold me back. I dressed warmly with a water proof jacket over my clothes and proceeded to enjoy the most satisfying ride imaginable. About an hour later, the rain started to taper off and a beautiful, perfect rainbow appeared from horizon to horizon. The rainbow seemed to appear for *me* and for me alone. It was *mine*! I was now about to turn over a new leaf. I was for the first time, coming to grips with myself that my post heart attack era would never be the same as my pre heart attack life.

I fully believed that at the time but it would be another six months before the accumulated effects of the medications would prove once again that they were stronger than my own will power and my ability to continue on the same course.

After every weekend and no matter how enjoyable, there is always another Sunday which is the start of another work week in Israel. There is no doubt that Sunday's meeting with my boss would have been more difficult had it occurred before

Thursday. I would have known how to start the conversation but I am not certain where I would have gone from there.

I came away from the talk we had on Sunday knowing exactly where I stood and was pleased with the outcome of our meeting. The session I had with my boss was quite frank and pleasant to boot. I put everything on the table and suggested that this might be the right time to pass the baton to my assistant. It was though we would transfer responsibilities to the next generation who would run with the ball to new horizons. He would then be able to move me to one of his other crews in a different capacity.

While he did not negate the idea of some other position in one of his other departments, he said that Mike at eighty percent or even sixty percent of the previous Mike still knew how to lead his small department and meet all of its deadlines on time no matter what the obstacles along the way were. The harmony in which we as a unit performed without personal friction between us is something that was lacking in some of his other crews. As far as he was concerned, he preferred to stick with the new Mike at the helm. Regarding that new project around the corner, he would see to it that I had an outside source accompany me as far as technical guidance is concerned.

The new project turned out to be considerably more involved that anyone had anticipated and all of its development was out-sourced.

In January 2003 I had my next semiannual checkup. This occurred a month after the talk with my boss. Because of my improved stamina and overall fitness from bike riding, I had wrongfully assumed that the dosage for some of the pills that I had been taken would be drastically reduced or eliminated entirely as with the case of the Beta Blocker. The results of my stress test were very good. Despite a strong exercise regimen, my LDL (bad cholesterol) had again risen to slightly over 100 which is a red line for cardiologists. I had been strongly advised to keep my LDL reading below 100 even though my total cholesterol level was satisfactory. As a result of this report, all of the medications I was taking were destined to remain the same. There would be no reduction in dosage nor would any of the medication be eliminated.

Needless to say, I was disappointed with the check-up results. Although I had fully accepted the fact that that Mike 2003 has fewer features than Mike 2001, there was still a bit of the Mike 2001 in me that was yearning to think clearly, recoup my evasive memory that had previously functioned successfully on all four cylinders and last but not least, get back my emotional feelings that had been taken away from me.

I have always accepted my cardiologist's/professor's analysis of my condition as unquestionably sound. After all, I did have a heart attack, I did acquire a stent implant and he did postpone the time I would be joining my ancestors. Medicine is not my vocation, it is his. It belongs to the 'Professionals' that burn the midnight oil studying long after a four year B.A. or B.Sc. degree is earned by the average college graduate, an internship at a hospital, etc. So who am I to question what medication is mandatory for me to extend my newly borrowed time that was just given to me?

Since I was not about to lie down and roll over, I was determined to improve my health by increasing my exercise. When the next six month stress test rolls around, the test results should reflect my increased activity in a positive way. What better way to accomplish this then to increase my bike riding distances. I installed front and back lights on the bike and by five-fifteen a.m.I was out accumulating the mileage/km. As it turned out, I lost nothing by not waiting for my January checkup before having that big talk with the boss.

I have reached a new plateau in life. I am happy to be alive and realize that I will have to live with lapse of memory, inability to learn new things, difficulty in making simple decisions, continue to have lack of emotions and mood changes. All of these characteristics now belong to post-attack Mike. This is now as good as it gets!

10

Current Diary?

Today is **Saturday, March 15, 2003** about nine-thirty in the morning. I am on my morning bike ride and since this is the weekend, I did not have to get up very early as there was no work scheduled today. Hence there wasn't any timing conflict. It just occurred to me that last night Sagi mentioned that he needed the video camera for this afternoon as he was going to a party and wanted to film the event.

Chalk up another memory loss! Instead of focusing on the battery to make certain that it was fully charged, Sagi's request simply went in one ear and out the other. At least now there is still time to ride home, put the smaller battery into the charger, and send him off on time on his way. I stop off at home, take care of the battery and continue my ride.

A thought came to mind about my own health situation and others suffering from the same problem. Since heart disease is one of the world's most prevalent health problems, could it be that I was the only one that was not able to bounce back mentally and emotionally to my pre heart attack era? Perhaps there are others experiencing the same doldrums that I am going thru and are unaware that there are others out there in the same predicament.

Hey, maybe I should write a book or something, something regarding the joys and benefits of bike riding for the post heart attack patient! Now that's a laugh – I never had any intention, neither as a youth, nor as a grownup, to write a book. Nevertheless, I felt obligated to share my experiences with other heart attack victims; to let them know the strong factor bike riding played in bouncing back from both the mental and physical disabilities I had incurred following my attack.

The more I thought of recapping my experiences in my post heart attack period, the more I was inclined to start accumulating data that was pertinent to events that enfolded in my struggle to regain my place in society. It is amazing the things we take for granted when we are feeling good. By the time I finished my morning ride, my mind was made up. I was determined to put into print the phases I went thru in my post heart attack period.

I was off to a good start. The title of this book would be called *"Surviving a Successful Heart Attack"*. All I have to do now is to fill in the space from cover to cover! My adrenalin flow was kicked up a notch as I put my bike into the shed, removed the empty water bottle as well as the speedometer/odometer. I recorded the odometer reading, the time and date, mileage, etc. The odometer reading in particular reflected just how far I went in my physical rehab program as well as the progress I made in my mental/emotional advances.

Time:	10:09
Date:	March 15, 2003
Max Speed for the Day	51km/hour (31.6 mph)
Distance for the Day	26.50km (16.4 miles)
Cumulative odometer reading since April 5, 2002	4788.3km (2873 miles)

I guess I should mention that you readers should no longer be bothered by not exactly understanding the 'hieroglyphics' in the first chapter.

The clock is now ticking. There are still twenty days to go for me to reach my goal of 5,000km (3,000 miles) by April 4, 2003. I am only 211.7km (132 miles) short of this goal. This should not be a problem because my daily average in the past several months has been significantly higher than what is required for me in the next twenty days. Had it not been for a case of the flu, followed by a week of extra harsh wintry weather, I surely would have reached the 5,000km milestone by now.

March 16th and before going to work, my new total is now 4,801km. This evening I have an appointment with a holistic doctor. My first appointment with him was several weeks ago. He is not the average type of holistic doctor that seems to be prevalent today (several months of alternative medicine courses for the layman, and boom, you are a doctor). Before going into his holistic practice, he was an internist in one of the major hospitals in Israel. He combines his experience in conventional medicine with his expertise in various alternative solutions. Esty and I attended one of his lectures. Esty was so impressed that she made an appointment to see him during his private practice hours. She had several recurring chronic health problems that had haunted her since childhood and unfortunately she had only partial relief from standard medicine.

Why all this about Esty's health Curriculum Vitae? After receiving treatment from this holistic doctor, her chronic health problems seemed to have melted away. I was anxious to hear what he would say about my condition and in particular what side effects my medication might be causing and how this would affect my overall health.

During my first appointment with the holistic doctor, as with any first time visit to a doctor's office, the usual

102

paperwork had to be completed; the medical history of myself and family, medication I was now taking, recent test results for stress, blood analysis, echo, etc. The Mike file was now officially opened in his office. He did mention the particular blockage I had in layman's terms was known as the *widow maker artery*. No further explanation needed. Another appointment was scheduled. He wanted to review my file thoroughly at his leisure. In the meantime he assigned some homework for me that entailed obtaining information on the internet regarding:

- E.E.C.P Therapy – which is short for Enhanced External Counterpulation (that clears everything up, doesn't it??)

- EDTA — Ethylene-Diamine-Tetra-Acetate, a.k.a. Chelating Therapy. Chelation comes from the Greek word Chele – which means to *bind*.

The EECP website (http://www.eecp.com) defines EECP Therapy as:

> *"Enhanced External Counterpulsation treatment is a noninvasive, outpatient procedure to relieve angina by improving perfusion in areas of the heart deprived of adequate blood supply."*

In layman's terms, EECP Therapy increases blood circulation and reduces or eliminates the frequency of chest pains and angina.

EDTA Chelating Therapy is a procedure associated with the cleansing of heavy metals from the body. And what is the origin of these metallic pollutants in the body? It runs the gamut from the air we breathe to the amalgam fillings in our teeth. Claims that this type of therapy for successfully treating cardiovascular disease is controversial and has provoked a fair amount of backlash.

The PROS and CONS of this type of therapy are quite striking. The PROS claim that in many cases the treatment does reduce plaque that has built up over a period of many years. The PROS are also divided into two camps regarding the best way to apply this treatment. One group claims the only efficient treatment is the standard intravenous procedure. The other group claims that a much simpler treatment should be administered orally. On the other hand, the CONS claim that the process is very expensive, time consuming and last but not least, this type of remedy has not been proven in the laboratory.

At my second appointment with the holistic doctor, the first thing he asked was whether or not I had checked out the two procedures that he had mentioned to me. I was eager to display the data that I pulled up on the internet which answered his question. He then stated that the reason he assigned me this task was two fold. I did have a heart attack and secondly he felt that I would find this information very interesting. He also felt that in all probability these procedures would not have been discussed in my rehabilitation program. He was right on both counts.

Regarding the EECP therapy, I was already getting the benefits of this therapy by riding my bike every day. This type of therapy is in reality an exercise workout program for individuals that do not or are unable to exercise. In regards to the Chelating Therapy, he would not recommend this procedure for me at this time but wanted me to be aware of this option since it had positive results for many people.

As the conversation continued, I realized that I now have an additional dietary option to ponder over: the Ornish approach of low fat and high complex carbohydrates; the Atkins approach of low carbohydrates and high fat; and now a system based on three balanced meals. The latter approach put a ceiling on carbs and also imposed limits on fat intake. Proteins, moderate amounts of carbs and salads were recommended coupled with the Franz X. Mayr[7] approach on *how* to eat.

The Mayr system was developed by the Austrian physician Franz Mayr who lived from 1875 – 1965. He claimed that many of our ailments have their roots in our digestive system or more specifically, our own misuse of our digestive systems which causes havoc in our intestinal tract. His analysis of the problem can be summed up as follows:

1. We eat too quickly and do not chew our food thoroughly. This practice short changes our digestive system as it does not allow enough time to mix with an adequate amount of saliva which is crucial in the first stages in the digestive system. Since we do not masticate our food properly, we place a disproportionate amount of stress on our intestines.

2. We overeat. (enough said.....)

3. We eat too frequently. Before our system can fully digest a meal, we have a tendency to load the system down with additional food.

4. We ignore the clock and eat at the wrong time. Our digestive system is running at its peak performance both in the morning and afternoon. In the event that we load up our system at night, digestion takes longer and is often incomplete. Remember: Breakfast like an Emperor; Lunch like a King; Dinner like a Beggar.

5. We eat when we are not hungry, upset and/or annoyed.

The complete Mayr system involves considerably more activities than just correcting the eating problems listed above. It includes a detoxification process called Colon Hydrotherapy, light fasting, etc.

Regarding my current medication, he strongly suggested that my aspirin regimen be continued. He also indicated that he wanted to check the printout of my recent tests that could possibly allow him to reduce or eliminate the Tritace medication. He thought it best at the present time to continue with this medication. The only change he suggested was to reduce the Lipidal dosage for two months and follow this up with a blood test for a cholesterol analysis.

Today is **March 17, 2003** and I tacked on another 15.15km on my odometer for a grand total of 4,816.6km. The following day I was unable to bike ride because of inclement weather.

It is now **March 19th** and it happens to be a holiday in Israel called Purim. I decided to take the day off as this had the makings of a hectic day. President George W. Bush's ultimatum to Saddam Hussein expires this evening and I have a fair amount of work to do on the family shelter to bring it up to level for sustained use in case of an emergency. We have enough food and water stored for the family requirements.

There is a number of urgent chores that still has to be taken care of such as sealing the windows and doors, hook up a phone line and TV antenna similar to the situation we went thru in 1991, during the first Gulf War. This allowed us to know what was going on in the outside world and talk on the telephone while wearing gas masks. I also packed a month's supply of medication in the event we had to stay that length of time in the shelter. The medication included a small box of Cordil. These are the nitroglycerin pills that should be taken immediately in event of a heart attack. I always carry three of them in my wallet and another three pills in a small envelope whenever I am out on the bike.

Esty and Rakefet also made very good use of the free day to get the rest of the house in order. Rakefet does an extremely good job in the computer room. This room doubles as an additional bedroom when needed. It is also used for ironing, library, storing laundry before ironing and generally speaking, it is also known as our utility room.

I am usually up and ready to start the day quite early in the morning. The first thing on my agenda is the early morning bike ride before heading off to work. In my haste to get out of the house as quickly as possible, I have been known to disturb Esty's sleep while getting dressed and/or looking for the paraphernalia that is part of my riding equipment. The window ledges in the utility room have now become the holding area for these things which include the electronic speedometer/odometer, pulse meter, three Cordil pills that are always in reach and a wool hat and scarf for cold mornings.

One of the many attributes of Rakefet is her ability to tidy up any room in the house in record breaking time. Unfortunately my three Cordil pills that were stapled closed in an envelope succumbed to the whirlwind cleanup and were tossed out with the trash thus becoming the first and only casualty of the day. I usually pocket the envelope before the early morning ride but no real harm was done as I mentioned earlier, I always have three of these pills in my wallet wherever I go. (We will return to the thrown out pills shortly.)

The weather had not been favorable for bike riding this past week. Today is **the 21ˢᵗ** and my gloves are still wet from my last bike ride. It is a cold morning but not raining and I decided it was good enough to go out and add some mileage to my odometer. About 10km (6 miles) later my hands are extremely cold and I decide to return home and have some breakfast while my gloves dry out over a heater.

After warming up and satisfying my hunger growls, I am back on the bike again. It wasn't too long before I discovered that I had left my scarf somewhere in the house. I had left it draped over a chair adjacent to the front door so I would not forget it on the way out of the house. I am still amazed that I can look at an object and it simply does not register in my mind. It is as if I am not focusing on what I just saw and don't know what to do with this bit of information that I just acquired. I place the scarf around my neck and continued my ride until I finish at 4,863km.

Saturday, **March 22ⁿᵈ** and it is a weekend and a day off from work. Today my bike ride will be longer than the pre work day bike ride. My normal weekday routine after dressing in the morning is to place my cellular phone in my right front pocket and the speedometer/odometer plus the envelope with the Cordil pills in my left front pocket.

This is the daily ritual that I had been following for months. Instead of preparing a new envelope to replace the Cordil pills that had been inadvertently thrown out by Rakefet, I changed my daily routine and take the Cordil pills that are kept in my wallet at all times in the event of an emergency. This may not sound as though I made a significant change in my daily ritual in making preparations for my bike ride. However, it was enough to upset my apple cart in the sequence of things I had programmed myself to do before my daily bike ride. Tampering with my daily routine usually evokes unexpected surprises that are not too far away.

This morning, functional misbehavior again raised its ugly head. After removing the Cordil pills from my wallet, the sequence of events resembled that of the Keystone Cops of another era. I took my water bottle from the kitchen and headed downstairs to the bicycle shed. I felt that something was missing and then it came to me as I approached the bottom of the stairs. It was the key to the shed. As of late, I have become accustomed to periods of forgetfulness and I took this latest episode in stride. I was back to the house for the key to the bicycle shed. I was now riding my bike and still thinking about the key and then I realized my bike helmet was still back in the shed. I was not too upset about this latest memory lapse but was somewhat surprised how easy it had become to mix up and forget routine activities when I am not thinking about them constantly.

March 23rd - I have now ridden past the 4,900km mark. My goal of 5,000km (3,000 miles) is definitely within reach. Can I make it to my more ambitious goal of 5,215km - which translates to exactly 100 kilometers/week (61 miles/week) average for the entire year? A quick calculation – twelve days yet to go until April 4th - and another 312 kilometers (195 miles) - that comes out to an average of 26km (16¼ miles) a day - OUCH! That's a good bit above my daily average. If, however, I have two productive Friday rides, let's say 70km each Friday, that leaves 172km over ten days which is   17.2 kilometers/day - p-o-s-s-i-b-l-e………. and that's assuming no breaks.

It is now the **24**th and I am at 4,926km. The weather forecast for the following day is cold and rainy.

Perhaps it was a lucky guess, but the weather forecaster hit the nail on the head. It was indeed cold and raining on **March 25**th, and I lost a valuable day in my quest to reach my revised km/mileage figures. All is not lost as I would now devote some quality time to my piano which has now become the runner up form of my relaxation time.

I am now back at work in the real world. In the early afternoon, I notice a man and a woman entering a room off a hallway for a meeting that was very close to my office. As I passed the woman, our eyes met and there something familiar about this woman, yet I could not remember just where we had met previously. She broke the silence with "Mike, how are you doing"? She does look familiar, and apparently notices by the expression in my eyes that I have not exactly recognized her – to this she answers with a smile, "I'm your boss's wife." Keep in mind that I had been invited to their home on a number of occasions and also seen them together at social functions. Running in to her at my place of work where she had come to for a meeting automatically made me try to associate her with someone I deal with at work.

Under normal circumstances, this would have been an embarrassing situation. Since I had become acclimated to these mental shortcomings, I developed somewhat of a thick skin and did not give this awkward situation a second thought. Several months ago I had bumped into her at a gas station and recognized her at first glance.

A similar situation popped up that same evening. Tuval has been studying Karate for a number of years and a final annual event is held for individual national championships. In addition, the participants demonstrate a certain Kata which is a series of moves simulating combat against multiple opponents. At the end of the evening's activities just as Tuval and I were approaching the exit of the auditorium, someone called me from behind, "Mike, what are you doing here?" I turned around and looked at someone who seemed vaguely familiar. Unfortunately I could not place him immediately. Tuval was still dressed in his white Karate outfit. I then blurted out "I came to see my son". "That's great," he replied and "What did you think of *my* Kata?" When he said that, I realized that he was one of the judges in the Karate competition. During one of the intermissions between bouts, his name was announced over the loud speaker as he had performed solo one of the more advanced Katas. I told him that I thought that he put on a very good show while wondering where do I know him from since he knows me well enough to call me by name.

It wasn't until we reached the car when it hit me! He works at the same firm as I do but at a different location in the city. *Several days earlier he met with me in my office for an entire hour* to discuss a project that my staff and I had to process for him in the months ahead. Seeing him in an entirely different context (dressed in a white Karate outfit) outside of the environment that I would normally see him in did not trigger any recognition on my part. I thought there was a familiar ring to his name when it came over the loud speaker and yet, I could not make the connection at that time or when we spoke face to face

March 26th began like the previous day. It was going to be another cold and rainy day. I had no inclination to exercise the piano keys this morning since yesterday was Sagi's birthday and several of his friends slept over. Quite frankly, I did not want to torture his guests with a wake up call from my musical apparatus which would probably not be in tune with their morning sleep.

The 27th – another cold day but even though the rain had stopped, I take the day off from riding. Tomorrow is Friday, the day of my long rides, and I can make up the difference.

However, with my unwillingness to ride this morning, I more or less resign myself to the thought, "Well, the main intention was to get to 5,000km – and I'll indeed reach it." For three weeks my bike riding suffered because of my bout with the flu and the inclement weather I unexpectedly encountered. Both of these factors weighed heavily against raising the bar for a greater achievement - 5,215km (100km /week average for the entire year).

Yogli and I were both inclined to do a long bike ride. His busy schedule left him sans bicycle for several weeks and it has been quite some time that we had ridden together. We decided on a trip that would start in Jerusalem and finish at Herzliya. For the past three months, Yogli spent most of his time in his Tel Aviv office and not in the Jerusalem office. I let him know of my strong wish to exceed the 74km (44 mile) distance and it was appropriate for him to be riding along side of me on this occasion. After all, he had been my riding companion this past year.

Thursdays are usually upbeat days for several reasons. It is the last day of the work week and also a good chance that Naamah will have leave from the army and she will be able to join us at home for the weekend. She would normally arrive in Jerusalem from her army base about the same time I leave the office in the evening. I would meet her at the bus station and we would drive home together.

This particular Thursday happened to be a very busy day. I was tied up at the office when Naamah phoned and I still had a minimum of thirty minutes of work that had to be taken care of before I left the office for the weekend. I told her to wait for me rather than having to carry her heavy gear from bus to bus for the trip back home. About thirty minutes later I phoned her and let her know that I was on my way to pick her up. I told her to wait outside at our usual rendezvous spot and I would be there in about ten minutes. After watering my plants, I left the office, got into my car and I was on my way. It had been a hectic day and my thoughts were still wrapped up with the day's activities

Its is only after I am already on the expressway going home, it pops into my mind that Naamah is waiting for me at the main bus station, and I'm already on my out of Jerusalem. I changed lanes just in time to catch an exit that would put me back on track to the bus station. Again, my memory is playing tricks on me and I am still at a loss how to fully cope with this situation.

This evening (**27th**) is the last day before the start of Daylight Savings Time. I will be getting one hour less sleep and I will start the day when it will be pitch black outside. I set the alarm on my cell phone; however I immediately think to myself "the exact time that is displayed on the screen is not set manually by me – it is data that is regulated/received automatically from the cell phone headquarters. If they do not revise the correct hour on time, then the phone may not ring at the proper time."

I also do a back-up plan – set the alarm on my wrist watch. However I am not exactly satisfied with this either, as I can remember a previous time that I thought that the wrist watch alarm was set, only to find out later that I had not done it correctly. As a back-up to the back-up, I also set the alarm on the bedroom clock behind Esty's head as the sure bet; but in order not to wake her, I set it for fifteen minutes later than the alarm times of my first and second choice. And as before all my Friday rides, Esty loads all the ingredients into the automatic bread maker, and sets the finish time for six a.m.

The next morning **(28th)** I awake to the beeps of the watch alarm. I did it correctly this time. It seems a bit strange that someone with a college degree would feel ecstatic because he/she was able to set the alarm function on this stupid wrist watch!!! I quickly checked my cell phone and notice that the new time does not appear. Needless to say, the backup hedge paid off handsomely. Later I discovered that the new time could be reset by shutting off the phone and then restarting it. No, this is not called rebooting the phone. As of this writing, this terminology is still reserved exclusively for computers and routers. Lastly I remember for a change to switch off the alarm of Esty's alarm clock.

I pack my bike on the car and arrive to the rendezvous point that Yogli and I had agreed upon, the Pancake House. Actually, for several months it has no longer been the House of Pancakes -- it had closed and has now been reopened as the Hummus House; or, as its officially called, the Lebanese Restaurant. However, everybody still refers to this location as the Pancake House. It is located at the Shoeva /Shoresh junction on the main Tel-Aviv – Jerusalem Highway, known as Route 1. Yogli lives only eight kilometers from there and he arrives by bicycle.

Our trek starts our on the very scenic route in the direction of Bet Shemesh along the Kisaron River route, mostly down hill thru bumpy mountainous trails, but that's the fun of trail bikes. Once we hit the main (paved) road leading to Bet Shemesh we turn west at the Shimshon junction, and at the Nachshon junction, stop off to grab a bite at a gas station. This is not the official breakfast stop where we cut into Esty's bread. But a break is a break, Yogli orders a coffee and I order a slice of apple pie that is on the counter and seems to have my name written all over it. I pick up the tab and tell Yogli that he can pick up the Herzliya tab, as he has his favorite coffee stop in Herzliya already picked out.

We continue on our way thru Ramle, Tzrifin, Nachshon and to a place called Azur. After several hours of bike riding, Azur seemed like an oasis. It was a good place to pounce on Esty's bread and once again, Esty's bread came thru with flying colors. What is unique about her bread is that one never knows what to expect. It could very well contain berries, other fruits, nuts, edible seeds or a host of other surprises. Whatever the ingredients, the one thing you can count on is that it will always be yummy.

After arriving at Azur, I checked my cell phone for missed calls and saw that Esty had tried to reach me. She had asked about our current location and knew that we were going to Tel Aviv. There was a special bakery not too far off our planned route and she was hoping that we could drop in on them for one of their outstanding specialties called a mun cake. The English translation is called a poppy seed cake. I passed Esty's request on to Yogli who is the official navigator for our party of two.

We arrive to the old city of Jaffa and ride along the boardwalk which runs along the seashore. The official name of Tel Aviv is Tel Aviv-Jaffa and it is located on the Mediterranean Sea. Our ride on the boardwalk covers its entire length and culminates at the Reading Power Plant in north Tel Aviv. From there we continue into Ramat Aviv. Because our previous breaks were longer than anticipated, we decided not to continue riding north to Herzliya and felt that it was prudent to change directions and head towards Yogli's car which was parked in south Tel Aviv. Needless to say, the bakery that Esty mentioned was next on the agenda.

Yogli also set his sights at reaching 80km (48 miles) for the day's ride. We did ride eighty kilometers one day when we circled the Sea of Galilee (a.k.a. Lake Tiberias, a huge reservoir/lake further north in the country) together on a previous ride. Unfortunately on the break that we took at the end the lake, and before deciding to continue a bit more, he inadvertently reset his odometer. As a result, he finished that

114

particular day with only an 18km reading staring back at him from the handle-bars.

We find the bakery on King George Street which is adjacent to Shenkin Street and it reminds me of the Village (Greenwich Village to you non New Yorkers). For those not familiar with Greenwich Village, it is inhabited by a young crowd of mostly locals that are strongly independent and dress on the wild side, can sport a multi-colored hair do, skin piercing, tattoos, etc. (I WAS also young once.) Although it's late Friday afternoon and most businesses in the country are already closed for the Sabbath weekend, everything in this area seems to be open, except of course Esty's bakery - ☹.

Yogli has a place in mind for the drink he still owes me. I am now approaching 76km (44.4 miles) and switch the mode on my odometer from the daily total to the accumulative total. As we stop for a red light on Ibn Givriol Street at the corner of Arlozarov Street, my odometer reads 4,999.9km. The time is 2:40 p.m. The light turns green and as I pass thru the intersection, I read 5,000km (3,000 miles). I did it!

Why was it that a tremendous feeling of jubilation escaped me? After all, I had reached this goal that had its genesis over six months ago and yet, I did not feel **"WOW!!! I DID IT!!! I DID IT!!!** I should have experienced the feeling similar to the fireworks one encounters after an orgasm but this feeling of accomplishment just wasn't there.

I can think of two reasons why I did not feel the expected thrill of this achievement. First and foremost, 'my inner feelings are dead' syndrome that I had been experiencing since July, 2001 and secondly, perhaps it was revising my original goal of 5,000km to a higher level and the original distance was no longer considered an outstanding accomplishment.

We arrive to Yogli's coffee spot, I sit outside to watch the bikes and he goes in to order his coffee and my tea. I take out a pen and paper and start calculating what's left for me to do to reach 5,215km (3,130 miles) by April 4th. Seven days left

– about 215 kilometers to go – that averages to about 30km (18 miles) per day. These figures do not seem to be realistic as I have a heavy workload coming up this week. If I plan on a big ride next Friday, let's say 100 kilometers, then that would leave me with about 20km (12 miles) per day, which seems doable.

Lately I have been riding fifteen kilometers before work, and occasionally even twenty, so it IS possible. Yogli comes back with the drinks, likes the idea of a long ride next week and the 5,215 goal is again on. We finish the drinks, and when I go into the men's room to take a leak, Yogli uses the time to take a complementary postcard from the coffee shop. He writes "LeMike – Mazal Tov leSiyum haMasa shel 5000 kilometer bPahot meShana! - Yogev" which means "To Mike – Congratulations on your trek of 5000 kilometers in less than a year! - Yogev" and shoves it deep into my backpack while I am still in the men's room.

I finish the day at 5,004.6km.

One of the best parts of a long ride like this one, especially after not doing such a long ride for a while, is the feeling of total exhaustion that comes in the evening. And better yet, the feeling that this is going to be one of the most restful nights in a long time. And indeed it was.

In fact, I am still in bed this morning (29th) until about eight thirty – and with the feeling – ooooh – too much time lying down, and the back and legs feeling a little stiff. I decide to take a short ride and loosen up a bit. Since Tuval was up and dressed, he joined me for a ride around the neighborhood. After riding 10km, Tuval had enough for one day and headed back to our house. I'm feeling really good, no more aches and pains like at wake-up moment, and finish with about thirty and new total of 5,035.8km. The race to 5,215 is on!

The ride of the 30th finds me contemplating the time schedule for the rest of the week. Last night we attended an Outlook party. En route to the party, strange sounds were coming from the wheels whenever I put a little pressure on the brake pedal. This couldn't have happened at a worse time. The car had to go into the shop as soon as possible. I decide that I do not want to take the time this morning to first go to the shop, which does not open especially early, and then get a cab, which does not always happen too quickly, and then reverse the whole process when the car is ready.

So the plan is: I will go to work as usual, rendezvous with Esty at the garage when she finishes working and leave the car overnight so he can work on it tomorrow. Tomorrow morning I will drop Esty off at her work and take her car. When she finishes work at the end of the day, she'll release my car from the shop, which is in her part of town.

Good plan -- if it fits her schedule of course. I am really impressed with myself that I was able to come up with such an intricate plan! The only problem is how much I will be able to ride the next morning, because we have to leave the house fairly early together. As she should be getting ready to leave the house to go to work, I return home from my ride to confirm the plan and continue with the rest of my day. As I wheel the bike into the shed, I note of course my total – 5,057.2km.

Sometimes plans work out, sometimes they do not. This particular plan actually worked out as well as possible. One of our neighbors works very near to Esty's place of work. In the evening she calls him to find out when he is leaving the house, and if he is driving directly to work in the morning. The results: I do not have to leave the house early with Esty to drop her off to work, and I up the total to 5,077.3.

Yogli phoned later that evening and wanted to know whether or not we are still in the 'go mode' for Friday. The weather predicted for Friday could be a problem. Very dry hot air called a Hamsin is expected to roll in from the desert tomorrow (Tuesday) and will be with us for another day. Thursday is expected to be cooler and on Saturday we probably will be hit by another Hamsin. Hamsin days can be extremely uncomfortable if you are outdoors and more so if you are exerting yourself by doing manual labor or simply partaking in any type of outdoor sporting event. Riding a bike during a Hamsin when it can be avoided is not something that you would like to be included in your resume. Friday is still far off and weather forecasters have been known to err on their weather predictions. In the meantime, I intend to add another twenty kilometers tomorrow morning. Esty and I are going out this evening and hopefully we will be back at the house at a decent time.

April 1st – or April Fools Day if I remember correctly. Unfortunately, I have not yet adjusted to daylight savings time as my biological clock is not in tune with the new local time. My cell phone alarm is still programmed for 5:10 a.m. and my wake up call reflects a slightly darker morning because of the time change. My immediate thought was about racking up an additional twenty kilometers for the morning, but as I'm so close to a round number (5,100km), I continue another couple of kilometers, and ultimately finish the morning at 5,101.1. The master plan is to ride another fifteen - twenty kilometers tomorrow morning (Wednesday), rest up on Thursday, which leaves approximately 100 kilometers (61 miles) left for Friday – deadline day.

Later in the day, at work, I check the internet for the weather forecasts for Friday. The two alternatives that Yogli and I have tentatively decided on are Jerusalem– Herzliya (which we did not really get to last week), or an even longer ride, Jerusalem – Beer Sheva. The latter choice would definitely take us over the 100km mark for the day; an exciting fitting finish! The winning choice will undoubtedly be the trip that is least hot. The internet however has conflicting information regarding which destination will be hotter on Friday. The local sites have the Tel-Aviv area (just south of Herzliya) as reaching 30°C (86°F), and Beer Sheva reaching 31°C (88°F) I call up Yogli, and he is in full agreement that the best route is the one with the more comfortable weather conditions.

Yogli phoned me later that evening on his was home from Tel Aviv and was quite concerned about a revised weather forecast he had picked up on the radio. Extremely high temperatures are now expected for Friday and temperatures could climb to 40°C (104°F) This was a revolting development and we agreed to discuss this further at the office in Jerusalem the following day. Several minutes after hanging up the phone, I see the forecast on TV: unseasonably high temperatures starting tomorrow with a linear line going up and up thru Saturday.

I realize that a long ride on Friday will not be feasible and decide to change the riding plan for the week a bit. I cancel the planned resting day scheduled for Thursday and decide to start riding in the evening as well to make up the difference -- starting **right now**.

I almost forgot how nice it is to ride after the sun goes down. I phoned Yogli while I am riding to inform him that the long ride on Friday is officially out and left the message on his answering machine to this effect. He was probably in bed for the night. I return home, jump into bed with a new accumulative total for the day 5,118.2, just under 100 kilometers (60 miles) to go, and another three days to do it.

Despite the long ride on Friday being scratched, it now appears that the remaining distance will be a 'cake walk'. The contract with myself that I had concocted months ago will be fulfilled! All that is left to decide on is how much earlier I want to set the alarm for tomorrow. I decide on five a.m..

Apparently my biological clock is starting to get used to daylight saving time, or subconsciously the goal is pushing me forward, or maybe a combination of both. On Wednesday, **April 2nd** I wake up automatically at four-thirty a.m. I switch off the alarm, and kind of just lie in bed recuperating for fifteen minutes. At five a.m., I am already outside and two hours and 30km (18 miles) later, I return; I'm at 5148.8km.

Unfortunately my good spirits are short lived when I realized that my driver's license will expire in about two weeks. It is now no longer subject to an automatic renewal status. I had inadvertently omitted forwarding the results of a physical checkup which should have accompanied the renewal form. I vaguely remember receiving the official notice months ago but it got lost in the shuffle of things to be done. As we approach the end of the licensing validation period, a deliberate work slow down is now underway in all government ministries. Assuming that I can locate the physical checkup form and pass the subsequent examination, I am not certain whether or not the government employees working in the licensing department have finished playing games or are now back at work.

After work I start looking for the form. I take a break to eat dinner, and then I play the part of taxi driver (either Esty or I have to go bring Tuval back from his Karate class). We come back, I change my clothes, and I plan to do a nice leisurely fifteen or so kilometers (9 miles) – in the end its more like 17 (10 miles). I'm up to 5,166.3 – or only 49 kilometers (30 miles) short with two days to go. Not a bad day, 47 kilometers (29 miles), and that was around a very full day at work. And finally I find the form; it was in my briefcase the whole time!

Pressure is now mounting. The time necessary to procure signatures from my primary physician and the optometrist is competing with the time I need to push my odometer over the finish line within the time frame allotted for this year long challenge. Yesterday, Esty just happened to have a check up at the doctor's and of course could have signed her there. About a month ago, I changed the lenses in my glasses and could have signed the optometrist then. The problem is that I do not know if my doctor and also the optometrist work morning-afternoon shifts or afternoon-evening shifts tomorrow.

It is now Thursday, **April 3**[rd] and my wake up call had been programmed to sound off at four-fifty a.m. I had planned to be out of the house and on my bike shortly afterwards. My legs are a bit sore from riding last night and I remained in bed for another five minutes. It was five-fifteen before I left the house. This morning's ride was not as relaxing as usual and when I returned the bike to the shed, the new odometer reading was 5,189km (3,113 miles). I am pressed for time and the medical form is uppermost in my mind. The national work union is threatening a nation wide strike on Monday which could hold up my driver's license renewal well past its expiration date.

From a patient's standpoint, going to the health clinic is usually a hassle. I am very satisfied with my physician but waiting your turn for the one on one meeting with your doctor can be quite frustrating. There is usually a last minute emergency which plays havoc with your scheduled appointment or the individual who jumps the line informing the belligerent onlookers that only a signature is needed and exits the doctor's office twenty – thirty minutes later.

I phoned the clinic inquiring whether my doctor had the morning or afternoon shift and was told that she was presently in her office and she would see patients with an urgent situation without an appointment until eight-thirty a.m. I am certain that she would not have any objections if I pop in just for a moment and have her sign the medical questionnaire for the Department of Motor Vehicles. Arriving at the clinic, I was pleasantly surprised to find no one in line to see my doctor nor were there any patients presently in her office.

I was out of the doctor's office within minutes and made my way to the mall across the street for the optometrist's signature only to find out that the office would not be open until ten a.m. Since it was only eight-thirty, I decided to go to my office and catch the optometrist on the way home from work.

I began to have second thoughts about waiting until the afternoon for a rendezvous with the optometrist for the eye examination. At ten a.m., I decide to check out of the office and head for the nearest shopping mall. I found an optometrist just as he was opening, had my eye examination and was back at work by ten-thirty.

I faxed the completed medical form with attachments to the Department of Motor Vehicles together with information as to how they can reach me by phone, cell phone or e-mail. Shortly afterwards I received an e-mail reply confirming my fax was received and it had been forwarded to the department doctor for his approval. Several hours later I received a phone call from the department that my application had been reviewed and approved and that my operator's license should be in the mail by Sunday.

It doesn't get much better than this. I am really on a roll today and it seems that I can do no wrong. The idea did cross my mind to purchase a lotto ticket and somehow the odds of winning appeared to be gaining momentum but common sense prevailed and it was now time for me to carry my load at the office. The rest of the day was quite hectic and I finished work much later than I had anticipated.

I dash home and have time for only a quick supper; tonight Rakefet's dance group is appearing. She has been learning for years and I want to get there early enough so we can catch decent seats as I will be videotaping the show. It was a great show! The event ended at ten p.m. I checked my cell phone after the program ended and noticed that Yogli had tried to reach me. I returned his call which was about the bike ride for tomorrow and he advised me that it was going to be extremely hot and uncomfortable all day tomorrow.

We decide to do our usual route – the very scenic Jerusalem-Bet Shemesh ride thru the mountain trail along the Sorek River. Because of the extremely hot weather forecast for tomorrow, we decide to start extremely early and to rendezvous in Bet Shemesh at six a.m. in order to leave one of the cars.

I would have to leave my house tomorrow at five a.m. and preparations for the upcoming trip would have to be done this previous evening. While Esty is adding her ingredient mix to the bread making machine, I am outside attaching the bike rack to my car in order to save another couple of minutes in the morning. I set the alarm for four-thirty and go to sleep.

I am definitely happy that even despite the very hot day tomorrow, I will reach my goal NOT on a typical early morning ride in my own neighborhood before work in the morning. Like last week's 5,000 km mark, it will be accomplished on a Friday fun ride with my standard Friday riding partner.

Friday morning, **April 4th**, four-thirty a.m.: The alarm clock does its thing on time and I can hear that the bread making machine is making its usual operational moans and groans followed by a beeping sound that alerts anyone in the area that the bread is now ready. Perfect timing! It is also time for me to leave my nice comfortable bed and get moving if I want to make this a day to remember. I worked hard this past twelve months, both physically and mentally and my unwavering perseverance is about to pay off.

My quick breakfast consists of a glass of orange juice with a tablespoon of olive oil, a grapefruit and a banana. I load the bike on the car and head for Bet Shemesh to meet up with Yogli. I arrive before Yogli and make preparation to transfer my bike and other equipment to his vehicle for the trip back to Jerusalem.

While waiting for Yogli to arrive, I use the time to readjust my helmet, as it will be a hot ride, and I am used to riding with a wool cap which also covers my ears beneath the helmet. Last week, on the ride to Tel-Aviv (without the wool cap), the helmet was quite loose and annoying. It wasn't long before Yogli arrived. The bikes and equipment needed were quickly loaded into his car.

This will be my first ride of the season with only my riding pants and T-shirt. There will be no sweat shirt or sweat pants on this trip. On our long Friday bike rides, I have been taking two liter size bottles of water in addition to the two water bottles attached to the bike. With the temperature expected to soar today, I have replaced the two liter sized bottles in my backpack with two larger one-and-a-half liter bottles. The extra weight of water would be inconsequential compared to running out of water during the anticipated record breaking heat. I finish adjusting my helmet en route to Jerusalem. At our starting point, we do some stretching exercises, put on our back packs, mount our bikes and we are now officially off and riding

The initial run is down hill on a paved road. We pick up a fair amount of speed before we reach the mountain trail which is about 5km (3 miles) from our starting point. It was uncomfortably cold speeding down the hill in our summer time riding clothes. The sun had not yet risen to saturate the area with the blistering heat predicted for today. It is still quite nippy when we reach the start of the trail at the bottom of the hill at which time we have to start pedaling. This is good because it means that a good part of our trip will be behind us before the sun's heat will start to take its toll.

The route is exceptionally scenic today. The daisies, calendula, poppies and other wild spring flowers are in bloom. These will remain in bloom until the summer sun bakes the land and this beautiful site will be laid to rest for another year. In the meantime, Yogli and I will enjoy their fragrance and beauty along the mountain trail. About 27km (16 mikes) down the trail, Yogli pulls over for a pit stop. It is getting much warmer now and the chilly weather we encountered earlier is now well behind us.

The euphoric feeling of accomplishment crossing the 5,215km finish line should be getting very close now and I switch the adjust button on my odometer from today's total to accumulative total. The odometer must have smiled at me because the new reading was 5,215.3km (3,129.2 miles). **Mission accomplished!** My reaction was similar to last week when another milestone was reached. I did not see fireworks and get all excited. I believe Yogli was more excited than I was! However, I did note the time. It was exactly 8:25 a.m.

Ironically, both Yogli and I had stopped at approximately the same spot last summer when he took a picture of me. We were both coming from the opposite direction at the time. That picture can now be seen on the back cover of this book. In the background of the picture is the route of the old Jerusalem – Tel Aviv train line that is presently being rebuilt. Yogli felt that in honor of this occasion, this would be an appropriate place to take our breakfast break. Unfortunately the noise generated from the heavy construction equipment negated the serenity around us and we decided to postpone our breakfast until we reached a more tranquil area.

We continue riding, and decide to eat breakfast at a small public area several kilometers after the main entrance of Bet Shemesh. It is already starting to get much warmer, but we find a table in a very shaded wooded area. Yogli starts slicing up the apples he brought, I start slicing up Esty's bread, as we both are curious to see what she's added this time to her whole wheat bread. This time around it is dried tomatoes and Marjoram.

Yogli jokes that if I would have done this *historic* ride in my neighborhood, then when the time comes and I have grandchildren, I could boast that "here next to the neighborhood garbage dumpster, I made my famous ride." Needless to say, crossing the finish line on the mountain trail will undoubtedly earn me a few more points with the future grandkids.

After eating our quota of apples and bread which was covered with Esty's homemade kumquat jam made from the fruit of a tree from our garden, we ride several kilometers back to my car. It is now about eleven a.m. and the weather forecasters called it right this time. It is now extremely hot outdoors and getting an early start this morning really paid off. We load the bikes on to the car and the year long bike riding venture is officially over. As I remove the digital odometer from the bike, it reads 5,230 km (3,138 miles). This averages out to 100.6km (60.4 miles) / per week for the entire year.

In order to reach this goal, I rode 304 kilometers (190 miles) in the last eight days. This was less than two years after my heart attack and during a full week of work, as opposed to the vacation when Tuval and I took our bikes and tent up north last summer.

Friday is still Friday and despite crossing the finish line earlier today, there are still numerous chores around the house that have to be addressed. Although I returned earlier than usual from a Friday bike ride, I am anxious to get started. Upon removing the lawn mower from the shed, I notice the grass catcher is still hooked up to the mower. That seemed odd as I usually empty the grass catcher every week and leave it disconnected for the next grass cutting day. It slowly dawned on me why the grass catcher was still connected. I forgot to empty it last week!

This was another subtle reminder that I am no longer able to do simple repetitive functions automatically and I now have to concentrate more on what I am doing at the time I am doing it. I did not dwell too long on the lawn mower episode and it surely did not dampen my upbeat feeling earlier in the day when Yogli and I crossed the finish line.

It is now time to get the outdoor barbecue ready. This type of meal is always the family favorite and today Esty wanted something extra special to commemorate the grand finale of the year long bike ride. That's right, I'm still a heart patient, and have to watch what I consume. However I'm still flesh and blood, and one of life's little pleasures is to sit over a hot grill after two beers, and stuff a piece of turkey breast or steak or some kebabs into a pita bread already lined with mustard and onions –

ISN'T LIFE GREAT??

(or so I thought then…………….).

11

Post 1 - The real book actually starts here

The purpose of writing this book was to record my own experience of what it was like to undergo a heart attack and subsequently how I dealt with this life threatening experience. I specifically had in mind other heart patients that may have experienced the same negative side effects that I encountered from medications taken in the post operative period. It was also my intention for the post heart attack victim to receive some encouragement from this book and to emphasize all the positive effects that the bike riding had on me.

For a brief period of time the reader may have been inclined to assume from the early chapters that I was heading in the direction of an autobiography. In reality, it was the post operative period that caused me the most grief and I learned that I did not have a monopoly on this type of malady. This phase of my recuperative period is what this book is all about.

I have become considerably more knowledgeable regarding heart disease since my heart attack as evidenced by the extensive array of supportive information that can found after Chapter 16. In addition, I thought it apropos for the reader to become familiar with some fundamental medical terms concerning heart disease in order that he/she could better understand the magnitude of their heart problem.

It had taken a fair amount of time to elapse before I was able to accept the fact that Mike year 2002/2003 model had less operating features than Mike year 2001 model. Bike riding therapy probably put me in my best physical shape during my lifetime. I was slim, trim and had the physique and stamina of a much younger man. To the uninformed or casual acquaintance I appeared to be in peak condition and a person to be envied. Hidden from view was my inability to cope with my power of concentration and the intermittent memory loss that seemed to follow me. Most disturbing was the feeling of apathy at work and at home and at times experiencing negative mood changes for no apparent reason. I was cognizant that I had become insensitive to my immediate surroundings and almost seemed helpless to remedy this situation.

Just about all of the medical professionals that I had taken my problems to agreed that it probably was the Ace Inhibitor that was causing me this grief. It was also strongly suggested that I do not discontinue taking this medication since the dosage was minimal and it would be in my best interest to continue taking it as prescribed. In regards to other medications I have been taking, both the low dosage of aspirin and Lipidal (Pravastatin), a cholesterol lowering drug, have been used extensively worldwide in combating heart disease. Aspirin is even taken by healthy people as preventative medicine

Earlier I explained in layman's terms the prescriptions I was given and what function each performed. I was of the opinion that articles written by experts in their field would be somewhat congruous with findings by other so called experts in the same field. This is not necessarily true as evidenced earlier by the so called experts in the various weight control and/or diet programs. You may recall the recommendations of some of the so called pros were diametrically opposite of other best selling authors on the same subject. A somewhat similar situation can exist with the literature found with prescription medication. The problem here is that not all pertinent information listed in the fine print descriptive literature included with the dispensed medication includes *all* of the possible side effects that one may encounter in taking these drugs.

While focusing on my cholesterol lowering drug called Lipidal (Pravastatin), a member of the statin family of medications, I made a startling discovery. Up until now, the vast majority of doctors and the public, myself included, were of the opinion that the lower the cholesterol level, the lower the chance of a heart attack. The lower the better! During the past twenty odd years, statins were considered to be the cornerstone in fighting heart disease and not too much thought was given to side effects resulting from very low levels of cholesterol.

I learned of a research program[8] currently being conducted on this very subject of very low levels of cholesterol and possible negative side effects of this condition brought on by the use of statins. This study was being funded by the National Institute of Health (NIH) and chaired by Beatrice A. Golomb, M.D., PhD, Assistant Professor of Medicine at the University of California in San Diego.

Common complaints in this study included memory loss; personality changes; irritability; aching muscle pain; weakness; fatigue; cognitive problems; sleep deprivation; neuropathy and erectile dysfunction. The discovery of this research program was truly mind blowing! Here was a study being performed and it was all about my own personal problems. **Had I finally found the roots of my disconnection from society? Was it really the cholesterol lowering drug that was causing my nightmare that gave me the feeling of being in suspended animation?** Then the culprit was not the Ace Inhibitor that I was led to believe!

I was truly amazed when reading this? Actually *amazed* is a gross understatement because you can be amazed by something, but still subsequently carry on with the 'status-quo'.

Finding Dr. Golomb's research study was for me more like the opening of a Pandora's Box, although in an opposite positive sense to what Pandora's Box usually represents. It was similar in effect to my initial reaction when discovering Dr. Ornish. The point with Dr. Ornish is not whether he was right or not, it represented a change in my own conception of right and wrong. Eventually from Dr. Ornish I continued in new directions, even totally contradicting most of Ornish's doctrines regarding health and food. However without that first stepping stone that Dr. Ornish provided me, I may have never continued in trying to find healthier ways to run my life.

The generally accepted notion of lay people has been that cholesterol is bad and the lower the cholesterol readings, the better. Cardiologists were obsessed in lowering their patient's cholesterol levels. Now this researcher, Dr. Beatrice Golomb has delved into the negative side effects of low levels of cholesterol that had previously been considered to be acceptable and in many instances an optimum target. Her interim findings were that prescription induced low levels of cholesterol are causing problems almost identical to problems that I am now experiencing.

Is it possible that the generally accepted theory of very low levels of cholesterol being preferred is now being challenged? Since Dr. Golomb's research introduced me to the world of statins, the glowing reports that had flowed initially from this type of medication are now being called into question. Baycol, a cholesterol lowering statin was pulled from the market after being linked to more than one hundred fatalities from a rare muscle wasting condition called rhabdomyolysis. The American Academy of Neurology published a Danish study[9] that reported long term exposure to statins may substantially increase the risk of polyneuropathy, a nerve disorder.

Post 1 - The real book actually starts here

During our fruit harvesting months, I usually start my breakfast in the morning with a home grown grapefruit. Our grapefruit tree has been furnishing our family with copious quantities of superb quality pink fruit for a number of years. I have yet to find any comparable quality fruit in any supermarket or open market.

As it turns out, grapefruits and in particular grapefruit juice, alters the effects of dozens of medicines!!! This was discovered by accident in 1989 by Dr. David Bailey[10] and associates at the University of Western Ontario, Canada, as a surprise observation during a drug interaction study between a blood pressure medication, felodipine and ethanol (ethyl alcohol). Double-strength grapefruit juice was used to cover the taste of the alcohol in a test control group. Felodipine, when administered with grapefruit juice, raised the blood levels of felodipine dramatically.

Further studies have determined that some prescribed statins namely Lovastatin[11] and Simvastatin[12], react unfavorably with grapefruit juice. There is no need to discuss Cervastatin which had been marketed under the name of Baycol in lieu of the fact that Baycol has been recalled and is no longer available. A French study[13] has concluded that Fluvastatin does not react unfavorably with grapefruit juice while two other studies, one in Finland[14] and one in Japan[15] have concluded that Atorvastatin does react adversely with grapefruit juice. The two latter studies also found that Pravastatin, a medication that I am taking, does not act unfavorably with grapefruit juice.

Just how potent is grapefruit juice with some of these statins? A study[16] comparing taking Simvastatin with a high concentrate of grapefruit juice, or taking it with water, showed that the blood level of Simvastatin was thirteen times higher when taken with the highly concentrated grapefruit juice!!!

Was this simply my good luck? Not everyone in my rehab class was taking the same cholesterol lowering medication that was that was prescribed for me.

Former astronaut and USAF flight surgeon Dr. Duane Graveline[17] had two serious bouts of amnesia. The first occasion occurred when he could not recognize his wife and other family members and on the second occasion he was unable to remember anything after he had attended high school. The amnesia was attributed to his taking Atorvastatin which is marketed under the name of Lipitor.

When I mentioned these findings to some of my doctors, their replies ranged from "oh, I think I read about that somewhere" to "stick to writing computer programs and leave the doctoring to doctors".

Since we are discussing statins and cholesterol levels, I thought it apropos to delve deeper into the bogy substance called cholesterol which has become a nemesis to those with less than desirable eating habits. Health foods have been with us for a number of years but as of late, a growing amount of shelf space is being allocated in supermarkets for "cholesterol free" items. Despite the negative handle that has become attached to the word called cholesterol, I was surprised to learn that cholesterol is one of the most common organic molecules in the brain. Researchers have theorized that blocking cholesterol production inhibits the brain's performance causing muddled thinking and memory loss.

From the statin family of drugs, I became aware of the connection between low cholesterol levels and the belief that these low levels may result in a reduced serotonin[18] level of activity in the brain. Studies conducted in the past decades have indicated that individuals with cholesterol levels considered to be below normal have a tendency to suffer from violent and/or depressed moods.[19] The reasons for these reactions have not been fully understood. Serotonin is a brain neurotransmitter that regulates mood, appetite, and impulse control. It is also a sleep related hormone. Its dysfunction in the brain can lead to major depression and is associated with suicidal behavior.

Autopsies performed on suicide victims almost always indicate very low levels of serotonin in the blood.[20]

Dr. Emile Bliznakov,[21] an authority on Coenzyme Q_{10} (also known as CoQ_{10}) has stated that statins can block the synthesis of CoQ_{10} in the body which results in sub optimal levels of the coenzyme. It is not in the scope of this book to delve deeper into CoQ_{10} other than to state it can be found in every cell of the body and researchers believe that it prevents the oxidation of LDL. It is interesting to note that when LDL is oxidized it can damage the lining of the arteries which is a precursor of heart disease. Dr. Bliznakov was not alone in linking usage of statins to reduced levels of CoQ_{10}. Dr. Peter Langsjoen[22] of the CoQ_{10} Association has not only confirmed this but has also researched the benefits of CoQ_{10} in heart patients.

Another interesting topic that I uncovered regarded the widespread use of amalgam fillings to fill tooth cavities. Amalgam fillings are actually mercury fillings, and I was never aware exactly how lethal mercury can be to the body and to the environment in general.[23] Hard core evidence indicates the down side of amalgam fillings. Studies have shown that mercury vapors originating in amalgam fillings are readily absorbed into the body via inhalation and swallowing.[24] Excessive levels of this element will cause one's blood pressure to rise.[25] A number of years prior to my heart attack, my blood pressure had been abnormally higher than it should have been. This despite the fact that I was a non-smoker, maintained a normal weight and did a fair amount of exercise that included swimming, bicycle riding, hiking and gardening. Incidentally, my first amalgam filling was performed when I was 28 years old.

A study[26] at the University of Kuopio, Finland concluded that the excess risk of MI (heart attack) could be best related to high mercury levels in the hair, and that

> *"mercury accumulation in the human body is associated with accelerated progression of carotid[*] atherosclerosis"*

In June of 2003 I had a prescheduled meeting / checkup with my Professor of Cardiology. From a cardiologist's viewpoint, the results of my blood tests were excellent. Total cholesterol was down to 150 and my LDL was down to 88.   I was anxious to share with my professor my current dysfunction mode and I wanted to discuss with him my cholesterol numbers.

As luck would have it, my appointment with the Professor of Cardiology was sidetracked as he was involved with another patient in the emergency ward. Needless to say, the patient in the emergency ward had a much higher priority than my routine checkup. He did assign a doctor from his department to fill in for his out patients that were lined up in the waiting room. The doctor I saw that day was quite pleased with the results of my recent blood tests I had taken. He felt that there was no reason to reduce any of my daily medications --ideal numbers as far as cardiology is concerned!

When I discussed the results of these blood tests with my family doctor (who ultimately is the one who writes the prescription), she agreed with the doctor that had reviewed my blood tests with me. Apparently, medication overkill is preferable and safer than taking responsibility of reducing the dosage, despite the latter route may not be advantageous to the patient's quality of life. After all, I did not just have **a** heart

---

[*] carotid – pertaining to the 2 main arteries in the neck that convey blood to the head

attack, I had **three** within a twelve hour period; I have to be handled with kid gloves..........

I realize that I'm one of the more fortunate survivors of a heart attack and I have nothing but accolades for Professor Weiss and his dedicated staff in getting me thru that critical weekend. The one complaint I harbor is the range of numbers assigned to both the LDL and HDL cholesterol readings. Keep the LDL (bad cholesterol) below 100 and keep the good HDL (good cholesterol) above 40. Sort of like stretch socks – one size fits all.

I often wondered how these same figures could apply to a couch potato and to an individual like myself who bike rides an average of 120km (72 miles) per week.

Common sense would suggest that an individual involved in daily aerobics and who is physically active would have a different set of bodily needs to cope with his different life style. I discussed this with my family doctor.

She initially objected to my holistic doctor's suggestion that I reduce my daily Lipidal / Pravastatin medication from 20mg to 10mg. She was also unable to explain why someone like me who recently rode 185km (112 miles - three complete rides around Lake Tiberias) in a twenty hour period (a twenty-four hour marathon ride around the lake to raise money for child victims of terrorist activities) should be required to conform to the 'industry fixed' recommended rates for cholesterol levels which are also the same for the inactive couch potato.

After inundating her with much literature from my personal research and in particular, Dr. Golomb's NIH Statin Study, she reluctantly relented and went along with the reduction in the Lipidal dosage. A month trial without the benefits of Lipidal was deemed to be worthwhile in order to learn whether or not there would be a change in my mood swings, my general apathy and the effect it would have on my cholesterol numbers.

I mentioned earlier, that in the mental and emotional state that I had been living, it was as if I was alone in my own Matrix world – very similar, yet different from the real world. And now, suddenly I'm in a different movie altogether. In Terminator II, the out loud thoughts of John Connor's mother Sara on the way to the Cyberdyne building to destroy the chip were

> *"The future, always so clear to me, had become like a black highway at night. We were in uncharted territory now... making up history as we went along."*

For the reader that did not see the movie, it alluded to a future event that was considered to be inevitable, but the tables have now turned. The past realization that because of my attack I would now be required to live out the rest of my life as a zombie was now something that *could* be changed. I, like Sara, was about to embark on a new road, destination unknown.

According to the material that I had found regarding the statins, I expected that when discontinuing them, a feeling of normalcy would occur over an extended period of time. I was totally surprised, no, totally amazed that after only a couple of days my mood simply improved. This included the feeling of a revival of something resembling a normal sex drive, something that was definitely a pleasant surprise after what seemed to be such a long period of time.

I was after my morning ride, the piano and coming out of the shower when Esty came back from her morning walk. She had the day off from work. It was eight-thirty a.m., which means I'm late if I planned on getting to work by nine a.m., however I simply had the feeling *the hell with work* and for the first time in a long time it was me who started with Esty instead of the opposite (pleasant surprise for her – so what if I finally arrived to work at 9:45). An even a bigger surprise for *both* of us came that night with an 'instant replay' of what happened that morning. It was probably the first time since Paris two years earlier that we had 'intimate episodes' twice in one day.

Later the same month, I visited my holistic doctor for a follow up visit. I showed him the blood test results and how life just seems to have turned around after getting off of the Lipidal. He suggested that because the Tritace is a low dosage, that I could start gradually fazing that out also. He recommended that I continue to monitor my progress (periodic blood checks and blood pressure readings, and of course the annual stress test).

Regarding the information I had found regarding EDTA Chelating Therapy, he said that all the medications that I had been taking until now were intended to protect the status quo following the stent insertion. The medications were NOT intended to reduce the existing accumulated plaque in my arteries and to reverse this accumulated potential danger. It is something that I should be aware of for future reference. However, this was all starting to sound like freedom at last!

I know that the Tritace (ACE inhibitor) was prescribed for me in part to keep my blood pressure level within limits, this I could follow up myself as I have the apparatus to measure BP at home. I also made a mental commitment to myself to do a better job on eating less junk, which I do sneak in on occasion, possibly too often. Furthermore I planned to raise my daily rides from fifteen to 20km (12½ miles).

Two weeks later, after being off the Lipidal and Tritace altogether, I had my blood rechecked. I probably should have waited another week or so, as the blood check was shortly after returning from a romantic week vacation with Esty. This vacation included of course a bit too much of restaurant type food that I would not normally eat for obvious reasons, and not the usual daily sport routine. (It did of course include the typical 'sport activities' that one does on a vacation with his/her mate. It probably does not burn off the same amount of calories as a nice long bike ride -- but it does have other advantages.........)

As my holistic doctor had predicted, my Cholesterol readings did make a big jump. The HDL maintained a good level at 51, the LDL took a big jump to 117 and my total cholesterol had jumped to 182. What was surprising was a significantly below normal rate for sodium (salt). Apparently drinking loads of water during biking was simply washing out my body's salt supplies.

About the same time as my lower than normal sodium results returned, I came across some interesting articles by a Dr. Fereydoon Batmanghelidj, who claims that many of today's ailments are not really actual diseases, but rather the results of simple dehydration. He claims that the western world seems to prefer prescribing medicines instead of using the ultimate medicine – water! After all that I had gone through with my standard prescribed medicines, I found his approach to be quite refreshing. In particular, according to Dr. Batmanghelidj,[27] the foundation of having *heart disease* can be further divided into:

- high blood pressure and
- high cholesterol in the blood stream and
  build up on artery walls.

Regarding the former, Dr. Batmanghelidj claims that the state of body dehydration causes an imbalance between the water located inside of our body cells and the water located around the surrounding cells. One of the results of the body countering this imbalance is by the cell membranes utilizing a less than ideal quantity of water in the system which results in the increase in blood pressure.

Regarding the accumulation of cholesterol on the artery linings, Dr. Batmanghelidj claims that this is due to cell damage on the artery linings caused by – body dehydration. The linings become 'cracked' so to speak and the body's way of curing this problem is to coat the damaged tissues with a greasy bandage; the substance is cholesterol!

Unfortunately, modern medicine has come to consider cholesterol as the source of the problem, and not as the body's own first aid solution. As a result, we are treated for the symptoms and not for the root of the problem. We are prescribed cholesterol lowering **drugs** –and here I emphasize the word **drugs** to be interpreted according to the street definition of the term.

Up until now, I have covered only half of Dr. Batmanghelidj's claim to fame and discussed his general ideas regarding dehydration in the body. His *second half* becomes very interesting when related to my recent very low sodium blood levels.

It's *common knowledge* that anyone suffering from high blood pressure should curb, as far as possible, the use of salt in their diets. We have witnessed the marketing of various salt-free products in the supermarket in order to address this very serious problem of a significant part of the population suffering from hypertension (high blood pressure). In fact, today you can even buy *salt free* salt! Although apparently is not quite the ultimate invention as it may sound. I do remember from my rehab course that anyone taking ACE Inhibitors should definitely **NOT** be using the sodium free salt. Once again we come to an apparent conflict of accepted conceptions. Is salt (like cholesterol) really evil??

Dr. Batmanghelidj claims not. Moreover, it is mandatory to consume a certain amount of salt, directly relative to the quantity of water consumed. For starters, remember the imbalance between the internal part of our cells and the surrounding area? Salt helps maintain the quantity of water in this surrounding area. Dr. Batmanghelidj contends that salt is not only *a* vital element to the body; it is ranked in importance in the impressive number 3 spot – immediately following water and oxygen.

Drinking sizeable quantities of water alone simply washes the sodium and other elements out of our bodies, a subject I'll address shortly. Water, salt, and sugar infusions are commonplace in hospitals. Why do we have to ingest salt intravenously, when oral rehydration is possible?

The lower than normal sodium blood level also brought to mind several events that I remember from my past that had to do with drinking a significant amount of water on very hot days. The 'you can not drink too much water' adage which implies that at some stage you simply just urinate more now has taken on a new meaning.

I remember that on some bike rides in the middle of the summer, I would finish a bit light headed with the feeling of being overheated, and this in spite of drinking water at every opportunity! As per the rules, I was urinating a great deal, however I was sure that all the required water was being circulated through my body radiator and therefore everything was O.K.

I remember one stint of guard duty while in the reserves in the Negev (desert area in the south) in the middle of a summer over ten years ago. I was hospitalized for heat stroke, or at least that's what they called it; and this despite drinking loads of water and even periodically washing off my face and head with water to cool myself off.

This brings us to a new medical term, Hyponatremia, which means a low concentration of sodium in the blood. What does this have to do with bike riding on a hot day, or any other sport for that matter? When we sweat, we lose water AND salt. The more we sweat, and the more plain water we drink, the more we increase an imbalance of water and sodium in our systems. Our remaining sodium simply becomes more and more diluted. What is important is not the total amount of sodium, but rather the concentration of sodium.

The sodium plays a major role in water balance in the body. It is required to draw water through permeable membranes, thereby distributing the fluids throughout the body. Without the sodium, you can drink as much as you are able to, however the water just accumulates like an expanding water balloon in your stomach. It does not make it to the bloodstream.

I was not able to find numerous serious research papers that Dr. Batmanghelidj has published in respectable medical journals as I had found, for example, regarding Dr. Golomb. Besides the books he has written, I did find two articles he had published in journals over twenty years ago. After being disillusioned by standard medicine, I decided I had nothing to lose by trying the Dr. Batmanghelidj water/salt cure for a limited time while keeping tabs on its effect by more periodic blood testing and keeping track of my blood pressure.

At this point, you must be thinking that there is 'something wrong with Mike' – discontinuing the cholesterol lowering medication!!! - replacing the amalgam fillings!!! - drinking salt!!! He's crazy! The point is that desperate people tend to do desperate things. The quality of life under the influence of the statins had fallen to such a frustrating level, that none of the possible consequences resulting from the discontinuation of taking them seemed to deter me any longer. It was almost as if I had decided to *risk* living less years at a higher quality, rather than more years at near zero quality. I had already crossed a personal red-line when I stopped the statins. Trying the salt now seemed like small change. Was I really *crazy*? Maybe, but in order to define *crazy*, you first must be able to define *normal*, and what really **is** *normal* in today's insane world??

I also decided to have my homocysteine level tested. *The hospitals are full of people with high cholesterol; the cemeteries are full of people with high homocysteine,* so I read.

Or, in other words there are those doctors who now seem to believe that cholesterol stats by themselves are inconclusive and misleading at best. This is in direct contrast to those that still believe the term cholesterol to be sort of a long four letter word, just as saturated fat was until Dr. Atkins starting blaming sugar and over insulination for heart disease.

And what exactly is homocysteine? Homocysteine is an amino acid (a building block of protein) that is produced in the human body. It may irritate blood vessels, leading to atherosclerosis. High homocysteine levels in the blood can also cause cholesterol to change to oxidized low-density lipoprotein, which is considered to be very damaging to the arteries. In addition, high homocysteine levels can make blood clot more easily than it should, increasing the risk of blood vessel blockages.

One of the research pioneers linking homocysteine levels with heart disease is Dr. Kilmer McCully.[28] In 1969, while at Harvard University and Massachusetts General Hospital, he developed his theory that homocysteine is the real cause of atherosclerosis, and that accumulated cholesterol is merely a **symptom** and **not a cause** of heart disease. His ideas at the time were not embraced with open arms by his colleagues, as happens often when going against the accepted current school of thought. Later studies[29] verified the causal effect of homocysteine on Heart Disease.

In the Norwegian Hordaland Homocysteine Study, (which involved over 16,000 people, 1992-1993) it was shown that lifestyle factors influence homocysteine levels. It concluded that

> *"elevated plasma homocysteine level was associated with major components of the cardiovascular risk profile, i.e., male sex, old age, smoking, high blood pressure, elevated cholesterol level, and lack of exercise."*[30]

Post 1 - The real book actually starts here

I am sort of curious as to what the conclusion meant regarding "elevated plasma homocysteine level being associated with..... elevated cholesterol level". The other factors listed in the conclusion, male sex, old age, smoking, high blood pressure, and lack of exercise all seem to be some *causes* and not *effects* of elevated plasma homocysteine level. After all, I assume that it was not the intention to imply that high homocysteine level will cause someone to start smoking, or even determine his sex in later years!! Was cholesterol really isolated from other risk factors and determined to be a cause, or was it really an effect caused by higher homocysteine?

Unfortunately, my health clinic does not include homocysteine testing within its basket of paid-for blood tests. I had to pay for the test to be done at the hospital privately, which was not exactly cheap! The result of the test was 14.2. Most literature lists the top normal level to be not exceeding 15, and I have found literature mentioning 12 to be a recommended upper limit for people with heart related problems.

After a month or so of drinking *natural* salt dissolved in three liters of water during the work day, I had my blood retested. Drinking the three liters was spread out over the entire day, as opposed to drinking one liter three times a day. Before going further, I would like to stress that I am not referring to adding regular dry, white table salt to water and drinking it.

Commercial salt that is white and dry contains only Sodium and Chloride. All the other healthy minerals have been factory baked out. This reminds me of the difference between whole wheat bread and bleached white bread; all the healthy ingredients have been bleached out. This also goes for what is labeled as 'sea salt', which is definitely misleading.

Practically all salt originated along the way in the sea. The real sea salt Dr. Batmanghelidj is referring to is neither white nor dry; it's sort of grayish, generally larger crystals than table salt and is damp. If you are not sure if you have the real

143

sun dried material or the manufactured factory heated/dried types – put a teaspoon of salt in a glass of water before going to bed, stir it up, and check it in the morning. The authentic salt dissolves in water, and does not accumulate at the bottom of the glass, as does regular common table salt.

Indeed, after a month or two, my sodium level did rise; however it rose to 138 which is just over the minimum lower limit but less than half way on the total scale. Contrary to popular belief, the increase of sodium in my daily diet did NOT cause any significant change in blood pressure.

In addition to my sodium increase, I did experience a decrease in cholesterol; not a significant change, however a small change in the *right* direction. Total cholesterol dropped from 181 to 174, LDL from 117 to 114 and the HDL remained at a reasonable level of 49.

While we are on the subject of water and Dr. Batmanghelidj's cure for whatever it is that ails you; there also is a downside to water, or more specifically, the chemicals that we ourselves have put into the water supply. Dr. Joseph Price an opponent of the still existing practice of disinfecting public water supplies with chlorine wrote a highly controversial book in 1969 entitled "Coronaries/Cholesterol/Chlorine". He concluded that:

> *"Nothing can negate the incontrovertible fact, the basic cause of atherosclerosis and resulting entities such as heart attacks and stroke, is chlorine."*

He also points out that the addition of chlorine to our drinking water began in the late 1800s and by 1904, it was the standard in water treatment. Heart disease was virtually unknown until the twentieth century.

(If drinking chlorinated water is bad, exposure to chlorine due to inhalation of steam and skin absorption while showering certainly does not sound healthy, however that is WAY out of the scope of this book).

Chlorinated water is not the only alternative (even if little known) explanation that scientists have come up with in explaining the source of heart disease. According to Dr. Leslie Klevay, Professor of Internal Medicine, University of North Dakota School of Medicine and Health Sciences:

"Copper deficiency is offered as the simplest and most general explanation for ischemic heart disease." [31]

Dr. Klevay points out that copper deficiency in the body has adverse effects on electrocardiograms, impairs glucose tolerance which promotes thrombosis and oxidative damage, and increases blood pressure and cholesterol. His research does not end with copper alone. When copper deficiency is coupled with a high ratio of zinc to copper, Dr. Klevay claims that this imbalance results in hypercholesterolemia and increased mortality due to coronary heart disease.

"the ratio of zinc to copper may be the preponderant factor in the etiology of coronary heart disease." [32]

Another not well publicized indicator of potential heart disease is elevated levels of a certain protein known as CRP (C-reactive protein). CRP was discovered seventy years ago, and for the last several decades, doctors have noticed that after a heart attack, CRP levels would rise. This led researchers to believe that increased CRP levels in healthy individuals might serve as an early warning signal for an approaching heart attack. Dr. Paul Ridker of Brigham and Women's Hospital in Boston states:

"Several reports have linked inflammation and cardiovascular risk, particularly a novel acute inflammatory peptide, C-reactive protein (CRP), with future risk of coronary events independent of the traditional coronary artery disease risk factors. To this end, many studies suggest that

CRP may be used as a marker of sub-clinical atherosclerosis and cardiovascular risk. Specifically, CRP has been positively linked to future cardiovascular events in healthy women, healthy men, elderly patients, and high-risk individuals".[33]

The international medical community still seems to give a high priority in reducing high LDL Cholesterol levels as the best prevention against developing heart disease, and even more so for the post heart attack patient. However Dr. Michael Miller, Director of the Center for Preventive Cardiology, University of Maryland Medical Center emphasizes the importance of raising low HDL cholesterol levels:

The body of evidence showing an inverse relationship between HDL-C levels and risk for coronary heart disease (CHD) has grown large. Low HDL-C is the most common lipoprotein abnormality in patients with CHD and is predictive of subsequent CHD events, even when total cholesterol is within the desirable range. The National Cholesterol Education Program's ATP III report clearly defines a serum HDL-C level less than 40 mg/dL as an independent risk factor for CHD.[34]

Dr. J. Michael Gaziano of the Brigham and Women's Hospital in Boston brought the maximum levels of HDL argument in a new direction altogether, when comparing HDL to the level of triglycerides in the blood stream. Dr. Gaziano's main purpose was to study the affects of triglycerides, which are compounds in the blood made up of fatty acids that bind to proteins and form LDL. Triglycerides can adhere to the arteries in the form of fatty plaque. The results of Dr. Gaziano's study indicated that the ratio of triglycerides to HDL was the best predictor of a potential heart attack (the lower the ratio, the better).

> *.....Furthermore, the ratio of triglycerides to HDL was a strong predictor of myocardial infarction ....Conclusions Our data indicate that fasting triglycerides, as a marker for triglyceride-rich lipoproteins, may provide valuable information about the atherogenic potential of the lipoprotein profile, particularly when considered in context of HDL levels.*[35]

It of course is not my intention to endorse the views of Dr. Batmanghelidj (water cure), Dr. Price (chlorinated water) Dr. Klevay (copper), Dr. Ridker (CRP), Dr Miller (HDL) or Dr. Gaziano (Triglycerides/HDL). I am not medically qualified to do so. However, having my heart attack was caused by *something.* According to the alarming statistics regarding so many other people also having heart attacks, it does seem that mainstream medical thought has not yet exactly zeroed in on that *specific something.*

November 2003 – It has been a couple of months since my last writing. At this stage of the book it was not my intention to make this like a diary. The original intention was to finish the year end goal of 5,000 kilometers, which was the original natural end to this book, and continue with life just as before. However as the draining effects of the statins kept wearing me down, so I continued writing, and still continue now.

Something small, but for me, significant happened this week. It may seem totally ridiculous to the normal reader, and I almost feel embarrassed to write about it. It certainly may be appreciated by someone still at some stage or other of the mental-drugged stage that I wrote about earlier.

My cellular phone (like most I would assume) has one hundred memory allocations for phone numbers from which I can search alphabetically. It also has a feature that allows me to see past calls in the order that they arrived – listed with a name in the event that the caller is defined in one of the one-hundred slots. Sometimes towards the end of a work day, Rakefet would call from her boyfriend's house (regular phone) and request that I pick her up on the way home. As I would never know how much traffic I would hit along the way, I would give her a ring five minutes before arrival. Usually, while driving, I would page through the alphabetic listing, unless she was one of the recent callers, which would allow me to find the number faster.

The frustrating part would be that while driving. I would be half looking at the road, half hitting buttons on the phone. I would ultimately get a busy signal, which would require redoing all the button hitting and searching again; half concentrating on the road and half on the telephone.

This week when she called requesting a ride home -- it just automatically hit me -- a much better way to call. It was so obvious, something that I've been doing every time I call Esty or one of the kids, but until now **it simply never occurred to me** that I can call Rakefet at her boy friend's house in exactly the same fashion.

Every one of the phone number cells in memory is identifiable by its actual number in memory. For instance my house is two, Esty is three, Sagi is four, etc. One long press on the three would automatically call Esty. Simple, right? The 'small insignificant event' that happened to me this week was realizing that I could ring Rakefet's boyfriends house automatically in the same fashion!

Instead of half driving, half searching the cell phone all at the same time, I could simply hit the shortened number code for his house. Indeed, before leaving work, I searched for his name on my address book, saw that he was defined in cell number eighty-six, and five minutes before arriving to his neighborhood I hit the 'eight' button and then a l-o-n-g 'six', and lo and behold his phone started ringing!

And why did this *extraordinary* feat all of a sudden increase my good spirits? It was just another one of several very small daily items occurring to me recently that were now forming a trend as per by Dr. Golomb's article regarding the recovery over a period of months from the use of statin type cholesterol reducing drugs.

I was very surprised at how fast my emotions had started to reawaken within a couple of days after stopping the Lipidal (statin medication) several months ago, even if my mental thinking abilities still seemed to be impaired. Now, finally, I was witnessing – no – not just witnessing – actually experiencing a return to the pre-statin thinking/analyzing/focusing abilities that I had been missing now for close to two years.

As much as something so insignificant as entering a code to call on a cell phone instead of looking up the number in the directory would be for most people automatic, even ridiculously automatic, for me it was like a major breakthrough – I was now able to think again!!!

My daily morning routine has now also changed a bit from what it had been for the last year or so. The mornings would always start out with my bike ride and then a twenty minute - half hour piano playing session. This was followed of course by getting my act together and going to work. Still being ever conscious that stopping the Tritace (ACE inhibitor) and Lipidal (cholesterol) is nevertheless somewhat of a calculated risk, my bike riding routine in the mornings has not only retained its prime importance, it has also expanded to a daily routine of an hour and a half. This unfortunately does not leave any time whatsoever for the piano, which I now try to squeeze in the evenings, but now no longer every day.

Something definitely worth mentioning now that I have been off of the statins for half a year: During the past few months I have also noticed a change in my attitude towards my normal Friday routine that I had been following for the last two years or so. My Friday ritual for the day would be a nice long ride somewhere. I would leave the house very early in the morning, regardless of whether I was going on a ride with friends, or riding alone. As I mentioned earlier, the bike riding had become more than just a tool for physical rehabilitation. It had become an obsession, my eloquent reason to just *get away by myself*. By the time I would return in the late afternoon, my Friday, practically speaking, would be about over as far as getting anything else done before supper time.

I've noticed during the last couple of months that I felt less of the need to get away by myself for a ride, especially if my riding buddies were not available. I started doing my Friday rides early in my local neighborhood, without of course the restriction of time that I have in the morning before work. This still enabled me to get in a good Friday ride and leave me with the whole Friday ahead of me for....... whatever. During the last couple of months, the *whatever* of some of these Fridays has become light shopping/window shopping/hanging out with Esty in Jerusalem, usually also accompanied by sitting somewhere over a cup of something (coffee for Esty, anything else for me) and not infrequently a light lunch.

This may seem like a normal thing for a couple to do together, but for a long time it definitely was not something that I would enjoy doing, and especially not totally willingly. While still taking the statins I had the urge every week to get away and ride on Fridays, which was the high point of my week and what I'd be waiting for the entire week. Over the last couple months this desire to get away, especially by myself, has started losing its appeal and importance. In fact, now I look forward to the couple of hours of getting out with Esty on Friday mornings/early afternoons outside of our daily home environment routine.

Even under normal conditions, the relationship between a couple can be an intricate, sometimes complicated matter. Any couple who has 'made it' to at least twenty years together knows that there have been ups and downs -- obviously preferably more ups than downs. Since the descent and landing from my statins trip, my relationship with Esty has surpassed our own routine normalcy that had characterized our relationship even during the years preceding my heart attack.

I wish that I could write a list of reasons explaining why our relationship seems to be much stronger now than it has been in years; maybe even more than the newlywed's period of the early 1980's. Life is more complicated than that and it's not really possible to 'isolate' individual causes.

Coming out of a very bad period (the dark two statin years) is certainly not a foolproof recipe for the successful rebirth of a relationship; the exact opposite could have just as easily happened. In retrospect, I suspect that the Outlook Seminars that we both attended several years ago are now paying us back dividends, especially now that my head is functioning normally again. In fact, I also now wonder if I had not gone thru the 'Outlook Process', if this book would even have been written. I imagine that only someone who has experienced the seminars will really understand this last statement -- my apologies to the rest of the world...........

December 7th had a bit more personal significance for me this year. Unfortunately, I'm afraid that some of the younger readers might not even know what December 7th represents in American history. After reaching the first year goal of 100km/week average I purposely have not been boring you readers with more bike stats. This does not mean however that I had abandoned keeping track of the kilometers/mileage -- just the opposite. December 7th just happened to be the day that the odometer turned over. This may not be as '*exciting* as watching an older model car odometer go from 99,999.9 miles/kilometers and reset to 0; however I definitely felt that it was quite an accomplishment that after a year and eight months to see

9999.9 turn over to 0 - my 10,000[th] kilometer (6,200 miles) bike riding.

In order to drive the point home on how I keep track of the mileage, I bought a new battery about two weeks before my scheduled 10,000th kilometer, in order to replace the existing battery with a new one exactly at the 0 kilometer turnover. This prevented the unwanted situation of having the battery expire somewhere within the next 10,000km, which would make keeping track of the accumulated mileage more complicated. Obviously not exactly a life/death situation, however knowing exactly how much I am riding is an excellent way to encourage me to keep up the ritual.

Later on that month (December 2003), there was a rehab reunion meeting with my Cardiology Professor and us veterans; those who had our heart attacks two - three years ago. The professor and the head nurse of the rehab program updated us on what's new in the world of having a heart attack, and the changes in caring and rehab over the last couple of years:

- A change in the procedure regarding patients arriving to the emergency ward currently going thru a heart attack. Way back during my time, the routine was to stabilize the patient if possible (clot dissolving, expansion of arteries etc) and wait to do an angiogram only after the patient was stabilized (obviously emergency cases received emergency treatment where necessary). The new trend is to do the angiogram as soon as possible after admittance and to perform the angioplasty procedure immediately and if necessary, the stent insertion. This is significant in my case because we arrived to the closer Mount Scopus branch of Hadassah hospital when I had my attack. After being stabilized (two days later), I was sent by ambulance to the Ein Kerem branch of Hadassah to have the angiogram performed; this procedure is not done at Mount Scopus. The very direct hint to us at rehab was that if we have a recurring attack, we would be better off by saving time and getting directly to Ein Kerem if possible.

- The importance of watching our diets, and again stressing the foods to avoid, or at least eat in moderation, for instance foods containing high cholesterol, and food containing a high percentage of saturated fat, such as red meat, eggs and rich cheeses.

- The importance and the advantages of the prescriptions we have to take, and urging us NOT to STOP taking them on our own personal discretion. He even went out of his way to emphasize the advantages of taking the cholesterol lowering statins, and keeping the LDL under 100.

- The importance of a regular exercise routine.

During this rehab session, we were all given forms to fill out: personal info, how we are feeling, what we are taking, eating habits, exercise habits, and the like. I listed on the form that I had stopped taking the Tritace and the Lipidal six months ago, and that I would definitely like to talk to him about this during my annual visit in January at the hospital.

A final incident at the end of December made me realize that I had FINALLY returned, as far as I can tell, to pre-heart attack levels of the ability to think and reason, and the ability to feel. Although I did start feeling a reawakening of emotions very shortly after stopping the statins, it was not yet complete. It was only now that I was able to cry real tears in response to a real situation. It's not that I'm a *chronic* crier, but

153

it's been years since I have been physically able to express myself in this manner. I was now complete again.

The upcoming checkup/visit for January 2004 will be very significant for me. Previous to the visit, I will have had a stress test done, as well as blood tests taken. These results will be scrutinized at the visit. Their significance for me is great. It will be a full half-year since taking myself off of the ACE Inhibitor and Cholesterol lowering drugs and increasing my bike riding. Time enough for a good indication as to whether I am really on the way to a true recovery or, that I ultimately was very irresponsible to myself and to my family by putting myself at increased health risks.

At the time, with my impaired judgment and impaired ability to feel things, I was so frustrated at going thru life as a total zombie. The choice of continuing until old age as a zombie, or getting my life back but risking an earlier departure was definitely not an automatic decision to accept the former. It's only now that I can appreciate the severity of the consequences of what I had then decided, and the realization that the results of my upcoming stress test and blood tests may possibly persuade me return to some form of medication. I have never been in jail, but I have the feeling that my situation is in a way similar to someone who HAS been in jail, has again tasted freedom and now stands before the possibility that he may be going back in.

Mid January Tests

The stress test actually was coming at a less than ideal time. My blood pressure levels during the last month or so have started becoming a bit erratic; sometimes O.K. and sometimes going too high. I had already cut back on the salt; even discontinued it except for the long bike rides when I drink non-stop. However the last couple of months of constant pressure at work may also have contributed to the erratic BP readings, in addition to eating habits which have gone astray over the last couple of months. As I had expected, the results of the stress test were fine. It took over twelve and a half minutes to reach my target pulse rate. The recommended minimum time to reach my target pulse rate is twelve minutes. The extra half minute that it took me means that I am considered to be very fit endurance-wise.

A week later, I had my blood test. The critical results as far as I was concerned were the cholesterol readings. Even before receiving the results I was already mad at myself for losing a good bit of self discipline over the last couple of months, especially the last couple of weeks as far as eating habits go.

I was not really gaining any weight these last couple of months, but who knows how some of the junk that I had resumed eating had affected my BP and cholesterol levels. After all, I should not have to be overly particular regarding what I eat…..., because I ride.......

Several days after having my blood tested, the results came in - a jump in the total cholesterol from 174 to 199 and a jump in the LDL for 114 to 137. At least my HDL remained a healthy over 50 at 51. I was definitely NOT looking forward to the upcoming hospital exam with these figures. My 137 LDL was starting to deviate too much from the text book upper limit of 100 that seems so holy in the cardiology world. My family doctor had told me when my LDL jumped to 114 that the "cardiologist will not like these figures."

At this stage, I did start to have second thoughts regarding my decision six months earlier to stop taking the ACE Inhibitor and the cholesterol controller. My blood pressure during the last month or so had not been stable and now with the higher cholesterol levels, were my convictions so wrong that my daily bike rides of twenty – twenty-five kilometers would be enough to keep the blood pressure and cholesterol reading in check??

I also had some flashbacks regarding two events of the past couple of years. We had eventually managed to receive an unofficial reason why the staff at Hadassah seemed to be so tense on the day that I was transferred from Mount Scopus to Ein Kerem, and the extra special treatment that I received in getting there. If you recall, my Mom went back and forth in rickety transit vehicles and she was seventy-five years old at the time. She was the one on her way to a quadruple bypass, and it was me who was transported in a fully equipped intensive unit ambulance.

A nurse that we know that also worked at Mount Scopus (in a different department) managed to learn that apparently my three attacks within twelve hours is not something that happens all the time. After the third attack I was then diluted to the maximum, and that an additional attack may have resulted in immediate emergency surgery.

They all knew it and were on alert, however because I and the rest of the family were in relatively good spirits during the entire ordeal, the staff did not want to dampen our spirits. They were hoping that I would remain stable enough to get to Ein Kerem and have the angioplasty calmly and routinely performed.

Regarding the second flashback – Dado, (Yossi's brother, the former soccer star who had a stent implanted about a year before me) also came to mind. It was not because of his heroics on the field but because he passed away suddenly this year. He was on vacation down at the Dead Sea with his wife, and had three attacks within a half an hour.

The first aid staff that was taking care of him succeeded in stabilizing him after the first two attacks. They were not able to save him after the third attack, even as an emergency helicopter was landing to evacuate him to the nearest hospital. He had told me a couple of years earlier that he was then only taking aspirin. I had no way of knowing if it was his doctors who had discontinued his other medications, or if he had discontinued them by himself, as I had done. His brother had later told me that Dado eventually continued his indiscriminant eating habits. Was it this lack of discipline that led him to another heart attack?

A question nagging me with no chance of an answer was "if Dado had continued taking certain medications, would they have prevented the attacks from occurring on that fateful day, or at least would they have protected him enough to survive them"?

I also now wondered if it was the doubling of my statin in January 2002 which pushed me over the *mental/emotional side effects* line. Would I have continued a normal life with the previous reduced dosage and not consciously feel any significant side effects? It can ultimately be said that every cloud does have its silver lining. It was because something had pushed me over the line that I started to read and research for myself where and why I went amiss. It might seem bizarre, but as a direct result of my two awful statin years, I may have found the way to a much higher quality, longer lasting life!

While I was quite unhappy with the numbers that I would be taking with me for the hospital exam, Esty was quick to point out that if I was not a heart patient, then the numbers would be considered to be quite excellent. All of the results were well within the normal zone, not to mention that because of my attack I am today generally much more health orientated than most others.

The first one to see me at the hospital checkup was a cardiologist whom I had not seen before. She 'debriefed' me before the professor also joined us. To my surprise, she was not alarmed by the LDL count; maybe not over pleased, but definitely not yet ready to hit the panic button. She definitely was in favor of keeping tabs on the numbers over the coming months.

She was much more concerned with the blood pressure not being static over the last couple of months. Her recommendation was to take Disothiazide, a diuretic (blood lowering medication) that works by removing excess water and salt from the body. She also recommended to consider the use of a Beta Blocker if need be. At this stage the Cardiology Professor entered and was briefed on all that I had experienced over the last six months and all the events leading up to my decision to stop the medications (except for the aspirin). He was not 'overly pleased' with the LDL readings; however I think that he now had the full picture regarding the side effects that I had experienced.

The next day I made an appointment with my family doctor to brief her as to what had transpired at the hospital and to fill the prescription for the start of my blood pressure problem. It was her opinion that a diuretic might further aggravate my blood fat balance and decided that an ACE Inhibitor would be better suited for me. She wrote me a prescription for Enaladex (enalapril maleate) for the coming month, and I was to keep track of BP at home.

I also felt that a diuretic was not in my best interests because of all the sport that I do. Especially in the summer, I will *need* the water and salt. It was also my feeling that my bad side effects from my previous medications were attributed to the statin, and NOT the ACE Inhibitor. Within a day or so, my blood pressure readings stopped the fluctuations that had characterized the last two months and leveled off at the 120/80 range.

The only side effect that Enaladex seemed to cause was an annoying dry cough, which is common with ACE Inhibitors. After a couple of months we replaced the Enaladex with Tritace which I had been taking before, and the cough disappeared and the blood pressure readings remained normal.

12

Post 2 - What's wrong with this book?

Actually, the real question is, *is there really something wrong with this book, or is the book really O.K. and is there is really something wrong with the rest of the world?* How could the book up until now not be O.K.? I related my *normal* childhood and upbringing and my definitely *normal* standards of American-style eating habits. Following these were my *normal* western world heart attack, and the *normal* standard treatment following my attack.

Although heart disease today is very widespread, is it really *normal, natural*; or are there other underlying hidden reasons that I as well as many others have heart disease and am no longer considered to be healthy?

Addictions to the wrong types of food were in part drilled into our heads by mass media and advertising. As long as we are on the subject of advertising and the disregard for health -- what about 'I'd walk a mile for a Camel' and the famous ride through 'Marlboro Country'. Who even remembers that two of the Marlboro Cowboys, Wayne McLaren and David McLean died from lung cancer? I even remember that I enjoyed the jingle for L&M cigarettes. I do not remember the melody or even the words, by I still remember that it was cute.

We consumers respond to advertising; we spend huge sums of money on food that ultimately brings catastrophe upon us, from obesity to a wide variety of diseases. Thereafter we would spend a fortune on medications and support the pharmaceutical industry for *solution*s to what our own eating has caused. We then spend even more money for even more medications to counteract the bad effects and side effects that the first medications were causing.

The pharmaceutical industry is a massive industry. It became massive because it obviously is responding to a demand; to supply us with all sorts of medications to fix what's wrong with us. Where exactly did we go wrong? Apparently we as homo-sapiens are not evolving as fast as today's ever changing technology dictates.

We humans have been roaming around this earth for thousands of years; however heart disease has only started to become a problem in the last one hundred years or so. One hundred years ago we did not own automobiles. They did exist, although only for the very rich. It was not until 1913 that the first Model-T Ford rolled off of what we now call an assembly line. This resulted in a considerable price drop for what was previously an individually built vehicle, which made it possible for us common folk to afford it. Up until then we walked, or rode horses; you get the picture. Most of us did not work in what's known as an office job. The work was much more physical.

We *used* our bodies. We worked hard to light our homes. There was no *click* on a light switch and then by magic......... light. We worked hard to heat our homes. There was no *click* on a thermostat and then by magic...... heat. And after a long day at the salt mines, there was no TV to sit back and enjoy. We worked hard and had 'strong hearts'.

In fact, it was not until 1929 that Dr. Paul Dudley White, later President Eisenhowers's personal physician, saw a heart attack for the first time. Interestingly, Dr. White himself was an enthusiastic bicyclist and when President Eisenhower suffered a heart attack while in office in 1955, Dr. White prescribed an exercise regimen featuring a stationary bicycle for the president. He believed even back then that bicycling provided significant cardiovascular benefits.

I was born in 1950, the same year that my folks bought their first TV. At least in those early days, one had to get off his/her butt in order to change the channel or adjust the volume. Later on, with the invention of the remote control, it became possible to watch TV for hours without ever getting off the couch.

Subsequently the VCR was introduced. You could watch any movie that you wanted without having to leave the house to go to a movie theatre. Think about the stereophonic music systems. You could enjoy a philharmonic concert while sitting in your living room without going to a concert hall. What's good for parents is good for kids.

Why go out and play baseball or something when you can stay in and watch a cartoon? Then came the computer age; I do not think that I've yet met a kid who is not capable of sitting for hours at a time at the computer playing any one of an infinite number of computer games. In fact, with e-mail you do not even have to go to a post office or mail box to send a letter.

The great technology age -- our wonderful bodies, which for thousands of years had evolved into marvelous working machines, were now becoming idle. What about the new fuel that we feed those marvelous idle working machines, our bodies? Trans fats, the byproduct of the hydrogenation process, something that was not significant until the twentieth century.

The hydrogenation process was developed for food oils and patented by chemist William Normann in 1903. The descendants of William Proctor, a candle maker and his brother-in-law, James Gamble, a soap-maker, (later "Proctor and Gamble") needed lard and tallow to make candles and soap. With the help of chemist E. C. Kayser, they utilized the new hydrogenation process to transform liquid cottonseed oil into a solid that resembled lard. This directly led to the development of Crisco. Crisco hit the market in 1911 and labeled itself as the *scientific discovery which will affect every kitchen* – they sure were right about that!

It was not until World War II that Crisco-like products, shortening and margarine, really caught on as a cheaper alternative to expensive, rationed butter. Later on in the 1980's, when the public was sure that it was the saturated fat that caused heart disease, the hydrogenated products market flourished even more, and partially hydrogenated oil/fat became very prevalent in a vast number of products that we purchased at our supermarkets, not to mention its wide use in the fast (junk) food industry.

Partially hydrogenated fats are created when liquid oils that are largely unsaturated are processed by adding hydrogen to it through a heat and pressure/chemical method which causes it to become a fat, solid or partial solid at room temperature. During hydrogenation, healthy unsaturated oil becomes more saturated and is modified to contain high levels of trans fats.

Trans fatty acids are, on the one hand, similar to natural fats and the body readily accepts them, however the high temperatures and pressure incurred in the hydrogenation process alter their chemical structure. This ultimately causes havoc with many necessary chemical reactions in the body, in addition to taking the place of the necessary good fats and prevents them from doing their jobs.

Why do food producers use hydrogenated oils? These oils give food a good, rich taste and not only are they good substitutes for tasty butter, but are considerably cheaper. In addition they also extend the supermarket shelf life of the products containing them. Even though we started eating hydrogenated oil products close to one hundred years ago, it was not until the 1950's that the first studies[36] started appearing regarding possible health hazards regarding the hydrogenation of vegetable oils.

The medical industry is definitely on the conservative side with regards to change. New ideas are not always readily embraced by colleagues; especially new ideas that cause serious conflicts with the existing way of doing things. Later studies were overwhelming in their causal linkage between trans fats and heart disease, for example:

- *"Metabolic and epidemiologic studies indicate an adverse effect of trans fatty acids on the risk of coronary heart disease"*[37]

- *"The combined results of metabolic and epidemiological studies provide strong evidence that trans fatty acid intake is causally related to risk of coronary disease. Because the consumption of partially hydrogenated fats is almost universal in the United States, the number of deaths attributable to such fats is likely to be substantial."*[38]

- *"On the basis of these metabolic effects and the known relation of blood lipid concentrations to risk of coronary artery disease, we estimate conservatively that 30,000 premature deaths/year in the United States are attributable to consumption of trans fatty acids."*[39]

It could be argued that until the twentieth century, we would die of a variety of natural causes before reaching old age, as death due to heart disease was **NOT** considered to be a problem of middle aged and younger people.

As early as 1950, an American doctor, John Gofman,[40] hypothesized that blood cholesterol was to blame for causing fatal heart attacks in *older* people. However, autopsies performed on soldiers killed in the Korean War[41] (early 1950's) showed that a significant percentage of these *young* soldiers suffered from some advanced degree of atherosclerosis.

Later during the Viet Nam War[42] (late 1960's 1970's), the autopsies performed on soldiers killed then revealed an alarming rate of young soldiers who suffered from advanced atherosclerosis. Coronary heart disease does not happen over night.

One of the conclusions of The Bogalusa Heart Study[43] was that the origins of adult heart disease, atherosclerosis, and coronary heart disease begin in childhood. Documented changes (for the worse) in the cardiovascular system occur by five to eight years of age!

So that's where we went wrong. We wrecked our heath by physically letting our bodies go to waste with inactivity. To make matters worse, we loaded up our digestive system with new man made materials (and even learned to deep fry in them!) that our systems were unable to process efficiently, if at all.

I now find that many of my own previous beliefs that I had grown up with regarding the existence of an absolute universally accepted conception of 'right' regarding medicine and health are no longer necessarily valid. The Dr. Ornish doctrine and the Dr. Atkins doctrine cannot be simultaneously absolutely correct; they contradict each other! They are both real doctors, have both sold a tremendous amount of books in the world, however they cannot be both simultaneously completely right!

Today, for me personally, the very wide use of statin drugs to lower cholesterol levels in the world while ruining the quality of life is a form of contradiction, not because I read about it, but rather from my own personal experience with it.

Is Canola oil the next best thing to monounsaturated olive oil and very healthy as we were taught in hospital rehab, or is it an unsaturated oil rich in trans fats[44] and that should be avoided at all costs?

If trans fats are detrimental to your health, why have they not appeared on food labeling like saturated fats?

Furthermore, if saturated fats are really so bad, why is it that heart disease has only been with us for about the last one hundred years only (like hydrogenated vegetable oil), while butter and lard have been with us for centuries?

In addition, if cholesterol is so important that our own bodies manufacture it, has it become the scapegoat for today's 'epidemic' of heart disease? The well documented Framingham Heart Disease Study[45] has itself produced ambiguous results. At the time, Framingham Study Director Dr. William Kannel[46] stated that "total plasma cholesterol is a powerful predictor of death related to coronary heart disease". A decade later, Dr. Kannel's successor, Dr. William Castelli,[47] stated "the more saturated fat one ate, the more cholesterol one ate, the more calories one ate, the lower people's serum cholesterol ... we found that the people who ate the most cholesterol, ate the most saturated fat, ate the most calories, weighed the least and were the most physically active." One study, two different study directors, two different conclusions – a gross contradiction!

I had grown up with the conception, not only my conception, but the universally accepted conception, that butter (highly saturated fat) is *bad*, and that margarine is *good*. It was not always like that. Do big business interests overwhelm the health aspects of the public in general? The Institute for Shortening and Edible Oils on their web site (http://www.iseo.org/faq4.htm) states:

"The hydrogenation process is very important to the food industry to achieve desired stability and physical properties in such food products as margarines, shortenings, frying fats, and specialty fats. Examples of enhanced stability provided by hydrogenation include increased shelf life of commercial snack foods and prolonged frying stability of food service deep frying fats. An example of a desired physical property is the semi-solid consistency at refrigerator and room temperatures of margarines and spreads."

If the Institute for Shortening and Edible Oils was simply an independent organization innocently representing the industries in its field, then one could say that this is legitimate. However in 1971, Mr. William Goodrich, the general counsel for the Food and Drug Administration (FDA), whose job it was to prosecute violations of FDA regulations, left the FDA to become president of - the Institute of Shortenings and Edible Oils!

And in the opposite direction, at about the same time Mr. Peter Hutt, who had been the legal representative of the edible oils companies, became the general counsel of the FDA!

Isn't this a bit of conflict of interests?

Unfortunately, this is not simply an isolated case. Industry pressure and industry sponsored studies had their effects on many governmental and quasi-governmental agencies that we expect to neutrally supply the public with unbiased scientific guidance. At various times throughout the years, agencies such as the U.S. Department of Agriculture (USDA), the American Heart Association (AHA), the American Medical Association (AMA), the National Cancer Institute, the American Dietetic Association, the Center of

Disease Control, and the National Heart Lung and Blood Institute all publicly promoted diets with vegetable oils, hydrogenated products and margarine instead of 'evil' saturated fat to reduce the risk of heart disease.[48]

The Institute for Shortening and Edible Oils / FDA case brings to mind a story regarding one of our less known former ministers by the name of Gonen Segev. Mr. Segev was elected to the Knesset as part of the now defunct Tzomet party in the mid 1990's. Tzomet did not enter the government, but was part of the opposition. When then Prime Minister Yitzhak Rabin was having trouble gaining the necessary support of his government to approve the Oslo agreements, he beefed up his coalition by luring Segev out of the opposition. The previously unknown Gonen Segev was named Minister of Energy and National Infrastructures in Rabin's government.

Okay, so politics has never been known to be a clean sport! However, at the end of his term as minister, he was immediately hired by the Eisenberg Group, a conglomerate deeply involved in the energy industry here in Israel. In other words, he immediately became a paid employee of a conglomerate that only a short time before was regulated and monitored on the government level by Segev himself! As a result of public uproar, his status with the Eisenberg Group was reduced from employee to outside consultant.

Eventually the Attorney General launched a police investigation against Segev on suspicion of advancing Eisenberg business while he was still Minister of Energy. The charges: Fraud and Violation of Public Trust. A direct result of the Segev episode in Israel: additional legislation requiring a cooling off period after leaving a government regulatory position.

And what does this interesting story have to do with us? While the connection between the Institute for Shortening and Edible Oils, definitely an interest group promoting the use of hydrogenated oils, and the FDA might not technically be illegal, however like oil that's gone rancid, it does stink.

When I decided to start researching what had really caused me to 'stop functioning' as a normal human being, and uncovered the Dr. Golomb study regarding statins, I realized that I was definitely not the only one in the world who was responding badly to the statin's side effects. Literally a whole new world opened up to me, as far as my interest in my own health, and then trying to comprehend fully how it was that I had a... heart attack.

And the more I read, the more some of the *self-evident truths* that I had been brought up on, were no longer so *absolute* – especially concerning fats and cholesterol. I started coming across more and more articles appearing in serious medical forums claiming that **cholesterol is NOT the real problem at all**, and at a time that butter and lard were the exclusive fats that we consumed, there was no significant heart disease; the real problem only started with the widespread use of vegetable oils and foods processed using hydrogenated oil!!

Remember Dr. Kilmer McCully of Harvard back in 1969? His views then regarding cholesterol as a *symptom* and not as a *cause* of heart disease resulted in his banishment[49] from Harvard University and Massachusetts General Hospital. He was denied a new position for more than two years because of his research.

Today, one of the leading advocates of the saturated fat/cholesterol myth trend of thought is a Swedish physician Dr. Uffe Ravnskov, who has an impressive list of credentials and publications accredited to his name. Dr. Ravnskov, author of "The Cholesterol Myth" has organized a group called the 'International Network of Cholesterol Skeptics'. In his own words

"The International Network of Cholesterol Skeptics (THINCS) is a steadily growing group of scientists, physicians, other academicians and science writers from various countries. Members of this group represent different views about the causation of atherosclerosis and cardiovascular disease, some of them are in conflict with others, but this is a normal part of science. What we all oppose is that animal fat and high cholesterol play a role. The aim with this website is to inform our colleagues and the public that this idea is not supported by scientific evidence; in fact, for many years a huge number of scientific studies have directly contradicted it."

The website can be found at http://www.thincs.org and contains an impressive list of scientists throughout the world and their respective publications/studies. To me, a layman, this trend of thought is of course revolutionary and contradictory to many self-evident truths that I had grown up with regarding nutrition. Throughout this book, I downplayed the eating of high cholesterol foods and the high fat (saturated) dairy products.

That was the world I was born into; that was the status quo; that was the right, the truth. Is this to say that I as a non-medical person can say which camp is correct? Obviously not, however it might just be that this other non-conforming camp holds the key for beating heart disease.

As a non-medical layman, my use of the terminology throughout this book regarding 'atherosclerosis' and 'coronary heart disease' may not have been entirely accurate. After all, in many medical publications, even real doctors tend to use the two terms synonymously. Dr. Kilmer McCulley[56] in "The Heart Revolution" defines arteriosclerosis as:

"...literally hardening of the wall of the arteries. The muscles cells of the artery multiply creating a toughened area often containing calcium deposits called plaque."

and defines atherosclerosis as:

"...advanced form of arteriosclerosis complicated by deposits of cholesterol fats and blood clots within the plaques of the artery walls"

The National Heart Lung and Blood Institute (web site) defines Heart Disease as

Heart disease is caused by narrowing of the coronary arteries that feed the heart...When the coronary arteries become narrowed or clogged by fat and cholesterol deposits and cannot supply enough blood to the heart, the result is coronary heart disease (CHD)...

Standard mainstream medicine has always emphasized the point that a person suffering from atherosclerosis has a much higher risk of developing heart disease and eventually having a heart attack. This is due to reduced blood flow thru impaired, smaller than ideal 'pipe diameters'. Atherosclerosis was always stated as being a cause, an important factor, preceding heart disease. It is not heart disease nor is it the result of a heart attack.

Logic dictates that if we lessen the circumstances that contribute to developing atherosclerosis, then we lessen the chance of eventually having a heart attack. We were urged to refrain from eating highly saturated fats and high cholesterol foods, universally accepted factors that contribute to atherosclerosis.

If this was so, one would expect to find that populations with low/no atherosclerosis to have a very low incidence of heart disease. A large scale study[50] done in 1968 involving 22,000 corpses throughout fourteen countries showed that the degree of atherosclerosis was irrespective of populations that were vegetarian, or meat eaters. Even more significant, there was no correlation between the degree of atherosclerosis and the incidence of heart disease! It concluded that the narrowing of the arteries is a natural phenomenon much too complex to be attributed to the single hypothesis of lipids (fats/cholesterol).

I stated in the introduction of this book that my intention was to write a layman's book of answers and that in part it evolved into book of *questions* – now you know why

But then again, the whole world we live in is full of contradictions and absurdities. There is still a dwindling number of living survivors of the Holocaust. It did happen, it was real. Yet today there are 'scholars' with their 'truths and proofs' who claim that the Holocaust never happened.

Possibly the most absurd of all is the coveted Nobel Peace prize, named in the honor of Alfred Nobel who invented **dynamite** in 1866. His dream:

> *"My dynamite will sooner lead to peace than a thousand world conventions. As soon as men will find that in one instant, whole armies can be utterly destroyed, they surely will abide by golden peace."*

I wonder what he would think today if he knew that flesh and blood human beings strap his wonderful invention to their own bodies in order to blow up other innocent flesh and blood human beings.

After all, for a long long time it was the sun that rotated around the earth, which was then also flat.

171

Anyway, I'll let someone else try to straighten out the rest of the world!

♥ ♥ ♥

I should also point out at this time, that although there is a growing camp of scientists denouncing the popular notion that 'high cholesterol *causes* heart disease', mainstream medical trend is still seemingly leaning to lowering the existing standards for LDL even further than what has up until now been in effect. For people suffering from heart disease and specifically post heart attack victims, present U.S. government guidelines advocate keeping LDL levels below 100.

Still where did this magic number of 100 originate from? Dr. Thomas Pearson, head of preventive medicine at the University of Rochester, helped write those guidelines. He stated:

The goal of less than 100 was an approximation using some very early data. It was the best guess at that moment. It may need some improvement.[51]

The New England Journal of Medicine in its April 8, 2004 issue contains a paper that was presented to the 2004 annual meeting of the American College of Cardiology entitled "Comparison of Intensive and Moderate Lipid Lowering with Statins after Acute Coronary Syndromes", headed by Dr. Christopher Cannon of Boston's Brigham and Women's Hospital. The paper reviews the results of a study involving over four thousand patients and comparing the effects of two popular statins: Pravachol (Pravastatin) and Lipitor (Atorvastatin). Follow up of the patients lasted from eighteen to thirty-six months. What I would like to point out is NOT which statin *won the contest* however the conclusions of the study.

"Among patients who have recently had an acute coronary syndrome, an intensive lipid-lowering

statin regimen provides greater protection against death or major cardiovascular events than does a standard regimen. These findings indicate that such patients benefit from early and continued lowering of LDL cholesterol to levels substantially below current target levels."

As we already know, the existing LDL target level is 100.

Confused??? We have the recent Dr. Cannon study maintaining that LDL should be kept significantly lower than 100 by the wider use of statins; exactly how low no one knows for sure. We have Dr. Golomb (NIH statin study) although pro-statin[52] herself, who warns against serious side effects resulting from use of statins to lower LDL. We have Dr. Ravnskov *(THINCS)*, Dr. McCully (homocysteine), Dr. Klevay (copper deficiency), and Dr. Batmanghelidj (water/salt) who claim that there is NO *causal* connection between cholesterol levels and heart disease whatsoever. They maintain that the mainstream medical establishment is simply grossly misinterpreting clinical findings regarding the causal correlation between cholesterol level and the causes of heart disease.

So how do we find a common denominator among all these very different approaches? Who is actually right? Let's start by examining the background as listed in Dr Cannon's recent study:

"Lipid-lowering therapy with statins reduces the risk of cardiovascular events, but the optimal level of low-density lipoprotein (LDL) cholesterol is unclear."

The common denominator between Dr. Cannon and Dr. Ravnskov is that *statins reduce the risk of cardiovascular*

173

events; however they greatly disagree on the reason. Dr. Cannon attributes the reduction in cardiovascular events to a reduction in *Lipid-lowering* (lower LDL levels), the lower the better. Dr. Ravnskov[53] acknowledges that the *effects* of statins do result in a lowering of cardiovascular events however the *cause* of the cardiovascular benefits is **not** due to the lower cholesterol levels. Statins inhibit the body's production of a substance called mevalonate,[54] which is a precursor of cholesterol.

As production of mevalonate declines, ultimately so does the production of cholesterol. Mevalonate is also a precursor of other substances in the body that control various other important biological functions. Dr. Ravnskov believes that it is interference with some of these other bodily functions which ultimately cause the benefits with respect to cardiovascular disease, totally independent of cholesterol level. Or in other words, statins do lower cardiovascular disease, **despite** their bad side effect of also lowering cholesterol levels!!!

Again, it is not my purpose to medically judge which side is valid. It is my purpose to state that many of the *self evident* truths regarding health and nutrition that we have grown up believing to be absolute, may not be true!.

13

Post 3 - Tips - Epilogue

This chapter more or less completes the circle that was started way back in the introduction, in which I stated that I am **not** a doctor. In the three years that have passed since having my heart attack and all that I have experienced since then, I still am not a doctor, and again stress to all you do-it-yourselfers that this is **not** a typical 'How to do' book. I definitely do **not** recommend making any changes in prescriptions being taken, and for that matter, drastic changes in any physical exercising habits without doing so with the full knowledge and instructions from a qualified, competent medical authority.

I am certain that critics of my reasons for the discontinuation of the statins will be quick to point out that there was really nothing scientific or clinical about my conclusions that it was the statins that were causing my mental/emotional disorientation. After all, I did discontinue the statins more or less at the same time as I discontinued the ACE Inhibitor, so how could I be so sure that it was the statins alone?

In retrospect, at the time I was in such a discouraged state, that I was not really interested in doing an exact medical

research study on myself. I simply wanted to find some .....
any solution .... that would help me crawl out of the
mental/emotional abyss I had somehow stumbled into.
Ultimately, the trick is to learn how to work *with* your doctor.

Procedures and medical policies are constantly changing
in tune with the technological advances and increased
knowledge in the field that occurs over time. The *hit* today that
was non existent several decades ago are the stents, and even
the stents have undergone improvements over the last couple of
years. Now they can be coated with an antibiotic material that
gives further protection against complications occurring in the
inserted area.

As far as my preferred type of daily exercise, I chose
bike riding. I do admit that at some point it became something
of an obsession for a variety of reasons, almost like an
addiction. I do have to say that there definitely are worse
things in life to become addicted to, such as drinking, gambling
and the like.

I had started to bike ride as a form of physical
rehabilitation. Ultimately, when the statins started taking over,
riding became more than just a physical obsession, it was also a
mental/emotional one. It was my way of escaping from the real
world – of getting away – of being by myself. Fortunately for
me, it was a healthy avenue of escape. If bike riding sounds like
it's for you, like any other exercise, the name of the game is to
start slowly. Do not start out over-enthusiastically as many
people start out dieting, and to proceed at a realistic rate.

Today I ride approximately 150 kilometers (94 miles)
per week – every week. This comes out to an average of
slightly over 20 kilometers (12½ miles) per day. Obviously the
normal daily routine of life also dictates restrictions from time
to time, such as weather conditions, getting into work for that
early scheduled meeting, having to drop one or more of the kids
off early for one reason or another, etc. In other words, there
are those days when I do not ride. Usually the weekly tally

balances out over the weekend when on at least one of the days I take my long ride out in the country.

Six weeks after my attack and stent insertion, I started out doing fifteen minute *circular* rides in a flat area, not more than 150 meters (164 yards) long. At a natural pace, I started increasing my daily ride and eventually graduated to adjoining areas which were not at all flat. I love the down hills, however in the long run you cannot fool Mother Nature. For every downhill, there is ultimately an opposing up hill approaching somewhere.....

The best way to monitor your progress is to actually measure it. An odometer/speedometer adds a whole new dimension to riding, and supplies a good solution for keeping you on track.

The twenty - twenty-five kilometers of daily riding translates to approximately one and a half hours of continuous riding. This has me outside on the saddle at 5 - 5:15 a.m. In other words, during a week in which I ride every morning, the hour and a half in the morning fills my quota. During weeks that I'm short several days, I still make every effort on the weekends to meet my current weekly quota of 150km.

It's good to set a long-term goal; for instance a certain amount of mileage to ride by the end of the year. Why am I now locked in on at least 150 kilometers average per week? Its because I revised my year end goal for this year to finish my riding year (which ends April 4th) at an overall average of 140 kilometers per week. I have about another three months to go, and my cumulative current weekly average meanwhile is close to 137.

This by the way is a good example on how to tackle **ALL** big projects in our lives. My long term goal is 7,320 kilometers (4,575 miles) for the year (20 kilometers per day times 366 days – hence 140km/ week -- do not forget that 2004 is a leap year). This 'huge' project seems unmanageable without a more detailed plan. The year plan was separated into fifty-two smaller projects, the weekly quota, which is something that can be comprehended and tackled.

The twenty - twenty-five kilometers per day is the basic unit. It is adjusted as need be to obtain the weekly quota, and meeting the weekly quotas ultimately results in meeting the distant yearly goal! The first problem of starting a *big project* is to……. actually *start* it. Once starting it, the next problem is to *continue* it.

How many times have you heard about people starting out on diets with much enthusiasm, only to eventually give up? Keep in mind that the actual **doing of something** as opposed to only **thinking of doing something** often leads to other directions/projects/hobbies/jobs that only materialize after actually physically **doing** in the first place. My very modest short rides in the morning have meanwhile led me to excellent physical stamina. This has enabled me to hold my own with other much younger riders on long organized treks out in the country, which I greatly enjoy. It has also led me to meet and spend time with new acquaintances. For example: a small very friendly group called the "Green wheelers" (http://www.geocities.com/greenwheelers/) that I sometimes ride with, not to mention the occasional, very large well organized national/popular rides, which attract hundreds of riders from all over the country. Who knows how in the future someone I'm yet to meet on a ride might very significantly influence my personal life!

As a parent, I have learned that part of educating a child is **not** done by demanding that he do this or that. A good bit of the real education of a child comes from the unspoken personal example. I am sure that my present basic healthy eating habits and deliberate daily physical activities will eventually have an impact on the kids as they mature into adulthood. They may not as yet put it to immediate use, but it definitely will be inscribed on their 'hard disks upstairs' between the ears.

In addition to giving an example that there **is** room for brisk physical activities in the post heart attack person, I also wanted to convey a particular message. Notwithstanding the hats off appreciation that us survivors want to express to the very dedicated doctors and medical staff who very likely saved our lives, or at the least minimized the damage, medicine is *not* an exact science. Medicines that work wonders with some patients cause havoc with others. We all respond differently to different medicines and drugs, and it's up to us patients on the receiving end to play an active part *with* our doctors in determining what works best for us.

I also gave other examples in this book regarding differences of opinion on a variety of other topics, such as what is the healthiest diet to follow. The hard fact is that some of the different doctrines are totally opposed to each other:

Dr. Dean Ornish – heavy on the complex carbohydrates, minimize the fats.

Dr. Robert Atkins – Heavy on the fats, stay off the carbohydrates.

Dr. Franz Mayr – Proper eating habits.

As far as Dr. Atkins is concerned, as I am writing these lines there seems to be a certain zigzag in the Atkins doctrine -- by Dr. Atkins himself. Shortly before Dr. Atkins died a year ago, he completed his 'next generation' book entitled "Atkins for Life" in which he gradually does reintroduce carbohydrates into the daily diet as opposed to his preaching over the last thirty years. In a four step process, the dieter is allowed to indulge him/herself under normal circumstances to 45 – 100 grams of *net* carbs per day. He defines net carbs as: *the total grams of carbohydrate minus grams of Fiber, Glycerine and Sugar alcohols.* In addition, in direct contrast to his earlier work, there is now a ceiling on the amount of saturated fat that is allowed.

Today there is still wide disagreement regarding the issue of whether margarine is really better/healthier than (saturated fat) butter. And again, is Canola oil really the best substitute for olive oil as we were taught at the hospital rehab program, or is it really very harmful due to its high trans-fat content?[44] I am not medically qualified to offer answers to any of these questions; I do however want you to at least be aware of the questions.

Following are some tips to get through the day for those of you that for a variety of reasons, have no alternative to taking various medicines, and as a result might be having trouble concentrating/thinking, or just feeling generally confused. First of all, before tackling a problem, you have to recognize that there indeed is a problem.

Because of the confusion, you want to be as totally organized as possible, which starts with the multiple bottles of all the pills to keep track of. There is nothing more frustrating than holding a prescription bottle and wondering, did I take that pill today, or was it really yesterday? The organized solution: buy one of those seven day pill organizers, and at the beginning of the week, fill it up with pills for the whole week. Some seven separate daily plastic pill containers are further subdivided into morning, lunch, dinner, bed time, so there is never a doubt if it was today, or yesterday...........

Take care of one small mission at a time. For example, if you are on your way to another room to take care of some small 'insignificant' task, do **not** get side tracked with something else that comes up along the way. If you take care of this new 'problem' first, you may find that the original mission is quickly forgotten. Carry a small pad and pen with you and do not be afraid to jot down errands, missions, in fact anything that you want to accomplish and do not want to forget.

And about those pills ....

For many of us, it became a physical necessity to take medications in order to be able to function normally (if you think about this sentence, it does sort of contain an absurdity). Whether we like it or not, medications have become an integral part of our lives. The problem is that by taking medications, as necessary as they may be, we are nevertheless in some way tampering with nature itself.

Believe me, in the long run, you **cannot** fool Mother Nature! All of our body systems are interrelated, that's simply the way we are. By regulating a particular internal process, we are automatically influencing other processes. Frequently, these are what we experience as side effects of that particular medication.

Ultimately all medications cause some type of side effect. Many may be unfelt by us and do not apparently seem to affect anything else, but others are strong enough to tremendously disrupt our normal lives. When taking medications, especially for the first time, READ THE FLYER that comes with the medication. Be aware of the potential effects that they can cause. Keep your doctor informed of all changes that occur with you. Many medications have similar substitutes, and a substitute medication may do the job and not cause those other undesirable effects.

If you are taking multiple medications, it pays to double check with your doctor which ones can literally be taken together at the same meal, and which ones should be taken at different separate times during the day. If there still is a conflict, find out which medication can be substituted for what. For instance, when I came home from the hospital with my 'shopping list' of pills to take, it went like this.

Morning: Beta Blocker

Noon: Aspirin, ACE Inhibitor, (and Plavix for additional 3 weeks)

181

Evening: Beta Blocker

Night before retiring: Statin (Cholesterol lowering)

I am presently taking the aspirin, and have recently resumed an ACE Inhibitor for blood pressure control. So what's the problem?[55] Aspirin benefits the cardiovascular system by keeping the blood thin and preventing the formation of blood clots. It also however inhibits the synthesis of a substance known as prostaglandin. Prostaglandin causes the muscles inside of blood vessels to relax and become less constricted which results in a decrease in blood pressure. ACE Inhibitors lower blood pressure by blocking an enzyme that constricts blood vessels.

The point is that simultaneous use of *large* dosages of aspirin and ACE Inhibitors may reduce the effects of the ACE Inhibitor to some extent, although up until now only preliminary studies have been done. The key in this particular case is *large doses* which is definitely not an objective term. We are all different; what is considered a large dose for someone may not be a large dose for someone else. My daily dosage of the aspirin is 100mg which is not considered to be large. However again, this is very subjective. It's just a point to be aware of. I recently decided to separate my simultaneous taking of aspirin and ACE Inhibitor; the aspirin I take in the morning, and the ACE Inhibitor with lunch.

And about that food.....................

While some of the more extreme eating programs might be beneficial for people wanting to start knocking off excess weight in a relatively short period (weeks-months), I ultimately adopted a more middle of the road approach. I did adapt something from each of the major conflicting nutritional doctrines.

From Dr. Ornish, I learned to cut out the deep fried foods, and became aware of the difference between simple and complex carbohydrates

From the Mayr system, I ultimately adapted a more balanced approach, and continued a 'light day' once a week. By balanced approach, I mean just that – balanced approach, as opposed to doctrines such as no/low fat or no/low carbohydrates.

A 'light day' (usually on Sunday, the first day of the work week) is basically eating a very small amount of something to supply me with just a minimum amount of sugar to get thru the day.

This accomplishes two basic things. First of all, it causes a clean break from the week-end's sometimes pig-like eating habits. It's a day off so to speak, so that the following day I am back on track. It basically is an insurance policy to not fall into a snowball effect ; starting to eat unwisely day after day after day.

Secondly, it gives my whole system an easy day that it does not have to deal with digesting food and body energy can be diverted to other functions. A typical 'light day meal': some small dry crackers/toast, eaten very slowly with a yogurt. The point is not eating to get the feeling of *stuffed up*, rather, just enough sugar intake to *get by*.

Balanced means having protein *and* carbs *and* fats at each meal, and not separating or eliminating them. There is another positive aspect to maintaining balanced eating habits. I already learned the hard way that all medications do cause side effects, some not consciously noticeable, some absolutely devastating. Our bodies are very intricate mechanisms; all of our inner processes are linked together. Similar to taking prescription drugs, when we artificially interfere with our own personal food requirements by over eating a certain type of food, or eliminating a total class of food altogether, we *risk* causing an internal reaction. This in turn creates another reaction someplace else, which in turn creates another reaction, and so on.

For instance, the source of vitamin B_{12} is from animal tissue. Vegetarians for instance, should be aware not to become B_{12} deficient. Why did I choose this particular example? Dr. McCully claims that one of the factors that can cause homocysteine levels to rise, is a deficiency of vitamin B_{12}.[56]

Examples of specific food/vitamin deficiencies are unlimited, causing unlimited types of health problems; potential calcium deficiency for people not eating diary products, etc. Specific elimination of certain foods or food types should be coordinated with a reputable medical source.

Today I steer away from simple sugars and prefer whole wheat flour over bleached flour. Research studies[57] definitely advocate the whole grains. However I have also learned that the whole grains must be properly prepared prior to consumption; for example I soak[58] the home made untoasted granola overnight which I eat the following morning in order to neutralize the phytic acid, which inhibits proper absorption of many minerals. I have become more selective regarding the oils/fats that I do consume, and stay as far as possibly away from anything containing hydrogenated/partially hydrogenated oil. This is not as easy as it sounds. Try looking at the labels of **everything** in your cupboards that you have been buying for years!

Recently the Food and Drug Administration finally issued a regulation which will require all manufacturers of food products to list the amount of trans fats contained in their products by January 2006. So until 2006, you have to read the labels. Stay away from anything containing hydrogenated oil, partially hydrogenated oil, hardened oil, and vegetable shortening. Unfortunately there still is a problem with what is labeled as *vegetable oil* as it is impossible to know which kind or how it has been produced.

And if you must fry, the oils that you put on salad are not necessarily the oils that you would want to heat and cook with, especially deep fry. In fact, if you, like me, grew up like most normal people believing that margarine and polyunsaturated oil are healthy, and not really being aware of the hydrogenation procedure, then the following statement might seem a bit shocking:

If you must deep fry, you may as well fry using saturated fat, which is chemically inert (stable), so does not transform into something worse via heating.

Sound strange? If you want to get the real facts regarding oils and fats, an excellent source of information is "Know Your Fats" by Dr. Mary Enig.

Exercise - How much is too little, how much is too much?

Today I average 150 kilometers of bike riding a week. How can I interpret the significance of this health wise? Basically the answer is to view this weekly physical activity in terms of how many calories I am burning, and how this compares to recommended standards. Keep in mind of course that recommended standards do not always exactly fit the very wide range of everyone's needs.

The American College of Sports Medicine (ACSM) recommends that we try, as a minimum to maintain a healthy body, to burn 1000 calories per week by moderately intensive exercise. Ideally, if our personal health permits, we should shoot for 2000 calories per week, which is considered to be an optimal physical activity level and it helps us to maintain proper weight.

According to the ACSM, the 1000 calorie burning can be accomplished by a simple thirty minute walk every (or almost) day. How is this calculated?

The calculation is:

Weekly Calorie burning = (weight in kilograms) * (time in hours) * METS.

To calculate the weight in kilograms, take your weight in pounds and divide it by 2.204

Time in hours: If you worked out 1 hour and forty minutes, that would be 1 + 40/60 which calculates to 1.66

MET (metabolic equivalent) is a way of expressing the rate of energy expenditure resulting from a given physical activity.

One MET is the basic unit of measurement and is based on the calorie expenditure/oxygen consumption while the body is at rest (such as sitting quietly) and is equal to 1 calorie burned per kilogram of body weight per hour. For example, my weight is approximately 66 kilos (145 lb), so for every hour of just sitting quietly, my body burns approximately sixty-six calories.

The Compendium of Physical Activities Tracking Guide is a comprehensive list of sport activities, as well as daily house/work functions, and their corresponding MET value. According to the guide, basic bicycle riding ranks 'eight' on the MET scale. Conservatively, let's assume that I ride at a rate of 'six'. Assuming that my daily rides fluctuate between six and eight, I will calculate calorie expenditure for both figures. I multiply

6 (METS) * 66 (my weight in Kilos) * 11 (rough approximation on how many hours I ride a week - sometimes more, sometimes less) and the calorie count is: 4356 calories.

8 (METS) * 66 (my weight in Kilos) * 11 (hours) and the calorie count is: 5808 calories.

The figures tell me that at the present I am burning between two to three times the ideal target of 2000 calories as recommended by the American College of Sports Medicine. This does basically coincide with their minimum recommendation of a half hour sport each day; I ride for an hour and a half each morning, which is three times the minimum recommendation. The question is 'Am I overdoing it?'

To this I do not have an answer; although just for the sake of comparison, let's go back to our ninety year old marathon runner, Abe Weintraub. At a head taller than me (at least that's how I remember him the last time I saw him twenty some years ago), let's assume that he weighs about 70 kilos (155 lbs). His record marathon runs have been in seven and a half hours. The MET rate for jogging is seven. According to these figures, 70 * 7 * 7½ comes out to 3675 calories burned off in one marathon run only! And what about the rest of the week's training sessions?

My major purpose for bike riding, as is the major purpose for other heart patients with their daily walking, is to perform some form of aerobic exercise to maintain good health. It is not to become an Olympic champion. So the question that remains is at what intensity should I ride in order to obtain maximum aerobic benefit?

Way back at rehab, we were taught that we do not want to exercise at an intensity that causes our pulse rate to exceed our maximum heart rate, which as a rule of thumb, is calculated by subtracting our present age from 220. As a general guideline, the best aerobic benefits are obtained by exercising at a starting pulse rate which is forty-five percent of our maximum heart rate, and over time as fitness and endurance improve, to reach a maximum of eighty percent of the maximum (the 45% - 80% is known as the target heart rate).

For example, I am fifty-four (actually I will be fifty-four by the time this is published) which sets my maximum heart rate at 220 − 54 = 166. So according to the simple rule of thumb, I would want to maintain my exercise at an intensity that would have my pulse rate between 75 (45%) and 133 (80%), depending of course on the duration of my intended riding session.

The name of the game is to *train and not strain* – do not overdo it! If exercise is not something that you have been doing, **it is imperative to first coordinate your intended exercise routine with your doctor!** Incidentally, if you are not exactly now in shape, no matter what your preferred workout is, biking, running, walking, swimming, some team sport, or whatever, you do not have to wait for a heart attack as a reason to start working out!!!

I'd like to offer a final bit of advice – for a healthy heart, try to live and enjoy each moment while it lasts, with family, with friends, at work, all the time; once each moment is gone, its gone.

Can I say that I myself live up to this? Unfortunately I am still more concerned with and worry about that future moment that nobody can even guarantee that I'll even get to, but it's definitely something worth aspiring to. Admittedly, I still view the world in black and white, even after my recovery, even after the seminars. I like what I like, I don't like what I don't like – very little middle ground – but I'm working on it.

For example, I leave the house in the morning in a hurry to get to work. This is not because I necessarily 'like' what I do; I'm in a hurry to get there, to accomplish what has to be accomplished, and return home as soon as possible. But once I do actually get home, do I really enjoy my time at home?? Probably not nearly as much as I could, because all my thinking is "oooooh – I still have to wait another four days until finally there will be another weekend". And do I really enjoy the weekend as much as I could? Again no! It's *only for two days,* and again I am waiting for that whole week vacation, which is months away.

When will I learn to live the moment all the time? That is definitely not a realistic question; it's not something that I may ever actually completely achieve, although it can definitely be aimed for – and by all of us. Believe me, the sooner, the better...............

April, 2004 – approaching the end

The book is now about finished – although I do have my own ideas as to what caused my heart attack, I must again stress for the umpteenth time that **I am not a doctor** and the reader should not make any exercise/eating/prescription changes solely based on this book without considering the input of a qualified medical source. My own gut feelings now regarding where I had fallen and what direction I see for myself in the future are just that – gut feelings. These are based upon what I personally have experienced these last three years and a good bit of reading and researching that I have been doing over the last six months. Where do I believe that I had fallen?

1. Food/eating habits for most of the years of my life: Today my conception of what *junk* food is has changed considerably from the traditional given reason of saturated fats/high cholesterol foods to the foods containing trans-fats and other highly processed foods.

   An interesting study 'close to home' also substantiates this claim. Israel, like the United States is a great *melting pot* for a wide spectrum of ethnic cultures (although after twenty-eight years in the country sometimes it feels more like a *pressure cooker* rather than a *melting pot*, but I will leave politics out of this book.......).

   One of Israel's ethnic groups is the Jews who emigrated from Yemen. A study[59] was done comparing new Yemenite immigrants, to Yemenites

189

who have been living in Israel for twenty-five or more years. The Yemenites living in Israel for twenty-five or more years had a significant increase in the incidence of atherosclerosis, ischemic heart disease and diabetes. What is the cause? The use of margarines and vegetable oils in the traditional Yemenite foods in place of the animal originated fats as in Yemen, which has been even further complicated by high sugar consumption for the Israeli group. (A later unrelated study[60] concluded that nearly three quarters of the fat in artery clogs is unsaturated – having their source from vegetable oils and not animal fats.)

Do you remember that as an adult I *graduated* from high saturated fat cream cheese to peanut butter? Have you read the list of ingredients lately on the jars of the leading brands of peanut butter? I am of course referring to the use of partially hydrogenated oil. I am now very conscious of the hydrogenated oil content in products when shopping and am no longer hysterical as in the past regarding the term saturated fat. However old habits die hard! It is only recently that I have resumed eating real butter, after years of eating that that 'wonderful modern substitute', margarine!!

At the beginning of this book, I mentioned that the hospital release report following my heart attack listed "existing heart disease is in the family" as background information regarding my own heart attack. If you recall, my mother suffered a heart attack and had a quadruple bypass operation performed three years before my own heart attack.

Let's analyze this *genetic argument*. My folks were married in 1948, and I, the oldest child, was born in 1950. My Mom grew up in a kosher household, eating traditionally prepared home cooked meals all her life. She married, moved out of the house and almost immediately started replacing her mother's kosher kitchen with the modern technology and western style foods. From her marriage in 1948 until her heart attack in 1998 - fifty years. From my birth year in 1950 until my heart attack in 2001 – fifty-one years. Although a generation apart, we both started eating modern junk foods at approximately the same time, and both had heart attacks about fifty years later!!!

2.   Poor personal stress management.

I don't know what caused my blood pressure to start becoming erratic several months ago. Was it really the salt I was then drinking? I tend to think not. I mentioned that at the time my eating habits had also gone astray. Was it a particular thing that I had resumed eating that contained something that was triggering the BP variations? Or was it simply normal daily stress again getting the better of me?

Sometimes it's hard to think of ways to reduce stress, and try to keep the lid on blood pressure during normal daily routines. We can influence to some degree, to what extent we allow our fuses to blow. For instance, even while driving, instead of always having to be in the fast left lane, and feeling that you are in competition with every other driver out there; you can simply stay in the slower right lane, and enjoy the good music. No matter how bad or even aggressive other drivers are, you simply cannot 'educate' them or 'teach them a lesson' so do not even get further upset by trying.

Will I someday consider chelation therapy to clean out my years of plaque which has accumulated in my system? Possibly!

Do I plan to continue bike riding? Definitely! And while on the subject of bike riding and physical exercise in general, I would like to point out that exercising alone does not provide any guarantee against heart attacks and/or an even worse scenario – *not* surviving a heart attack.

A recent event provided good proof of that. Brian Maxwell, the creator of Power Bars (convenient energy bars used by athletes to give them an energy boost while competing), died this week (April 2004) of a heart attack at the age of fifty-one. What is significant here is that he was a former world-class marathon runner. In 1977, Maxwell was ranked as the third best marathon runner in the world by Track and Field News.

While on the subject of runners, it was twenty years ago (1984) that Jim Fixx had a massive heart attack while jogging and died immediately. He was fifty-two at the time. It was Fixx's best selling book "Complete Book of Running" that started the big jogging craze in the seventies. (I guess there must be some consolation in that if *ya gotta go*, you may as well go quietly while doing something you enjoy ......).

One of the things that I did not like about walking (and for that matter, especially running) was that its constant – constant – constant. Even when feeling tired and slowing down, the legs are still working all the time, and the heart is still banging away even if it is a slower pace. The only way to really catch your breath is to slow down to a real snail's pace, or come to a complete stop.

What I like about bike riding for aerobic exercise, even on a long trip taking hours, is that by the sheer nature that bikes are wheeled vehicles, there are frequent very short automatic 'breathing breaks'. On only the slightest of declines, the bike continues to travel by itself and I go for the free ride. Often after a moving break of only several tens of seconds, I continue pedaling with a renewed refreshed feeling.

And in conclusion.........

Despite the fact that the Statins totally disrupted all aspects of my life for nearly two years, I am nevertheless thoroughly convinced that they do have a very significant benefit in minimizing the chance of a return heart attack for people like me, diagnosed with heart disease. I have simply accepted the 'opposition' arguments that the statin benefits are in spite of the resulting lower LDL Cholesterol levels, and not because of them.

Why is it that many, like myself, respond with significant side effects to Stains while many others apparently do not? I obviously do not have an answer to this. As a layman, I have no way of knowing for sure if the changes I have made in my life style offer me the same cardiologic benefits that I have knowingly forfeited when I discontinued taking them.

And a final note on my life changes:

- Dietary changes, with an emphasis on elimination of the trans-fats/hydrogenated oils from my diet, and abandoning the low/no fat agenda.

- Becoming more 'open', not letting work related stress accumulate, and appreciating more my domestic life at home with Esty – all these I chalk up to the Outlook seminars.

- My serious approach to daily physical exercise activity – which in my case is the hour and a half of daily bike riding.

And while on the subject of bike riding, we have reached the last chapter............

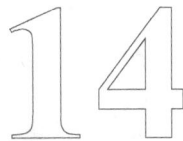

Happy Ending

April 4, 2004   (end of second riding year):

140.38km average per week[*] for the entire year.

Tomorrow starts a new year!!

ISN'T LIFE GREAT!!

.

---

[*] No, Yogli was not with me this time at the finish – not really critical;

Yes, this time it probably was near the trash bin – not really important;

Two year total – 12,570 km – now that's impressive! At least I think so.

15

After Happy Ending

Whew - writing a book is serious business – although it has been two months since officially finishing it, I have been rereading it, correcting here, correcting there, and now *finally* its ready for publication, taking me slightly longer than anticipated;

h o w e v e r

now that it is already the month of June, I recently had my biannual cholesterol blood test, and I must admit that in contrast to previous tests in which I waited to receive the results with apprehension, this time I would describe my wait as simple curiosity.

Contrary to the months preceding my last cholesterol test in December, these last several months I have made every effort to stay as far away as possible from anything with even a hint of containing hydrogenated ingredients. I have also abandoned the no/low fat dairy products, discovered butter again, and even usually add a soft boiled egg for breakfast. The result: my *total* cholesterol dropped from 199 to 181, the *bad*

LDL dropped from 139 to 114 and the *good* HDL is holding steady at 52.

And do you know what? I am not the least bit surprised!

16

One Year Later

July 2005: It has been a full year since releasing the original
version of "Surviving a Successful Heart Attack." I am
grateful for all the feedback I received. Some
correspondence was from other heart attack patients thanking me
for making my story known. Others raised questions regarding
data they felt needed further explanation. Hopefully this revision
gave them a better understanding of what I had gone through.

Now for the good news! I feel as though I am living a
full life again and not just *surviving*. Two years have gone by
since I discontinued my statin medication. The results of my
stress test taken six months ago show that I reached a
maximum level of 14.9 METS which is 59% above the
calculated maximum rate for me.

I realized that the subject matter I covered was going to
be controversial and I was well aware that as a lay person
without the benefit of an accredited medical background, the
content of my book could possibly raise some eyebrows in the
medical profession. Shortly after an initial distribution of
"Surviving", I was pleasantly surprised to receive an invitation

198

to address the staff of the Cardiology Department at Hadassah Hospital in Jerusalem.

It wasn't too long ago that I was sitting in a large lecture hall with approximately one hundred other post heart attack victims at a follow up rehabilitation session. We were the silent majority in the hall. On the podium were senior staff professionals that included the head of the Cardiology Department, the head of the Rehab Program and other senior staff members. Occasionally they would be joined by a guest lecturer. Talk about a change of places! That day it was me addressing the dedicated cardiology staff, the doctors, nurses, surgeons and the upper echelon of Hadassah Cardiology. I related my horrendous experiences the statins caused me and the extensive research I conducted which led to my decision to discontinue my prescribed statin medication.

I was also aware that my decision to abruptly discontinue the statin medication would not sit well with some of the cardiologists. After all, a computer geek lecturing cardiologists who have been prescribing statins for years could possibly have an abrasive effect and be somewhat counterproductive. There is a word in Hebrew that describes this type of behavior that I exhibited that day. It's called *hutzpa* and it has now seeped into a number of foreign languages. For those of you that never heard the term before, *hutzpa* is somewhere between *impudence* and *insolence.*

It was my hope that I might reach those few who still have open minds regarding the statin issue. Looking at some of the facial expressions in the audience, I realized I had reached a number of these professionals. In the discussion following my presentation, the department head asked his doctors if they had other patients that reacted adversely to statin medication. Almost sheepishly, several doctors stated they had patients that encountered negative side effects. It appears that negative side effects caused by statins are not issues doctors feel comfortable discussing.

Nevertheless, medicine today does offer a prescription alternative to statins that lower cholesterol levels in the bloodstream for those that experience negative side effects. The prescription is marketed under the name Ezetrol. Active ingredient is ezetimibe. According to the literature, it does not cause statin type side effects.

Statins reduce the amount of cholesterol in the blood stream by ultimately preventing its production in the liver. Ezetrol does not reduce the amount of cholesterol produced. It does however prevent the cholesterol from being absorbed from the small intestine into the bloodstream. During my presentation I stated my reason for refusing to try this latest medication. Simply put, I no longer believe that it was the cholesterol that caused my heart attack. I have totally accepted and adapted opposition views as represented by notables such Dr. Uffe Ravnskov – high cholesterol was *not* the culprit that *caused* my heart attack.

The following summary appeared on my blog: http://people.lulu.com/blogs/view.php?blog_id=1628

Mike Stone, author of Surviving a Successful Heart Attack was a guest speaker of the 'Journal Club' of Hadassah Hospital – Cardiology Department, Ein Kerem, Jerusalem.

On February 7, 2005, Mike Stone author of "Surviving a Successful Heart Attack" was the guest speaker of the Journal Club of Hadassah Hospital – Cardiology Department, Ein Kerem, Jerusalem. Mr. Stone discussed the two main themes of his book:

- The massive disruptions in his professional and personal life resulting from the statin medications he was given following his heart attack.

- His reason for discontinuing the statin medication, based upon published research works of Dr. Beatrice Golomb, Dr. Kilmer McCully, Dr. Uffe Ravnskov, Dr. Mary Enig, Ms. Sally Fallon president of the Weston A. Price Foundation and other reputable researchers.

Mr. Stone ended his presentation with a personal plea to cardiologists to be more receptive to those patients complaining about negative side effects after taking the prescribed statin medication. In addition he urged doctors and researchers to keep an open mind above and beyond standard reasons still being given as the major cause of heart disease – high LDL cholesterol levels.

A short discussion regarding statin side effects followed.

Life goes on! I am still making a concerted effort to prevent another heart attack from happening. No one knows for certain whether or not this may occur.

I continue to bike ride. My weekly target that I usually meet and/or exceed is currently 150km (94 miles). I am constantly striving to improve my eating habits and that of the Stone household. There is a sense of personal satisfaction when I see Esty or the kids looking over the ingredients listed on various food items. We now religiously weed out partially dehydrogenated ingredients and have abandoned the low fat agenda.

Lately I have been experimenting in the kitchen concocting various dishes which up until now, was considered an alien life style. It was not all that long ago that I had no idea whatsoever how the process occurs that magically transforms raw materials that are bought at the supermarket into a hot delicious meal in our dining room! It is amazing how one learns to innovate when a change of life style is thrust upon him.

My breakfast routine now includes a glass of homemade naturally fermented kefir. I make cheese Lebane by separating the whey from the fresh goat milk and then use the whey to make naturally fermented sauerkraut. I also use the whey in homemade whole wheat bread that I now bake. Believe me, these are things the pre heart attack Mike never attempted!

Finally, do I have the feeling that I outsmarted the doctors? My answer to that question is a resounding **NO!** I am reminded of this every time I have my semi-annual checkup at the hospital. On the one hand, I mentally have in my camp Dr. Ravnskov and his associates; I have Sally Fallon; I have their research, their papers, their articles -- theirs and many other sources and references mentioned throughout this book. On the other side of the scale I have my Professor of Cardiology sitting across his desk discussing my situation. His sincerity regarding my well being is overwhelming. Yet I can see the frustration in his eyes for his failure in not convincing me to get back on statins or at least to try the Ezetrol medication. He has been credited in saving hundreds of lives with case histories similar to my situation. I am not about to question his credentials or his devotion to each and every one of his past and present patients.

My professor certainly is not pleased with my cholesterol levels. Dr. Gaziano (chapter 11), with his emphasis on the Triglycerides to HDL ratio, would be. Interpretations of Dr. Gaziano's work indicate that the ratio of these two factors should be lower than 2. The lower the ratio, the healthier the patient. In May 2001, about the time of my mini heart attack in Paris, my Trig/HDL ratio was 3. Two weeks after my heart attack in July 2001, which included two weeks of continuous medication, my Trig/HDL ratio was down to 2.16, still above the red line of 2.0. In May of 2005 the ratio had dropped to 0.88! That's right, my HDL level was now higher than my Trigs level.

♥ ♥ ♥

Someone once asked me if I could turn back the clock, would I prefer NOT to have that heart attack. Needless to say, nobody wants to experience a life threatening heart attack. Ironically, because of my heart attack, I am now in the best physical shape of my life. I now have terrific endurance that I credit to my bike riding. In addition, I have totally changed my eating habits and I have learned to put a lid on stress. Yes, I also opened the door to the world around me.

Tough question indeed.......

Interesting Sources of Information

Some of these sources may be considered to be in dispute with current mainstream western medical doctrines, (but then again, the epidemic of heart attacks in the western world can also be considered to be in dispute with Mother Nature!)

Cholesterol – How Low?

Interview regarding National Institute of Health study conducted by Dr. Beatrice A. Golomb, regarding side effects of statin use for lowering cholesterol:
http://www.coloradohealthsite.org/topics/interviews/golomb.ht ml(if it was not for this article that opened my 'Pandora's box' – the second half of this book may never have been written)

B. A. Golomb, M. H. Criqui, H. White, and J. E. Dimsdale, Conceptual Foundations of the UCSD Statin Study: A Randomized Controlled Trial Assessing the Impact of Statins on Cognition, Behavior, and Biochemistry Archives of Internal Medicine, January 26, 2004; 164(2): 153 - 162.

Cholesterol-Drug Use Soars, Raising Questions About the Side Effects, The Wall Street Journal, Health Journal, February 1, 2002.

Water/Salt Cure

Dr. Fereydoon Batmanghelidj, "Your Body's Many Cries for Water",Global Health Solutions, (I don't think that standard cardiology will like this one too much.)

Cholesterol – good or bad?

Dr. Uffe Ravnskov , "The Cholesterol Myths", New Trends Publ.
(In my opinion this should be required reading for anyone going thru med school!)The International Network of Cholesterol Skeptics http://www.thincs.org

Oils and Fats

Dr. Mary G. Enig, "Know Your Fats", Bethesda Press(Still eating margarine and drinking skim milk? – try this book for size)

Cook Book

Sally Fallon, "Nourishing Traditions", New Trends Publ.(o.k. so you're back to butter, whole milk and eggs – what now?)

Calorie burning via exercise:

The Compendium of Physical Activities Tracking Guide (revised) - Ainsworth BE, Haskell WL, Whitt MC, Irwin ML, Swartz AM, Strath SJ, O'Brien WL, Bassett DR Jr, Schmitz KH, Emplaincourt PO, Jacobs DR Jr, Leon AS. Compendium of Physical Activities: An update of activity codes and MET intensities. Medicine and Science in Sports and Exercise, 2000;32 (Suppl):S498-S516.

Outlook Organization

Israel: http://www.outlook.org.il/english
England: http://www.outlooktraining.org
Spain: http://www.outlookandalucia.com/

The Internet

There is a wealth of information available on the internet, but at the same time a wealth of **dis**information. In contrast to articles submitted to respectable medical journals, which ultimately have to be approved by journal editors (including those which are in dispute among doctors and researchers), virtually anyone can 'publish' anything on the internet and immediately obtain worldwide exposure.

I encountered much information on the net that was even duplicated extensively from site to site verbatim -- which initially does give the impression of 'strength in numbers', 'widely published', 'must be right'. However when searching for confirmation of findings in legitimate medical journals, *NADA* – no mention. Not all that the internet has to offer is accurate, to say the least.

I stated at the beginning: "This book may now be finished, however my learning process still continues." Life long habits are indeed difficult to change, as are our own conceptions which govern our habits. If you are willing to have an *open mind*, to *think*, to be capable of accepting ideas and doctrines that contradict 'truths' that you were born into and grew up with, an excellent source of information can be found at the Weston A. Price Foundation (http://www.westonaprice.org) -- named for Dr. Weston A. Price, a dentist from Cleveland, who traveled the world over searching for evidence to substantiate his claims that tooth decay is a result of nutritional deficiencies.

His research showed that isolated populations throughout the world who enjoyed perfect health generation after generation were those who did not adopt modern western world eating habits (refined sugar, 'modern' vegetable oils, low fat – especially low *saturated* fat). They consumed nutrient-dense whole foods and the vital fat-soluble activators found exclusively in animal fats.

You do of course have an alternative to *thinking* – continue buying 'food' solely based on recommendations of TV commercials and other public media. But you may pay a heavy, heavy price…………..

Chronic Total Occlusion

After the Heart Attack,
the Statins
and Restenosis

Mike Stone

Heart Recovery Publishing
2028 Sawmill Road
River Ridge, La 70123

ISBN 1452836167

EAN-13 9781452836164.

Cover design by the author
    Front cover original photograph:
    http://www.heartrecovery.net/pictures.html
    Cross Golan bike trip April 3-4, 2009
    Golan Heights, Israel
    Heart borrowed from *Surviving a Successful Heart Attack*

Back Cover

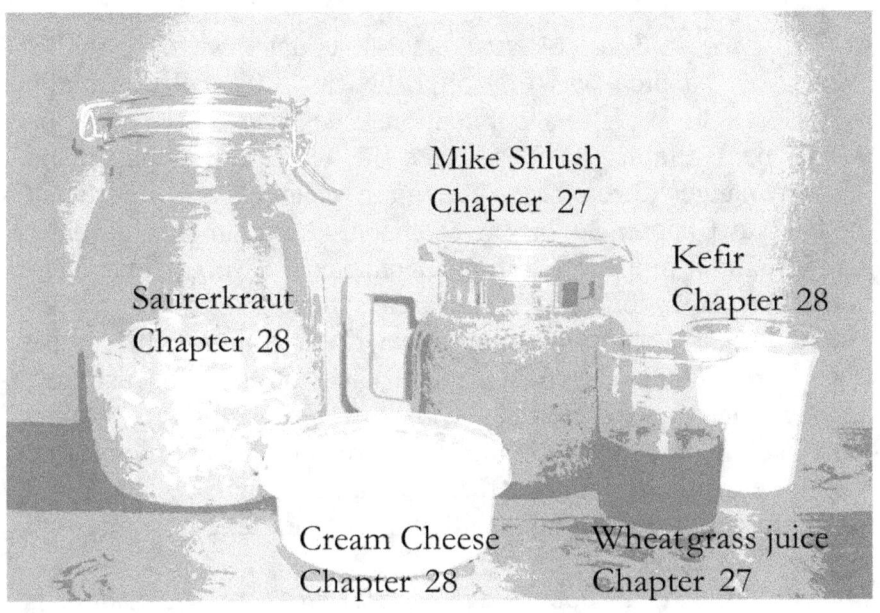

Mike Shlush
Chapter 27

Kefir
Chapter 28

Saurerkraut
Chapter 28

Cream Cheese
Chapter 28

Wheatgrass juice
Chapter 27

Yes, this is the actual color of my kitchen wall.

Arms and Hands Acknowledgements

Tuval – page 245, page 326
Limor – page 328

Author's Note

Chronic Total Occlusion is an updated version of *The Next 20,000* which was first published in 2007 and essentially supersedes it. With this publication, *The Next 20,000* will no longer be available. Besides a face lift, formatting changes and minor changes throughout, the main changes are significant updates to Chapter 34 (my ever changing and improving daily eating habits) and the addition of chapter 37. In Chapter 37, I introduce a new concept - 'Post Statin Syndrome'.

It was not my intention to rewrite and thoroughly revise *The Next 20,000*. For instance, in Chapter 26, I discuss new technologies and reference 20 different research papers published between 2006 and 2007 regarding the pleiotropic (cholesterol-independent) effects of statins. There was no point in reinforcing these findings with more of the same type research papers from 2009.

The Next 20,000, and now *Chronic Total Occlusion*, is the natural sequel to my *Surviving a Successful Heart Attack* first published in 2004 and later revised and distributed via the national networks in 2005. From hereafter, any reference to *Surviving a Successful Heart Attack* will be according to its initials SASHA. SASHA was written during a much more naive stage of my life. The term 'statin' and its true significance entered into my vocabulary only several years after my heart attack, as did the real significance of the term 'cholesterol'. What do I mean by naivety? In SASHA I stated

> *Again, it is not my purpose to medically judge which side is valid. It is my purpose to state that many of the self-evident truths regarding health and nutrition that we have grown up believing to be absolute, may not be true!*

'May not be true' is fitting for someone sitting on the fence, not knowing for sure which way to decide. *Chronic Total*

Occlusion starts out under the premise that cholesterol and saturated fat are not the causes of heart disease.* Period. End of story. Correlation, when occurring, does not indicate causation. All my life I have driven manual transmission vehicles. Several months before my heart attack in 2001, I started driving an automatic transmission car. Does that make automatic transmissions a risk factor for heart disease?

Anyone still needing further clarification regarding this subject should read the classic *The Cholesterol Myths* by Dr. Uffe Ravnskov and/or the more recent *The Great Cholesterol Con* by Anthony Colpo.

I had two main purposes when deciding to write this book. The first was to let the readers of SASHA know what has become of Mike and his stent after discontinuing the statins and recovering from the two difficult, statin-induced side-effect years. The second purpose of this book was to give a living example that it is possible to adapt to what may be conceived as unconventional health habits while still living in a conventional household.

Growing and juicing wheatgrass, preparing a daily glass of naturally fermented kefir and even cheese making are not rituals that can only be accomplished by the die-hard naturalist health freaks. They are not that difficult to do and can be integrated into normal routines and normal households.

Does that mean that all other family members have adopted my new habits? Unfortunately not. For most people, status quo evolves from an environment that one was born into. If I could turn back the clock 25 years, there are many things I would have done differently in raising the kids. I would have made English the language of the household. I would have also introduced them to my present eating habits from age 0. I guess that's what the Almighty invented grandkids for (when the eventually time comes).

---

* The premise that heart disease is caused by high cholesterol levels in the blood is known as the lipid (blood) hypothesis. This term will appear throughout the book.

213

This book is not a medical reference book in the classic sense. I am not medically trained. That said, I have recommended specific references throughout this book for people who do want further information from reliable sources.

Acknowledgements corner:

I am again indebted to Garry Borsi for his constant source of information and inspiration.

Thanks to Al Brandler for his assistance with the research.

Thanks to Tony Wiseman and Orit Josefi Wiseman of the Outlook Organization, for doing what they do.........

I greatly appreciate the unbound patience of our family physician Dr. Ayala Laufer.

I am also indebted to many individuals whom I have never met personally for the courtesy and time they took from busy schedules to personally answer the frequent questions I had regarding their published works. They really do care.

This list includes (in alphabetical order): Prof. Wilhelm Bloch, Mr. Anthony Colpo, Prof. John P. Cooke, Dr. Ron Grisanti, Dr. Duane Graveline, Prof. Jan Hoff, Dr. Joel Kauffman, Dr. Katharina Meyer, Dr. Ho-Jin Park, Prof Wolfgang Schaper, Dr. Ron Schmid, Prof. Ronald L Terjung, Prof. Axel Urhausen and Prof. Steve H.T. Yang.

Ultimately, the personal habits I have adopted over the last several years are of my own choosing and responsibility. They are not necessarily consistent with all the opinions of the fine people aforementioned, not in their published works nor in personal correspondence with me.

And of course, and foremost, a big hug and kiss to Esty who *still* puts up with me…… and to Naamah, Sagi, Rakefet and Tuval, who wound up with a dad that does things a little bit differently.

Mike Stone
July, 2007, *The Next 20,000*
March, 2010, *Chronic Total Occlusion*

Preface

From the back cover: Pick the one that's different from the others

Fereydoon Batmanghelidj	Ron Grisanti
Victoria Boutenko	Kilmer McCully
Anthony Colpo	Stephen Joseph
William Douglass II	Uffe Ravnskov
Mary Enig	Howard Roark
Sally Fallon Morell	Ron Schmid
Duane Graveline	Anne Wigmore

What do they all have in common?

How did you manage with the questionnaire on the back cover? The correct answer is Howard Roark. Howard Roark was a fictional character; he was the hero in Ayn Rand's epic *The Fountainhead*. He was an architect by profession and refused to lower his standards and accept the consensus ad hoc. As a result, he paid a heavy price in his personal and professional life.

The others are/were real-life personalities. They all promote health and dietary doctrines often conflicting with governmental health regulatory agencies, and ultimately the consensus accepted by the public at large. Some of them have also paid a heavy personal/professional price for advocating their beliefs.

Howard Roark was simply a fictional architect. He was not concerned about his fasting glucose level or the amount of trans-fat in his diet.

There is, however, a bit of Howard Roark in all of them.

The cure is secondary;
the key is prevention.

17

What Kind of Name is that for a Book?

What signifies knowing the Names, if you know not the Natures of things.
Benjamin Franklin[61]

The previous version of this book was titled *The Next 20,000*. What kind of name is that for a book, especially a book regarding life after a heart attack? This particular name has special personal significance for me. Those who have read SASHA can probably make an educated guess as to what the 20,000 represents. During the writing of this book, this significance changed somewhat even for me, as will be discussed later on.

A better name and one with Internet Search Engine Optimization significance could be something like 'How to Beat Heart Disease' assuming it hasn't already been taken. But no, this really is not a fitting title for a book authored by me simply because I am not a doctor, nor do I have any accredited medical training. This might be a fitting title if authored by Dr.

Christiaan Barnard, who performed the world's first heart transplant in Cape Town, South Africa in 1967.

Let me change this example around somewhat. If you were looking for a classy book about rebuilding your carburetor, would you buy a book called 'Overhauling Your Carburetor' by Dr. Christiaan Bernard, Heart Surgeon? Probably not. However, if the book was called 'Overhauling Your Carburetor' by John DeLorean, the developer of the original Pontiac GTO in the sixties, and the DeLorean car that starred in *Back to the Future* in the eighties, you just might buy it. So what if he was later arrested for drug trafficking -- he definitely knew his carburetors!

A better name yet, a name that I would be entitled to use, could be 'How I Beat Heart Disease'. Let's analyze this name for a moment. I had my heart attack at age 51 and discontinued the statins at age 53. If I succeed in living to the ripe old age of 93 without the statins, then no doubt I will have certainly earned the right to use that name. However, if I continue to lead a full life and make it to only 83 years old, what then? Yes, 83 is still considered to be a ripe old age, which would be 30 statin-less years. So again, I will have earned the right to use this title.

Let's take off another ten years. What if I lead a full life without the statin side effects until the age of 73? Now we are getting to a judgment call. Seventy-three is not considered to be especially old these days. How does one compare 20 years of full, no statin side effect years to 30 or more years of simple human existence without the ability to experience all that life has to offer? This is assuming of course that the statins would keep me alive longer as present cardiology guidelines dictate. And finally, if I only make it to 63, that is ten years of living and experiencing life as compared to possibly a couple of decades more of simple existence. Now that's a real tough call!

No, it is still much too early to pick 'How I Beat Heart Disease' for a title. At the time, I decided to stay with *The Next 20,000*.

18

What Really Worries Me

About half the men and women under sixty-five who have had a heart attack die within eight years of the precipitating event.
Dr. Louis J. Ignarro[62], Nobel Prize 1998 (medicine)

Statistics can be very misleading. Dr. Uffe Ravnskov proved this by his analysis of many research studies claiming to give legitimacy to the lipid hypothesis. The significance of results interpreted according to relative risks as opposed to absolute risks is very misleading and contradictory.[63]

Stats may be useful for analyzing the macro; however, they can be misleading at the micro level. Air travel is still statistically the safest way to travel. For anyone having the misfortune of being on one of those relatively few planes that do crash, his/her loss is a full 100%.

The chances of being killed due to a plane hitting a building you happen to be in approach zero. There are approximately 6.6 billion people in the world today. You figure out the odds of this happening. All lotteries offer you better odds than that, and when was the last time you won a major lottery? For those unfortunate 3,000 or so innocent victims killed on 9/11, the statistics are worthless.

Once a year, I have my annual outpatient rendezvous with the dedicated professor of cardiology who personally supervised my 'heart attack week'.[64] I come to the hospital prepared with the results of my blood tests taken at my local health clinic; I also bring the results of a recent (annual) stress test performed at the hospital associated with my health clinic.

The first order of business after presenting the nurse on duty with all the proper documentation from my health clinic is to undergo an immediate electrocardiogram. When my turn comes to enter his office, he is already reviewing his history notes in my patient file. The first entries were obviously all the events of the eight days of hospitalization in July, 2001, followed by my performance at his rehabilitation course I did at the hospital. He then goes over the original semi-annual monitoring of my condition, which has since been downgraded to an annual visit.

Over the last couple of annual visits, the dialogue starts the same.

"I have a problem with you," he opens.

"I know," is my reply.

"According to these cholesterol results you should go back on the statins."

The next few minutes are spent on his attempts to convince me to return to a statin, or as an alternative, at least to take Ezetrol[*], or a lower dose of a statin with the Ezetrol. When

---

[*]Ezetrol/Zetia (ezetimibe) does not reduce the amount of cholesterol produced like statins. It does, however, prevent the cholesterol from being absorbed from the small intestine into the bloodstream resulting in a decrease of cholesterol levels in the blood. Statins, despite well documented serious side effects at least do offer concrete cardio benefits. An article appearing in the New York Times March 31, 2008 entitled *Doubt Cast on 2 Drugs Used to Lower Cholesterol*, reported that ezetimibe 'failed

all attempts fail, he jots down a comment in my file – probably something to the effect 'patient refuses to take cholesterol lowering medication'. After all, if I do survive another heart attack, or worse yet, not survive another heart attack, he will have it documented that it was I who refused to take the his advice to lower my 'life threatening' cholesterol levels with statins. Bluntly stated, his butt will be covered. It was I who knowingly went against the cardiology world consensus.

He has been saving the lives of countless people over the last couple of decades. He was indoctrinated since his earliest days of medical school that cholesterol and fat are principal causes of heart disease. One would not expect that one Mike Stone would easily persuade a man of his stature that 'correlation when occurring is not causation' (regarding cholesterol and heart disease).

There is an important issue that the good professor never fails to bring up. It is also an issue that I have no rebuttal to offer him. The damage to my cardiovascular system resulting from 50 years of dietary abuse is a reality. The stent insertion did not cure my heart disease. It was simply a local solution to the most pressing problem to physically/mechanically open up a nearly completely blocked critical artery. The medications prescribed following my heart attack, including the statins, were not intended to cure the existing chronic medical condition. The sole intention of all of them was to help preserve the existing condition, and prevent further deterioration.

I also know as a non-medical person that this is the maximum that I can hope for even with all the changes I have made in my daily habits – the exercise, the dietary changes, reducing stress levels, etc. The elimination of trans-fats from my diet, being aware of omega-6 and omega-3 significance, less

---

to slow, and might have even sped up, the growth of fatty plaques in the arteries. Growth of those plaques is closely correlated with heart attacks and strokes.' Why am I not surprised??

cooked foods, the freshly squeezed wheatgrass juice every morning, kefir, rejuvelac and all the other changes I discuss in this book will not *reverse* the 50 years of damage I caused to my cardiovascular system.

My existing cardiovascular system is not in an ideal condition to prevent an additional event from happening. The existing accumulated plaque is potentially susceptible to rupture – a common cause of blood clots. The stent also has its inherent potential risks. It is not something that I was born with; for all of its benefits it still remains a foreign metal object located in a very delicate area.

I mentioned in SASHA that I may one day consider undergoing EDTA Chelating therapy to clean up the blockages, and in a sense turn back the clock on the existing damage accumulated over my first 50 years. The question remains, is it truly effective? It is still considered to be controversial. And if chelating therapy, would it be the traditional intravenous procedure, or would the alternative oral chelating therapy be just as effective?[65]

Therefore, the question that begs to be answered is: to what extent exactly have I slowed down the further deterioration of my cardiovascular system by my lifestyle changes over the last number of years? I truly believe that had I changed my exercise/eating habits 30 years ago, my cardiovascular system would be in a vastly different state today. That, however, is not the relevant point today.

Despite vast improvements in my current health agenda, I do not totally abstain from modern conventional foods. The fact that I consume less of them, have eliminated the trans-fats from my diet as much as possible, and have added more raw/unrefined food only means that the rate of deterioration of my system has slowed down; I doubt that it has entirely stopped. Even if the rate has significantly decreased, over the years it is still slowly advancing.

What is it that really bothers me? I am not in denial. I do know that it is a possibility I may meet my cardiology professor not at one of our annual reunions, but rather when he on his feet and me on the bed again. The problem would not be him personally telling me 'See, I told you so'.

What bothers me is that for him this would be further proof of the lipid hypothesis. When on the statins my LDL cholesterol was 88, and according to all the other medical testing (statin induced mental and emotional dysfunction are not part of laboratory 'medical testing') I was in great shape. When taking myself off the statins, my cholesterol levels rose, which 'resulted' in another heart attack. Another statistic for the consensus -- additional proof that 'correlation is causation'.

It bothers me that even in this hypothetical situation, deep inside I know that I am right.

19

Uh-Oh – What's Wrong?

*Within 6 years after a recognized heart attack (MI), 18% of men
will have another heart attack, about 22%
will be disabled with heart failure, 8%
will have a stroke and 7% will
experience sudden death.* [66]

These are not especially encouraging statistics for us men. The statistics for women are even gloomier. Should I be especially happy that I am quickly approaching my sixth anniversary of my July 2001 heart attack?

December 2006:

Annual test results: I was surprised by the electrocardiogram (a.k.a. ECG or EKG) results during my stress test, which showed signs of 'not normal' during the final higher stress stages of the test.

What could have possibly caused these declines? I do realize I have been riding less; however, I have been walking more. Instead of driving to the parking lot at work, I park a 15-minute - half-hour walk away, depending whether I leave my house on time. The walk to work is, of course, not at an overly intensive pace, however, I do believe my recent past activity would still be classified as 'active'.

Could there be an effect because of the change to the normal daytime hours I had been working for most of my life? Although I no longer work the graveyard shift like I did for the first half of this year, I still don't get to bed before one a.m. most days of the week. Long gone are the days when I would be out at five a.m. I do miss that previous schedule, but this is the present reality.

I long ago abandoned the low-fat agenda; have I been over exaggerating my higher-fat diet?

My cardiology professor recommended that I do a thallium heart scan. So back to my health clinic to make the request to have the scan done at the appropriate hospital affiliated with my clinic.

A thallium heart scan is used to evaluate the blood supply to the heart muscle. A small amount of radioactive substance is injected into the bloodstream and a special camera is used to make an image of the blood flow to the heart. The radioactive substance is a radioisotope of the element thallium (thallium-201). This scan can identify areas of the heart that may have a poor blood supply as a result of damage from a previous heart attack or blocked coronary arteries.

January 2007

On the appointed day, I arrived at the hospital ready for my heart scan after a three-hour fast. As per instructions, I came happily equipped with a chocolate bar; it was that or come with some sour cream -- I didn't yet know the reason for this. The first order of business was the insertion an intravenous needle (IV line) into the vein on my right arm just below the elbow, the kind of IV that allows for injecting fluids multiple times. I then started what seemed to be a normal stress test on the treadmill.

Towards the latter stage of the test, which was already at a very rapid pace, a small amount of thallium-201 was injected into my IV line. Shortly after finishing the treadmill walk, I lay down under a special camera called a gamma scintillation camera. It made photographs from the gamma rays emitted by the thallium.

The purpose of the chocolate or sour cream: Radioisotope thallium-201 is a radioactive form of the element thallium (half-life of 73 hours). It was explained that it is advisable to ingest the fats in order to pad the liver from the radioactive material now circulating in the body.

The thallium attaches itself to red blood cells and is transported throughout the body in the bloodstream. It enters the heart muscle by way of the coronary arteries. The thallium can therefore reach only those areas of the heart with an adequate blood supply.

After this first set of gamma photographs taken shortly after my fast treadmill walk, I was instructed to return in another five hours. After returning, I was again injected with an additional shot of thallium. Within an hour, I was back under the scintillation camera for another round of gamma photographs, this time to get an image of the resting heart.

A normal thallium heart scan shows healthy blood flow through the coronary arteries without 'cold spots', both at rest and during exercise. A cold spot is an area where the heart tissue has been damaged (previous heart attack) or suffers from impaired circulation due to a blockage in the coronary arteries. It is an area the thallium has not reached, therefore does not show up on the gamma ray photograph. During exercise, the heart has to work harder and has a greater demand for blood. Cold spots that appear during exercise and not at rest usually indicate some blockage of the coronary arteries. People in this category are considered to be at a greater risk for future cardiac events such as heart attacks.

Results of the Heart Scan

The computerized printout of the December stress test did not come back positive; however, it did contain some comments regarding irregularities that are 'probably insignificant'. It was the sharp eye of my cardiology professor that determined that some of the squiggly lines on the EKG printout were not so insignificant as far as he was concerned. And indeed, the results of the thallium heart scan were positive. His recommendation: undergo an angiogram in the near future to verify the cause of the positive results of the heart scans.

Since discontinuing the statins three and a half years ago, I have been exercising regularly. I have discontinued ingesting partially hydrogenated foods (as much as possible) and therefore trans-fats. I have also discontinued the low-fat dairy agenda, with all of the artificial ingredients contained in them to keep them edible and 'dairy'. I have been eating more live foods, from naturally fermented raw milk products to wheatgrass juice. Have I been deceiving myself and causing additional blockages in my cardiovascular system?

To be continued.............

20

Raw Food & Enzymes

*The length of life is inversely proportional to the rate of
exhaustion of the enzyme potential of an organism*
Dr. Edward Howell[67]

I n my generation the most important requirement regarding
healthy eating when growing up was to make sure we were
getting enough vitamins. Afraid of getting a cold? 'Drink
lots of orange juice because it has vitamin C' we were told. I
still remember a special kids' vitamin that was taken as a small
chocolate semi-sweet delicacy every morning. That may even
explain my long lasting love affair with chocolate. I loved
nearly every variation of chocolate that there was - with the
exception of any chocolate containing raisins. I think my
absolute favorite was Three Musketeers. That did not prevent
me from consuming the competition whenever available:
Hershey Bars, Nestle's Crunch, even the coconut filled Peter
Paul Mounds bar and the like.

The next technical term while growing up regarding
nutrition was minerals. What American kid did not start the day
off with cereal for breakfast? It was definitely reassuring to read

the message on the cereal box stating its contents were 'fortified' with vitamins and minerals.

I did not have any idea what the minerals were supposed to do, but having them supplied 'fortified' in my cereal definitely sounded reassuring. What kid could resist eating a 'fortified' cereal that had a picture of a baseball star printed on the front of the box? My favorite was mixing Wheaties and Cheerios together, letting them soak in the milk until mushy, and then eating it.

When growing up, how many times do you remember your mom telling you 'Eat your (whatever) to make sure you get enough enzymes'? Probably never. Enzymes? That sounds like a term for a chemist, or possibly a biologist. It was not for us laypeople, and definitely not a term that the average mom would be familiar with.

Why should I be concerned with enzymes? What you don't know can't hurt you, right? The problem is, by not knowing many things, I did have that heart attack at age 51, remember?

Merriam-Webster defines enzymes as 'any of numerous complex proteins that are produced by living cells and catalyze specific biochemical reactions at body temperatures'. In plain terms, 'catalyze specific biochemical reactions' translates to enzymes are the labor force of the body, catalyzing over 4,000 known biochemical reactions.[68] Enzymes are substances that make life possible. No mineral or vitamin can do any work without them. They are needed for **every** chemical reaction that takes place in our bodies.

Our bodies produce two types of enzymes:

Metabolic Enzymes

Metabolic enzymes run our bodies. A specific set of metabolic enzymes controls each organ in our bodies. These enzymes utilize the proteins, fats and carbohydrates that we eat to perform their functions.

231

Digestive Enzymes

Digestive enzymes have three main functions: to digest protein, carbohydrates and fat. Proteases are enzymes that digest protein, amylases digest carbohydrate, and lipases digest fat. Excessive production of digestive enzymes causes enlarged digestive organs, such as the pancreas.

There are hundreds of types of different known metabolic enzymes, and approximately two-dozen known digestive enzymes. Compared to vitamins and minerals, enzymes are the newest nutritional puzzle to be understood by nutritionists and scientists.

Many misconceptions apparently are still prevalent. Let's start with the basic Merriam-Webster definition: 'catalyze specific biochemical reactions'. A catalyst, by definition, is not consumed by the overall reaction. It accelerates or slows down the chemical reaction, nothing more.

It has been proven that the capacity of a living organism to make enzymes is limited and exhaustible. This negates the enzyme's status as a catalyst. It also follows that if the body is using its resources to produce digestive enzymes, it is at the expense of producing the metabolic enzymes. The best way to illustrate this would be to go back to my college days, and the famous Guns and Butter graph from Economics 101.

In a theoretical economy with the ability to produce two finite products and with a finite total production potential, a choice must be made between how much of each item to produce. In this example, as resources are used to produce more guns (military spending) the economy has less resources for the production of butter (domestic/food), and vice versa. The curve represents all possible choices the economy has at its disposal. The point here is that every choice has an opportunity cost; you can produce more of the first product only by giving up production of the second product.   Assuming a given finite production potential, you cannot produce outside the curve.

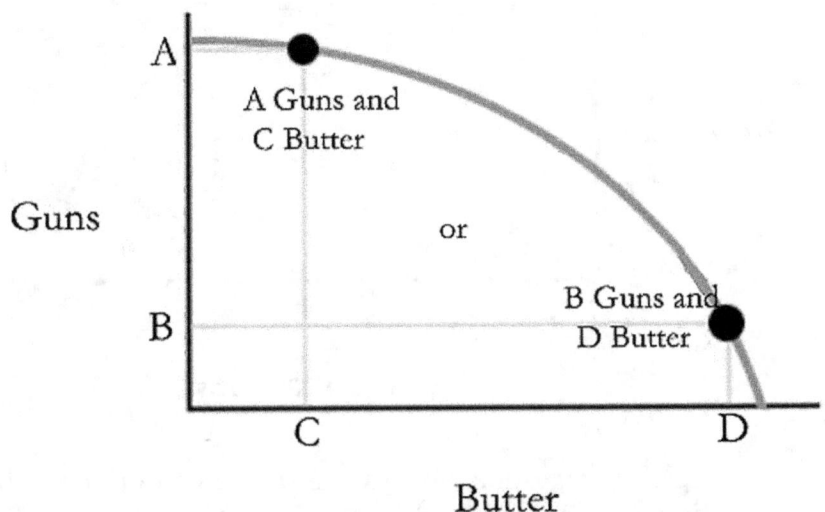

This model also demonstrates the production potential of body enzymes. When the body is forced to produce   digestive enzymes at a particular time, it is at the expense of producing metabolic enzymes.

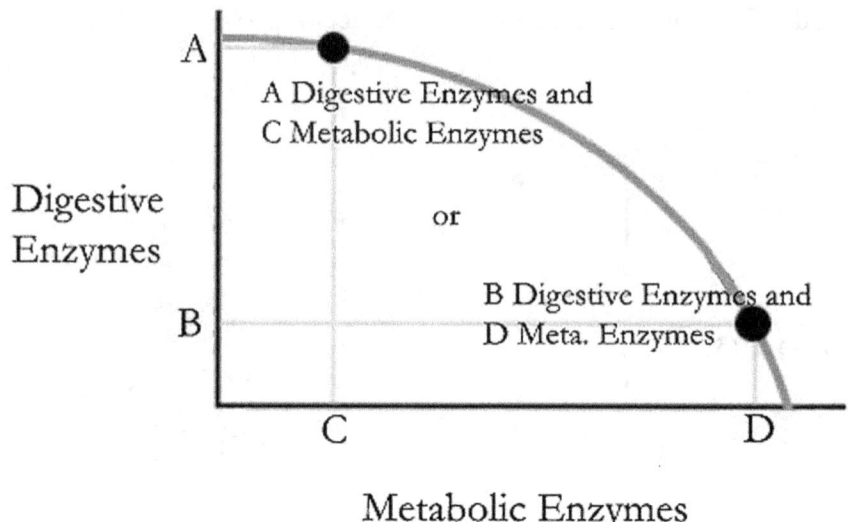

A

A Digestive Enzymes and
C Metabolic Enzymes

Digestive
Enzymes

or

B Digestive Enzymes and
D Meta. Enzymes

B

C

D

Metabolic Enzymes

Generally, digestion always has a high priority in the body's hierarchy of doing things. The production of the necessary digestive enzymes needed to digest the latest meal will have preference over the production of the hundreds of other metabolic enzymes necessary to run other important, if not critical, body processes.

Ultimately, man never comes out on top when tampering with nature. The case in point: tampering with the natural enzymes contained in raw food. Although our bodies are capable of producing digestive enzymes, it was not nature's intent that we do this function by ourselves. The enzymes contained in raw food play an important part in the pre-digestion of our food before it hits the stomach. This allows for a minimum production of supplementary   digestive enzymes, and allows for maximum production of the important metabolic enzymes.

How are we destroying the enzymes in our food supply? Very bluntly, we cook it, and this is in addition to commercial food processing, which is often performed at high temperatures. Any prolonged wet-heat temperature over 118°F (47.8°C) kills 100% of the enzymes. This statement is so important that I will say it again. **Any prolonged wet-heat over 118°F (47.8°C) kills 100% of the enzymes!**

How hot is 118°F? An item at 117°F can be held in the hand with no problem. At 118° it is already too hot to handle. It starts to burn. This is significantly less than normal cooking temperatures; water boils at 212°F (100°C) and normal baking is at 300°F (149°C) - 400°F (204°C) dry heat. Enzymes can survive higher dry-heat temperatures -- but nothing even close to normal baking temperatures.

The Law of Adaptive Secretion of Digestive Enzymes

The Law of Adaptive Secretion of Digestive Enzymes governs characteristics of digestive enzyme production. This law states that an organism values its finite supply of enzymes and will make no more than are needed to do the job. Accordingly, the body produces the exact type and quantity of enzymes needed according to the protein, carbohydrate and fat makeup of the food eaten. Stated a bit more technically, the greater the amount of exogenous (outside) digestive enzymes we consume, the less production of the endogenous (internal) enzymes is required.

It naturally follows according to this law, ingesting natural enzymes already contained in the food we consume means the enzyme potential in our bodies can allot less activity to producing digestive enzymes and more to producing metabolic enzymes.

A good example to see how this works is to take an example directly from nature. Wild animals have no enzymes in their saliva. The bulk of the digestive enzymes needed to digest their prey are the enzyme banks existing in the prey itself. They need no enzymes in their saliva to start the predigesting process; these are ingested with each bite of the prey.

On a more domestic level, family dogs and cats that eat raw food exclusively also have no enzymes in their saliva. When fed cooked food, enzymes start showing up in their saliva within about a week; this is in full accordance with the law of adaptive secretion of digestive enzymes.

Uncooked foods contain an abundance of food enzymes, which correspond to the nutritional highlights of the food. For example, seeds, nuts dairy foods contain fat and higher concentration of lipase. Grains contain higher concentrations of amylase.

♥ ♥ ♥

Is there a connection between the present state of my cardiovascular system and my own bodily enzyme activity? The two most potent enzymes secreted by the human body are amylase, which deals with the digestion of carbohydrates, and protease, which deals with the digestion of proteins. Our saliva contains a high concentration of amylase (how many times are we reminded to chew thoroughly?) while stomach juices contain protease.

Lipase, however, is present in weaker concentrations. As we grow older, enzyme activity grows weaker. Studies done over 50 years ago show a decrease in lipase levels and a definite alteration in the capacity of the aged human to handle fat.[69] Improvement in the fat utilization was exhibited by the subjects when later fed lipase. A later study demonstrated that there is a progressive decline of lipase in the blood of atherosclerosis patients with advancing middle and old age.[70] That certainly does not sound like good news for me. I am indeed considered to be an atherosclerosis patient and am now closer to 60 than to 50.

The easiest way to separate fat from its lipase enzyme is to destroy it by cooking. Without lipase to start the predigestion process, the fat remains unaltered for two to three hours in the stomach. All this occurs while the carbohydrates and proteins are being digested by the amylase and protease respectively.

Again, lipase is not present in saliva, so no pre-digestion of fats can take place. As stated earlier, a greater necessity to produce digestive enzymes comes at the expense of the production of metabolic enzymes. This is definitely not great news for the 98 distinct known (metabolic) enzymes working in the arteries, each with a particular job to do.

This leads to the speculation that fat not pre-digested may not be properly metabolized (unhydrolyzed/partially digested) when it later reaches body tissues; the result is aggravated arterial linings and hardening of the arteries. This is basically what heart disease is all about!

In SASHA, I discussed how I discovered Dr. Dean Ornish and his best-selling book *Dr. Dean Ornish's Plan for Reversing Heart Disease.* Today, Ornish's low fat/high complex carbohydrate regimen is considered to be the arch rival of Dr. Robert Atkin's high fat/low carbohydrate diet plan. This book, however, as its name implies, is not specifically a diet plan; it is Ornish's comprehensive plan to reverse heart disease.

After learning about the vital importance of enzymes, I was curious what Dr. Ornish had to say about enzymes in general, and in particular, about lipase. I searched in the index for the word 'enzymes' and was surprised that it wasn't listed! Maybe he was more specific and indexed enzymes according to specific name. I looked for 'lipase' in the index, and again, no entry.

Suddenly I understood the 'genius' of Ornish's plan to combat heart disease. Cardiovascular disease is the epidemic of the modern Western world. The ingesting of copious amounts of commercially processed fats devoid of enzymes in the Western diet is indeed a source of heart disease.

Dr. Ornish found an innovative solution to 'solve' this problem. For most people in today's modern world, obtaining and consuming necessary healthy fat in the form nature intended with enzymes intact is not feasible. His solution to circumvent the real problem: simply eliminate almost all the fats!

The emphasis in today's cardio world is not on prevention; it is on repair. And why not? Modern technologies can do wonders with our precious bodies with prescription medications and operations. Angiogram, angioplasty, stents and bypass operations are great tools to fix anyone who has managed to clog up his/her arteries, assuming of course that they make it to the hospital on time. What is sad is that this is considered 'normal' in our modern civilization.

Take someone with a Rolls Royce that gasses it up with kerosene instead of the proper octane gasoline. If it later does not run as it should, but he has a great mechanic who can fix it, would this seem normal? No? Why then is his Rolls more precious than our own precious bodies?

Would it not make more sense to consume foods with more live enzymes, or even supplement meals with enzymes rather than try and control the damage with medications or fix the problem later using intrusive medical procedures?

Are we like Pottenger's cats?

From 1932 to 1942, Dr. Francis Marion Pottenger, Jr. conducted a controlled experiment[71] on generations of cats (total 900 cats) to determine the effects of heat-processed food them. The cats were divided into groups. All the groups were supplied the same basic minimal diet (meat, milk and cod liver oil), but the major portions of the diets were varied. One group ate raw meat and raw milk exclusively, a natural food for cats. The other groups were fed processed milk: pasteurized, evaporated and condensed milk, with either raw or cooked meat.

All generations of the raw meat/milk groups remained healthy throughout their normal life spans. The first generation of all the other processed-food groups developed degenerative diseases and illnesses towards the end of their lives. The next generation of these groups developed degenerative diseases and illnesses in the middle of their lives and started losing their coordination. The third generation of the processed food groups developed degenerative diseases in the beginning of their lives and many died before six months of age. Bones became soft and the cats suffered from adverse personality changes. Males became docile, less interested in mating while females became more aggressive.

There was no fourth generation in any of the processed food groups. Either the third generation parents were sterile or the fourth generation cats died before birth. Again, this is in direct contrast to the fourth generation of the cats on the raw food/milk diet, which remained healthy throughout their normal lifespan.

Dr. Pottenger concluded that a diet consisting exclusively of raw milk and raw meat was the only adequate food that insured optimal health for the cats. Cats on the all-raw diet showed good bone structure with excellent bone density. They had wide palates with plenty of room for properly aligned teeth. They exhibited a shiny coat and were free of disease. In addition, these cats reproduced with ease and were gentle and easy to handle. The cats eating processed foods (meat/milk) developed physical degeneration that escalated with each successive generation.

Of special interest to those of you who do purchase and consume raw milk, Dr. Pottenger also showed that not all-raw milk is created equally.

> In comparing the experimental effects on cats of a diet including raw milk from fresh feed cows and those of a diet including raw milk from dry feed cows, we find that the cats fed raw milk from dry feed cows show similar deficiencies as those fed pasteurized milk.[72]

People are people, cats are cats, but…

Why should I be influenced by a study that was done on cats over 70 years ago? As in the computer era, 70 years is also a long time as far as medical advancement is concerned. In addition, how many people do you know that have received a kitten from a domesticated cat eating processed food and watched the kitten grow older and give birth to litter after litter of apparently healthy kittens? You probably know many people that fit this description; and those cats are all brought up on commercially processed food.

That said how is the research of Dr. Pottenger applicable to us today? I certainly have not noticed an abundance of domesticated malformed dying cats roaming around my own neighborhood. How were Pottenger's cats similar to us? How did they differ?

We are both warm-blooded. We are both mammals. We reproduce in a similar fashion, give birth after a fixed pregnancy period, and nurse the newborns.

On the other hand, we humans by nature are omnivores (capable of eating meat protein and vegetation). Cats are carnivores (meat eaters). This alone dictates that dietary requirements of humans will not be the same as cats.

This evolutionary development has resulted in more stringent nutritional requirements for cats than for omnivores such as the rat, dog, and man. [73]

The different dietary requirements are of course dictated by the differences in our biological systems. As an example, for us humans, taurine is a nonessential amino acid, meaning that it is manufactured from other amino acids in the liver. It does not have to be obtained directly through the diet. On the other hand, taurine, found only in animal products, is an important *essential* amino acid for the cat. [74]

Some of the abnormalities displayed by Pottenger's cats can possibly be attributed to taurine deficiency, such as poor reproductive performance and neurological abnormalities. This could possibly be explained by the cooking of the meat, which destroyed the taurine in the food fed to the cats. [75]

Dr. Pottenger studied cats. As stated previously, the cats eating raw food/milk were healthy and properly developed generation after generation.

Dr. Weston A. Price studied people throughout the whole world. The 'primitive' societies eating traditional foods were free of chronic disease and dental decay; they were strong and produced healthy children generation after generation. Dr. Price observed that modern civilization eating refined grains, canned foods, pasteurized milk and sugars suffered from degenerative illnesses, infertility, crooked teeth, narrowed faces, deformities of bone structure and susceptibility to every sort of medical problem.[76]

This same degeneration observed by Dr. Price in tribes and villages that had abandoned traditional foods was also observed by Dr. Pottenger for the cats eating heat-processed (cooked/pasteurized) food.

No, people are not cats; however Dr. Pottenger summed this up quite nicely:

> *While no attempt will be made to correlate the changes in the animals studied with malformations found in humans, **the similarity is so obvious that parallel pictures will suggest themselves.**[77]* (Bold emphasis is mine.)

What do **you** think?

How do we then conserve our finite potential of enzymes? Besides killing enzymes found in natural food by cooking, our own enzymes are used up faster during certain illnesses, during extremely hot or cold weather, and during strenuous exercise. We have all heard of Eskimos. Eskimos have been notorious for enjoying excellent health by eating a raw diet. The name 'Eskimo' itself is based on an American Indian language meaning 'he eats it raw' or 'eaters of raw meat', depending on which dialect is used. In the case of Eskimos, raw food means raw meat – their cholesterol levels are sky high, but heart disease if virtually non-existent.

A Western culture family that adapted eating raw food as the standard in the house, and not as the exception, is the Boutenko[78] family -- today known as the Raw Family. In the mid-nineties, different members of the Boutenko family suffered from a variety of illnesses, such as obesity, depression, rheumatoid arthritis, severe hyperthyroid, juvenile diabetes and asthma. After going on a totally raw diet, all those health problems were miraculously healed. We will return to the (Victoria) Boutenko family in chapter 27.

Is going on a 100% raw diet practical for most people? The answer is 'no' despite the enzyme conservation and other health benefits of doing so. Raw food is digested in less than half the time as cooked food. The extended hours of digestion creates rotting and intestinal illnesses.

What percentage of raw food in our diet should we strive for? 90%? 70%? How much? The natural health care nutritionist Hanna Kroeger[79] mentions figures of 50% raw and 50% cooked for fighting diseases. She also claims that enzyme supplements are just as valid as adding vitamins and minerals to our diets.

Do I even approach 100% raw food? Not even close. Although I do strive to increase this percentage, I cannot really say if I am at 30%, 40%, 50%, or 60%. It is the purpose of this book to show how small adjustments in our eating habits can make a big difference in improving these percentages.

21

Why is Raw Food so Unappealing?

I want my food dead. Not sick, not dying, dead.
Oscar Wilde

Why is it that so many people find the idea of eating raw food repelling? It all boils down to preconceptions of what we think food should look and smell like. As it turns out, these preconceptions are not at all objective; in fact they are very subjective.

There are many clichés out there – 'you can't judge a book by its cover', or 'beauty is in the eye of the beholder'. We even have a rhyming expression in Hebrew that says 'Ol Taam v-ol rai-och, ain ma lhitvaka-och' which translates literally to 'regarding taste and smell, there is nothing to argue about'. Stated more abruptly: one person's sense of what is aesthetic, smells nice or is tasty, may be utterly disgusting to someone else.

To prove my point, I have two actual examples involving real people. I won't mention the names and relationship to 'protect the innocent'. The first example involves something I consider to be a real delicacy, tongue. There are several different ways one can eat tongue.

243

One option: cut very, very thin, stacked nice and thick between two slices of fresh rye bread smeared with mustard -- literally heaven on Earth. One of my favorite places to eat a tongue sandwich when visiting New York was always the Second Avenue Kosher Delicatessen. The Second Ave Deli, as it was commonly known, had a long and interesting history. Abe Lebewohl, an Ukrainian immigrant who arrived in the United States in 1950, worked there as a waiter in what was then a 12-seat capacity coffee shop for several years.

In 1954, Mr. Lebewohl and several partners at the time purchased the delicatessen. As fate would have it, Mr. Lebewohl was murdered in 1996, a daylight robbery in which he was depositing the previous day's receipts. The restaurant doors were unfortunately closed for good in 2006 by its then owner, Jack Lebewohl, the younger brother of Abe. The closure was the result of a rent increase dispute with the building's new landlord.

I will state that there is a yearly ritual when we do eat tongue; it saves me the necessity of traveling all the way to New York just to have a tongue sandwich! Anyone who has ever participated in a Jewish Passover Seder[*] knows that before you get to the main meal, there is a long ceremony beforehand where various symbolic foods are blessed. In fact there is a special Passover plate that is divided in sections to hold the different symbolic items.

Here in Israel, it is the tradition in families of Sephardic origin[**] (Esty's family immigrated to Israel from Iraq in the

---

[*] The Passover Seder is a Jewish ritual feast which takes place on the first evening of Passover holiday in Israel, and on the first and second evenings of Passover in the Jewish Diaspora. The feast includes reading the Haggadah, which contains the complete Seder service.

[**]By strict definition a Sephardi is a Jew whose forefathers originated from Portugal or Spain. In a broader sense, the term has come to also include Jews of Arabic and Persian

244

early 1950's) to also have a ceremony preceding the festive Rosh Hashanah (New Year) meal. It is much shorter than the Passover ceremony; however, it does have various symbolic foods on which blessings are said. One of these blessings is:

yehi ratzon m'lifanecha adonoi elokanu v'elovei avoteinu sh-nehiye l'rosh v'lo l'znav.....

שֶׁנִּהְיֶה לְרֹאשׁ וְלֹא לְזָנָב

which basically translates to 'G-d willing we should all be like the head, and not the tail'. Following the blessing, we then eat something representing the 'head'. In our family it is a portion of boiled tongue, sliced into inch wide sections, a true delicacy.

What is all this leading to? This may seem like a benign point; however much of the food we consume on the plates in front of us doesn't always resemble what its raw material looks like before processing and packaging.

The case in point – real people, no names...we will refer to them as couple A and couple B. Couple A invited couple B over to dinner. Mrs. A was still in the kitchen when couple B arrived a bit early. Mrs. A still had a large tongue cooking in the pot.

It may seem redundant to state that tongue is called 'tongue' because it originates in a cow's mouth! When couple B saw the complete cow's tongue still in the pot and as yet uncut into individual portions, the sight of it sickened them. It simply ruined their appetite for the entire evening. What is interesting is this same couple B that could not stomach seeing a cooked cow's tongue in the pot loves eating lobsters.

---

backgrounds. In present day usage it has become an umbrella term for any Jewish person who is not Ashkenazi (Ashkenazis are descendants of Jews from Germany, Poland, Austria and Eastern Europe).

For those of you who may not be totally familiar with lobsters, they are undoubtedly one of the ugliest creatures on the planet. When I was younger, they would remind me of what a giant spider might look like, with armor and pinchers. The whole procedure of eating a lobster starts with its purchase, while it is alive and well, swimming in a glass-lined pool waiting to be bought. The buyer looks them all over, even looks the lobster straight in the eye, and decides, 'I want you'. Lobsters are tossed into a boiling red-hot pot for steaming, meaning that the first lobster to hit the pot has a good chance of hitting some boiling water before getting steamed live.

This procedure is accompanied with jokes to the tune of 'woo - listen to the lobster yelling'. I wonder if other lobsters do actually hear their comrades screaming from the pot. And of course, the culmination of this whole process -- the actual eating of the lobster.

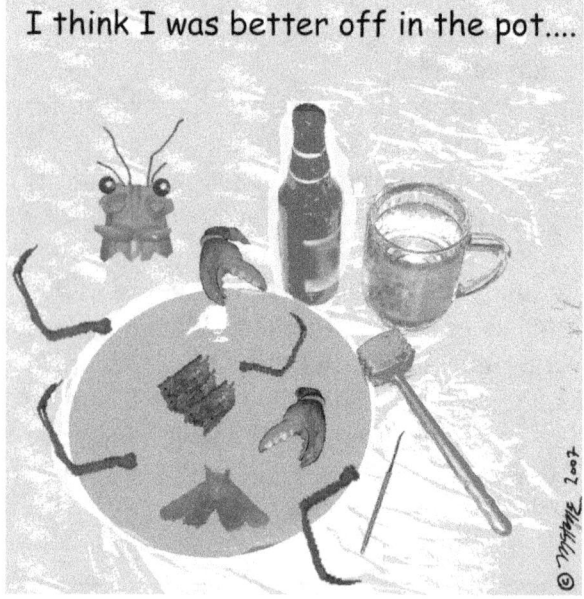

I think I was better off in the pot....

For someone who has never seen this ritual, it is grotesque. The process starts with literally ripping off its pinchers and its legs. To carve out the meat inside the armor you have something that resembles a nut clipper, and if you have trouble getting into the claw, you have a wooden hammer to crack the armored shell. Then of course there is opening up the lobster from its belly side, and scooping out the lobster meat from all of its dismembered parts. I did previously mention grotesque, didn't I? What's the point? To couple B, seeing a very natural complete cow's tongue cooking in a large pot was unbearable.

The whole process of purchasing, cooking live and then dismembering the lobster to them is an accepted way of preparing and eating food.

The second example is similar. Person C (yes, another name change) came over to Israel for a visit from the States. One evening Esty prepared a nice fish dinner. Again here we see the differences between different cultures, and how each views the same situation in different ways. It is very acceptable in Israel, in restaurants and in the home as well, to serve fish complete and intact. This is not to say that you cannot obtain a fish fillet that has been de-boned and sliced up into portions.

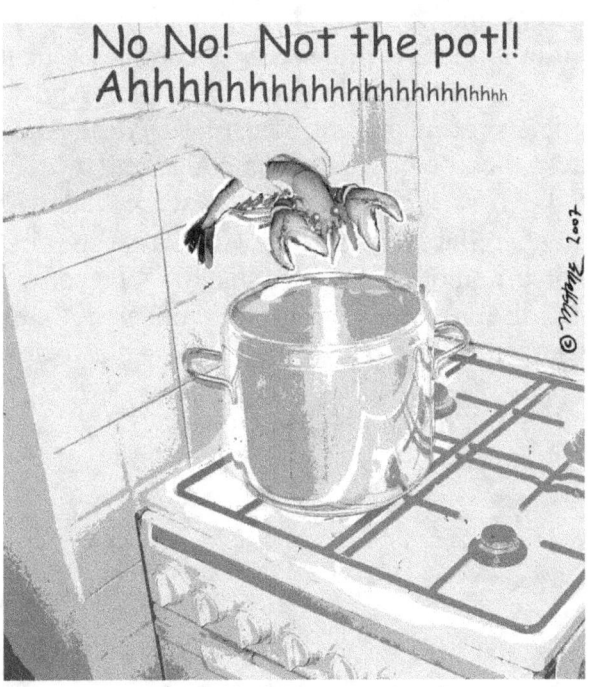

A complete fish means just that. It comes served with its head and eyes intact. When person C saw the cooked fish on the plate 'looking back at her', she simply freaked out. And what's special about this example? This particular person enjoys going out and ordering steamed crabs. The procedure for steaming, dismembering and eating crabs is similar to that described for lobsters -- and why not, they are in the same family known as crustaceans.

The standard procedure is going to a crab house with family or a bunch of friends. The table is lined with either newspapers, or a disposable paper tablecloth. What distinguishes a crab house from a steak house, for example, is that at a crab house everyone puts on bib.

No, I do not mean a napkin on the lap type of protection, but a bib that you tie around your neck to keep your shirt clean. Why the bib? When your neighbor on either side starts clobbering dismembered crab parts with the wooden hammer to break the outer armor shell, pieces of meat, shell and any other internal parts can start flying around the table.

Again, this to some people is a normal, pleasant, acceptable way of eating a meal, while seeing a complete uncut fish with its head still on is considered to be unbearable. And so it is with many people's preconceptions of eating anything raw for the first time 'Yuck! I can't eat that! It's not cooked!'

I admit that the first time I cut into a steak that was totally raw, I also had a similar feeling.[*] However, after the first small bite, chewing it up, and swallowing that first piece, the apprehension quickly disappeared. What we conceive to be aesthetic food and what isn't is all in the mind.

This concludes Introduction to Eating Raw Food 101.....

---

[*] Although cooking kills much of the healthy attributes of food, it also eliminates many harmful aspects, bacteria etc. Raw food must be 'prepared correctly' and obtained from reputable sources.

22

Pasteur – Hero or Villain?

The general public, however intelligent, are struck only by that
which it takes little trouble to understand
Antoine Béchamp[80]

Part 1: Louis Pasteur, Pasteurization – Brief Review

L ouis Pasteur, the famous French microbiogist and chemist, was born in 1822. He is best known for developing a system of heat application to control fermentation, which resulted in the non-spoilage of wine and beer. His heat application involved raising the temperature of wine to kill the specific living microorganisms that cause spoilage. This process, which ultimately immortalized his name universally and is today commonly associated with milk, is known as 'pasteurization'.

His other major claim to fame was his germ theory of disease, technically known as the pathogenic theory of medicine. The theory proposes that microorganisms are the cause of many diseases. Although highly controversial when first proposed, it is now a cornerstone of modern medicine and clinical microbiology, leading to widespread usage of prescription medicines and antibiotics. He also created the first vaccine for rabies.

His academic resume was impressive:

1848: Professor of Physics at Dijon Lycee
1849: Professor of Chemistry at Strasbourg University
1854: Dean of the College of Science in Lille.
1856: Administrator and director of scientific studies of the École Normale Supérieure.
1862: Member of French Academy of Science

Pasteur won the Leeuwenhoek medal, microbiology's highest honor, in 1895, the year of his death.

The remains of Pasteur are interred at the chapel of the Pasteur Institute, Marnes-la-Coquette, France. One of the walls of the chapel summarizes the accomplishments attributed to him.

1857: Fermentations
1862: So-called 'Spontaneous Generation'
1863: Studies in Wine
1865: Disease of Silkworms
1871: Studies in Beer
1877: Virulent Microbic Diseases
1880: Vaccinating Viruses
1885: Prophylaxis of Rabies

Interestingly, his list of accomplishments at the chapel does not include any specific reference to milk.

Pasteurization

Pasteurization is the process of heating food in order to kill harmful organisms such as bacteria, viruses, protozoa, molds, and yeasts. Pasteurization, unlike sterilization, is not intended to kill all microorganisms in the food; it aims to achieve a five-log reduction (0.00001 times the original) in the number of viable organisms, reducing their number so they are unlikely to cause disease.

This assumes of course that the pasteurized product is refrigerated and consumed before its expiration date. Today, pasteurization is typically associated with milk/milk products. The justification for pasteurizing milk was that it often became contaminated while being handled on its way to the consumer.

Pasteur became famous for saving the French wine industry when 'pasteurizing' wine to keep it from spoiling. The feat was immortalized on the chapel wall – 1863. Again, the wall contains no reference to milk! Interestingly, when was the last time you bought a bottle of wine labeled as 'pasteurized'?

Pasteurization methods for milk are usually standardized and controlled by national food safety agencies, such as the USDA in the United States and the Food Standards Agency in the United Kingdom.

Today, there are two widely used methods of pasteurizing milk:

HTST - High Temperature/Short Time

> HTST is by far the most common method. Milk labeled simply as pasteurized is usually treated with the HTST method. HTST involves holding the milk at a temperature of 145°F (62°C) for half an hour or 161.5°F (72°C) for at least 15 seconds. The HTST pasteurization processes must be designed so that the milk is heated evenly, and no part of the milk is subject to a shorter time or a lower temperature. HTST pasteurized milk typically has a refrigerated shelf life of two to three weeks.

UHT - Ultra-High Temperature

UHT involves holding the milk at a temperature of 280-285°F (138-141°C) for at least two seconds. This process actually sterilizes the milk. UHT pasteurized milk can last in the refrigerator for two to three months. When UHT pasteurization is combined with sterile handling and container technology, the milk can even be stored unrefrigerated for long periods. For those of you who like to drink UHT milk, Dr. Paul Kouchakoff determined in 1930 that the critical temperature above which milk becomes recognized by the white cells of the blood as an enemy of the body is only 88.3°C (191°F).[81]

There are different pasteurization standards for different dairy products, depending on the fat content and the intended usage. For example, the pasteurization standards for fluid milk differ from the standards for cream; the standards (heat used) for pasteurizing cheese are designed to preserve the phosphatase enzyme, which aids in curing the cheese.

Part 2: Pasteur and Pfizer – are there similarities?

"Louis Pasteur, one of the legendary figures in the history of science, lied about his research, stole ideas from a competitor and was deceitful in ways that would now be regarded as scientific misconduct if not fraud."[82] This is part of a book review that appeared in the New York Times reviewing *The Private Science of Louis Pasteur*, by Dr. Gerald L. Geison of Princeton University. Big deal! For 100 years since Pasteur's death until the publication of the New York Times article, Pasteur was a world hero, the scientist's scientist. So what if he cut some corners here and there. Why should that bother me?

Don't things like happen in other professions? For instance, let's look at some recent journalism scandals.

Who doesn't remember *Jimmy's World* a phony story about a child heroin addict? The story appeared in the Washington Post on September 29, 1980 and won a Pulitzer Prize for reporter Janet Cooke. The prize was later returned.

Newspaper reporter Jayson Blair resigned from the New York Times after admitting he faked and plagiarized dozens of stories. Jack Kelley, the ex-USA Today reporter resigned following allegations that he faked major stories.[83] I do not feel that Jack Kelley dramatically changed my life, or Jason Blair, or even Janet Cooke, who initially walked away with the Pulitzer. All of their events occurred within the last 30 years. Louis Pasteur died over 100 years ago. I should not have to be concerned if he plagiarized or lied about his research. Or should I be?

Louis Pasteur, while still alive, never released his laboratory notes. He left them to his family with instructions never to release them. With the death of his last male descendant, a grandson in 1975, they became the property of the French National Library.

Professor Geison was the first person to thoroughly review those notes; he spent 15 years studying more than 10,000 pages of lecture notes and lab workbooks.

It was not Geison's intent to discredit Pasteur or his contributions to science, but he did want to present the unadorned truth. The American Association for the History of Medicine awarded its 1996 William H. Welch Medal to Professor Geison for his suburb investigative work.

The question remains if humanity had to wait the 80 or so years following Pasteur's death to fully understand how he conducted and publicized his research. Does it significantly affect our lives today?

With today's modern technology, anyone, and I do mean anyone, can write and publish a book. You can find books on virtually every subject imaginable, with all views possible represented. Take for example the underlying subject matter of this book. There are almost an infinite number of books claiming to explain the 'real cause' of heart disease. There are a myriad of books siding with the current consensus that cholesterol is the main culprit in causing heart disease, and a growing number claiming exactly the opposite.

Anyone can write a book? I am a classic example. I am not connected to the medical profession, and here I am writing not my first book, but my second book regarding a very serious and relevant health issue. SASHA being a self-published paperback does not meet the requirements to appear on the New York Times bestseller list, nevertheless, it has obtained ranking on the major international sales outlets: Amazon, Amazon England, Amazon Germany, Barnes & Nobles, etc.

Yes, the electronic age has made it very easy for anyone not only to market a book, but for the actual writing as well. I remember when the first personal computers hit the market. The big key on the right-hand side of the keyboard was not marked with a '◄┘' as today, but with the letters 'CR'. Ask any 15-year-old computer whiz today what the CR stands for. I doubt that very few, if any, will give the correct answer. It stands for 'Carriage Return'.

For those of my generation, the CR will bring back the memory of those old Smith-Corona heavy typewriters, pounding away at those mechanical heavy keys, where each hit of the key moved the carriage physically one letter width to the right. You would arrive to the end of the line; a small bell would ring signaling for the typist to finish the present word being typed and then Trockkkk! The right-hand leaves the keyboard to slam the carriage return lever back to the left-hand side of the typewriter. The Trockkk would also advance the page to the next line according to the line spacing previously set mechanically, and the new line begins.

Pasteur – Hero or Villain?

OOOOOPS -- you made a mistake -- advance the paper forward, use your eraser shield to expose the misprinted letter and protect adjacent letters, erase it, move the paper back into the exact location on the page, and then retype the new letter.

Typewriters also advanced with technology. I remember when we had an IBM Selectric electric typewriter. Instead of having to hen peck the heavy keys, the electric touch made the actual act of typing similar to the light touch-typing of the modern computer keyboard. On the IBM Selectric, the paper remained static. There was a small metal ball embedded with all the letters, numbers and symbols that ran back and forth in place of the carriage and typed the letter. Even correcting errors became easier. Quick drying white correction fluid and the dry 'correct-o-type' sheets replaced the eraser shields and erasers.

Today, in the computer age, typing and basic editing have become a no-brainer. OOOOOPS, you made a mistake? No problem. Use your mouse to go directly to the error and retype. Change around the order? No problem. Simply 'cut and paste' and rearrange to your heart's content. Turn on the spell checker, and automatically some misprints and mistakes are clearly identified.

Writing and publishing a book was not always as easy as it is today. There was a time when a writer had to be extremely dedicated in order to present a finished manuscript in acceptable format. As a prerequisite, the subject matter of the book had to be worthy of the effort in order to find a reputable publisher.

No, humankind did not have to wait until the computer age and the Internet to read a book regarding Pasteur's method of science back in the 1800's. One of the first books published that took a serious look at the work of Pasteur in an unfavorable light was *Béchamp or Pasteur* by Ethel Douglas. The book was first published in 1923 and later revised and published in 1932 – that is more than half a century before Pasteur's lab notes were made public! Ms. Douglas had much to say regarding all of Pasteur's accomplishments listed on the wall of the chapel of the Pasteur Institute at Marnes-la-Coquette. For instance:

255

We have already seen, firstly, that in regard to fermentation in general and vinous fermentation in particular, as also in regard to silkworm disease, it is impossible to deny that Pasteur plagiarized Béchamp. Secondly, we have seen that Pasteur's experiments were insufficient to defeat the theory of spontaneous generation and that they never satisfied Sponteparists, such as Pouchet, LeBon and Batian.[84]

It is not my intention to go into any additional technical detail regarding her revelations; what bothers me is the monster that Pasteur ultimately created.

Pasteurism has become a vested interest, and one, unfortunately, supported by that powerful trade union – the Medical Fraternity[85]

Dr. Guylaine Lanctôt wrote a book called *The Medical Mafia*. The title is self-explanatory; she delves into numerous existing medical issues. Regarding her comments about Pasteur:

Pasteur was ambitious, an opportunist? He was also a genius in the art of promoting himself, and he plagiarized, and then vulgarized, the work of Béchamp. He stole the idea of small organisms being responsible, but he only revealed a small part of Béchamp's discoveries. Pasteur proclaimed that these small organisms only came from the outside. He forgot to mention that, once exposed to air, germs and other morbid (abnormal) microzymes lose their virulence very rapidly. ***And this deceit has been perpetuated ever since****.*[86] (Bold emphasis is mine.)

The point I am leading up to can best be described by Shelley and Denie Hiestand in *Electrical Nutrition: A revolutionary approach to eating that awakens the body*:

Béchamp, a man without public savvy, argued all his life that disease was caused by disharmony and imbalance of the body's natural microflora; but his boss, **Pasteur, who was being funded by his friends in the rapidly growing pharmaceutical industry**, *promoted the idea that bacteria caused disease and that bacteria could be killed by drugs.* ***Our entire germ-based microorganism-killing pharmaceutical industry grew from this erroneous scientific premise.***

On his deathbed, Pasteur apologized for deliberately taking Béchamp's research out of context so that **his institute could benefit from the funding that was coming from the newly emerging drug companies**. *In fact, he admitted that he was wrong and that Béchamp was right. By then, however,* **the drug companies and their 'kill-the-germs-at-all-cost' system is a direct legacy of this lie.**[87] (Bold emphasis is mine.)

What is the connection between Pasteur and Pfizer? Pfizer is the world's largest drug maker. Its 2006 revenues totaled over $48.3 billion.[89] Its research and development spending for the same year reached almost $7.6 Billion.[89] It manufactures Lipitor, the world's top-selling medicine, with almost $12.9 billion in annual sales.[90]

Lipitor (atorvastatin) is a member of the statin family of medicines. Statin sales in the world depend upon prolonging the 'validity' of the (blood) lipid hypothesis. Just as Pasteur benefited greatly from marketing erroneous scientific results, so has Pfizer been benefiting from the existing world belief that high cholesterol causes heart disease (lipid hypothesis).

Why did I particularly pick on Pfizer? No particular reason, simply because they are the largest and most well-known pharmaceutical company on the planet. Dr. Duane Graveline,[91] a flight surgeon and former astronaut, was a pioneer in publicizing the serious side effects caused by Lipitor which caused his two bouts of transient global amnesia (TGA).

I could have just as easily picked Merck, the manufacturer of Zocor (simvastatin) and Mevacor (lovastatin). I could have picked Bayer, the manufacturer of Baycol (cerivastatin), which was withdrawn from the market in 8/2001 due to too many fatalities; or Novartis, the manufacturer of Lescol (fluvastatin). I could have picked AstraZeneca, the manufacturer of Crestor (rosuvastatin).

I could have even picked my 'favorite', Bristol-Myers Squibb, the manufacturer of Pravachol (Pravastatin). It was a locally marketed version of Pravastatin known as Lipidal that so disrupted my professional and personal life and inspired the writing of SASHA.

23

Post Pasteur

There are two kinds of statistics, the kind you look up,
and the kind you make up.
Rex Stout

During my university days, I took several statistics courses, which included of course lessons regarding statistical testing. I remember the time when flash bulbs were still used when taking indoor pictures. The flash bulb was basically a very small light bulb; it could only be used once. The one time flash occurrence when taking the picture was the bulb's entire purpose of existence. One picture and that was it; then to the trash can and flash bulb heaven. As we learned in statistical testing, testing all the bulbs would certainly be counterproductive, as all the bulbs would be destroyed in the test.

Calcium

The successful test of pasteurization for milk is to verify that all of the enzyme phosphatase in the milk has been totally destroyed.[92] The one small problem with this test is that phosphatase is essential for the proper absorption of calcium. Do you wonder why you encounter more and more people that suffer from osteoporosis? Proper calcium levels in the body are essential for strong bones and teeth, regulating muscle and heart function among other functions. Sure, calcium is abundant in other food products besides dairy products. However, if they are also cooked, then the natural occurring phosphatase is still destroyed. Incidentally, eating foods 'fortified' with calcium doesn't guarantee that your body will automatically be able to absorb and process this form of calcium effectively. Synthetic nutrients can be toxic.[93]

Vitamins

It was stated as early as 1942 that the cows of the country produce as much vitamin C as does the entire national citrus crop, but most of it is lost as a result of pasteurization.[94] The vitamin C that does survive the pasteurization process is diluted even more in many supermarkets even before it reaches your refrigerator. Most milk is packaged in translucent plastic jugs. Many supermarkets market milk in refrigerated sections lighted by fluorescent lighting. Fluorescent lighting has been shown to destroy half of the vitamin C content of the milk.[95] Pasteurization has also been shown to destroy vitamin A (necessary to assimilate protein[96]) and greatly reduces the amount of vitamin B complex.[97]

Digestion of Fats

Pasteurization destroys lipase,[98] the enzyme that aids in the digestion of fats. Triglycerides are the main constituents of milk fat.[99] How often are we told after blood testing that our 'trigs are too high'? Carbohydrates and proteins start undergoing the pre-digestion process in the upper stomach thanks to salivary amylase and pepsin. While this is occurring, the fats, devoid of lipase, remain unaltered in the stomach for up to several hours after swallowing. When hitting the hydrochloric acid in the stomach without the benefit of pre-digestion, the fats may be improperly metabolized when they ultimately reach body tissues.[100]

Milk Sugar

Lactase is an enzyme that breaks down the milk sugar lactose into galactose and glucose.[101] Pasteurization inactivates the naturally occurring lactase in raw milk. It also destroys galactase, the enzyme needed to break down galactose. How often do we hear of people being 'lactose intolerant'?

Selenium

Selenium is an antioxidant mineral that helps regulate nitric oxide in the arteries, which is of prime importance in preventing heart disease.[102] Pasteurization reduces the availability of selenium in commercial cow's milk by 10%.[103]

Dirty, Dead Milk

Pasteurization is an excuse for the sale of low-quality, dirty milk. It discourages the effort to produce clean milk.[104] It all starts with the personal hygiene of the cow herself. As Dr. William Douglas II aptly stated, "A cow is not a cat...Cows are not neat. Their personal hygiene would embarrass a pig."[105] Producing clean milk would entail making the effort to physically clean up the teats of the cow properly before each milking. This takes time and money.

Truthfully, it is hard to blame the modern commercial dairy in this day and age. In order to survive, it has to maximize production and minimize costs. The nutritional quality of his final product is of little, if any, concern. And why should it be?

The dairyman's milk totally loses its personal identity once it leaves his diary and mixes with the milk of possibly hundreds of other diaries at the processing plant, some diaries likely much filthier than his own.

The pasteurization process involves raising the temperature of the milk to high temperatures not necessarily only once, but possibly several times to kill off all the harmful 'ingredients'. Some processes even involve steam cleaning.[106] Stated differently, due to the pasteurization process, most of the harmful junk in the milk that we would not want to drink is also dead by the time it hits our refrigerators. This is sort of like a built-in booby prize.

Pasteurized milk is therefore essentially dead milk. Pasteurization kills the natural enzymes present in raw milk and alters the protein[107] and fat. Raw milk sours when not refrigerated. Pasteurized milk, with all of its enzymes killed and protein and fat altered by the heating process, simply rots. It putrefies; it is dead before it reaches your refrigerator.

The Ultimate 'Cat' Scan

Who am I to state that raw milk is alive, and pasteurized milk is essentially dead? After all, what do I know? I am only human. In order to test this out, we will go to a non-human, however, a connoisseur of milk and milk products. This will be a true 'cat' scan, supervised by Nivi and Gray, two of the family's cats.

Nivi is intelligent as far as cats go. When hungry, instead of just meowing she jumps up to the kitchen window, stands on her hind legs and scratches continuously on the window while looking me straight in the eye. You can see Nivi in action at the bottom of web page http://www.heartrecovey.net/books2.html. Gray is Nivi's grandson (as far as I remember – it's easy to lose track…).

This 'cat' scan is opposed to the more familiar CAT (Computed Axial Tomography) scan where digital geometry processing is used to generate a three-dimensional image of internal organs.

For this particular cat scan, I prepared two glasses of milk. One glass was raw (unpasteurized) goat's milk; the other was a glass of standard HTST 3% carton milk purchased at the supermarket.

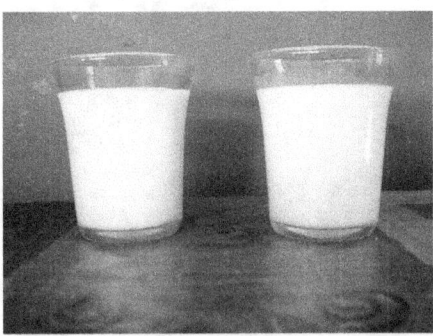

Day 1: On the left is standard 3% fresh pasteurized homogenized (cow) milk. On the right, fresh raw (unpasteurized) goat's milk. They look identical.

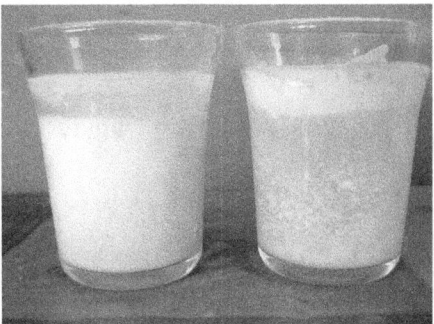

A week later at room temperature, the pasteurized milk has started to evaporate. The fresh goat's milk has separated into whey and cheese curds.

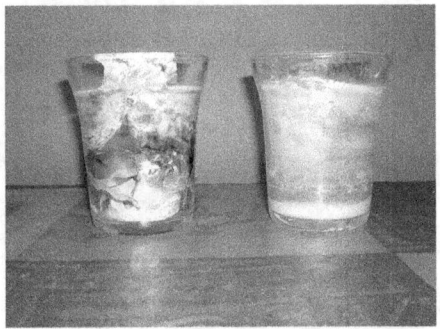

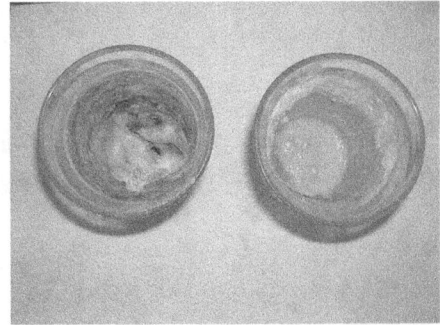

Close to two months later, the liquids have evaporated almost entirely from both glasses. What remains from the pasteurized milk is greenish/blackish 'rot'. The solids remaining from the raw goat's milk is a dry yellowish cheese.

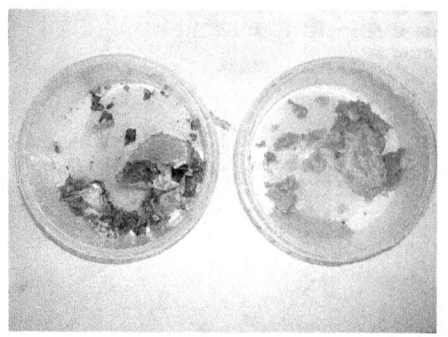
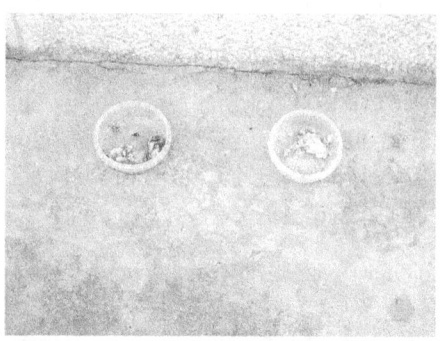

The solids are transferred to plastic bowls – bring on the cats!

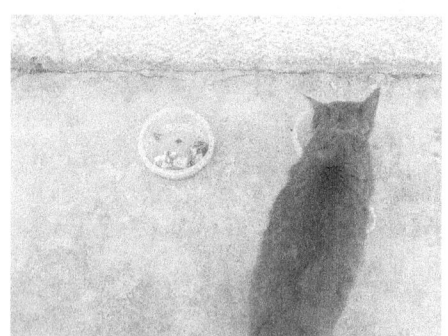
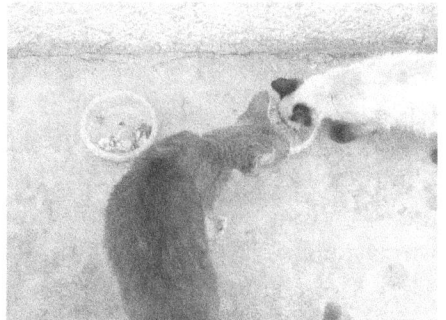

First to arrive is Gray…and one by one the 'word gets out'.

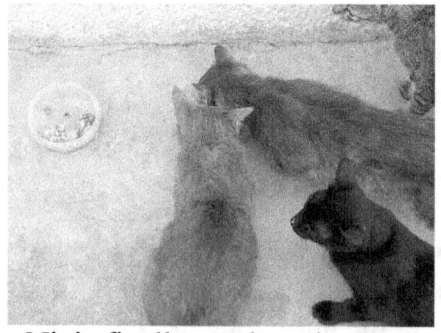
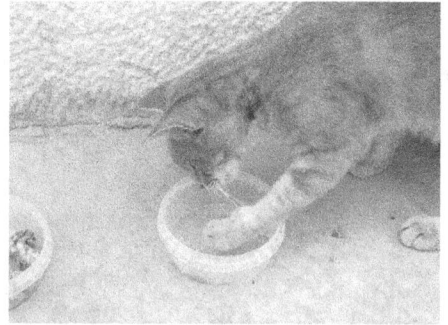

Nivi finally makes it (upper right)

Gray – finger lickin' good!

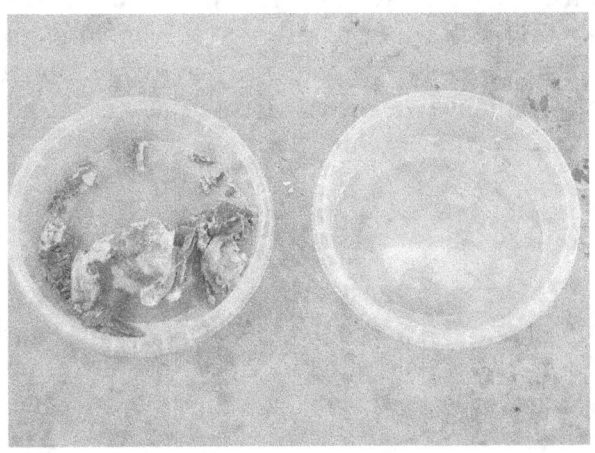

The bowl with the two-month old cheese from raw goat's milk has been licked clean. The green-black pasteurized rot remained untouched!

Why pasteurize in the first place?

Research overwhelmingly demonstrates that pasteurization creates higher rates of degenerative illnesses in both humans and in animal research.[108] For all of its heath detriments, why has pasteurization become the norm over the last 100 years? Shortly after the start of the twentieth century, the sloppy production methods, delivery through streets laden with fly infested horse manure, and lack of hygienic cool storage areas in many homes (later known as refrigerators) did result in the contamination of the raw milk. Drinking of the milk did cause a considerable amount of disease and death.

Pasteurization supplied a practical and economic solution to the ultimately disease-infected milk. It was necessary to prevent the spread of communicable disease. There was no simple way to enforce hygiene on so many small independent milk-producing farms, and then guarantee its safe delivery to the end user. As a result, the monster had overcome the creator. Once considered a wonder treatment (before pasteurization), medical literature today no longer advocates the use of raw milk diets[109] as a universal way to cure disease.

Raw milk cures have gone the route of the phonograph record and the manual typewriter. Pasteurized milk, however, is not used today to cure anything.

Epidemics and pasteurized milk

The proponents of pasteurization would have us believe that epidemics caused by milk became extinct with the widespread use of pasteurization. The U.S. government has documented numerous outbreaks of food-borne illness from pasteurized milk.[110]

1945	1,492 cases for the year in the U.S.
1945	One outbreak, 300 cases in Phoenix, Arizona
1945	Several outbreaks, 468 cases of gastroenteritis, nine deaths, in Great Bend, Kansas
1976	Outbreak of Yersinia enterocolitica in 36 children, 16 of them had appendectomies due to pasteurized chocolate milk
1978	One outbreak, 68 cases in Arizona
1982	Over 17,000 cases of Yersinia enterocolitica in Memphis, TN
1982	172 cases, with over 100 hospitalized from a three-Southern-state area
1983	One outbreak, 49 cases of Listeriosis in Massachusetts
1984	August, One outbreak S. typhimurium, approximately 200 cases, at one plant in Melrose Park, IL
1984	November, One outbreak S. typhimurium, at same plant in Melrose Park, IL
1985	March, One outbreak, 16,284 confirmed cases, at same plant in Melrose Park, IL
1985	197,000 cases of antimicrobial-resistant Salmonella

	infections from one dairy in California
1985	1,500+ cases, Salmonella culture confirmed in Northern Illinois
1987	Massive outbreak of over 16,000 culture-confirmed cases of antimicrobial-resistant Salmonella typhimurium traced to pasteurized milk in Georgia
1993	Two outbreaks statewide, 28 cases Salmonella infection
1994	Three outbreaks, 105 cases, E. Coli & Listeria in California
1993-1994	Outbreak of Salmonella enteritidis in over 200 due to pasteurized ice cream in Minnesota, South Dakota and Wisconsin
1995	1 outbreak, 3 cases in California
1995	Outbreak of Yersinia enterocolitica in ten children, three hospitalized due to post-pasteurization contamination
1996	Two outbreaks Campylobactor and Salmonella, 48 cases in California
1997	Two outbreaks, 28 cases Salmonella in California

Pasteurization is also not a magic wand able to neutralize harmful ingredients that find their way into the cows' commercial food sources. Ultimately they find their way into the milk supply...through pasteurization...to the dining room table.

The 1973 Michigan PBB (polybromylated biphenyl) disaster[111] is proof of this. PBBs are manmade chemicals that were used as fire retardants in plastics. At the time, one of the plants manufacturing PBB was the Michigan Chemical Company. The same St. Louis, Michigan plant also manufactured a magnesium oxide cattle feed supplement. According to the State of Michigan Department of Community Health, in 1973, 10 to 20 50-pound bags of PBB were accidentally sent to the Michigan Farm Bureau Service instead of the cattle feed supplement. Other sources are less conservative regarding the actual amount of PBB that made its way into cattle feed.

Five years after the contamination, about 97% of Michigan's residents showed measurable levels of the chemical. In August 1976, the Department of Public Health found that 22 of 26 samples of human breast milk from the general population in Michigan showed the presence of PBB. Later, a more scientific study detected PBB in the breast milk of 95% of nursing mothers tested in Michigan's Lower Peninsula.[112]

This is the real catastrophe of this disaster. Children who weren't even born at the time of the disaster have likely been exposed. The possible long-term health consequences remain a point of concern and uncertainty. There is no medical treatment that will lower PBB levels in the human body. Daniel Rosen from the Centers for Disease Control (CDC) in Atlanta, GA published a 1995 article in Environmental Health Perspectives citing approximately 10.8 years as the calculated half-life of PBBs within the human body.

Although not easy to calculate specific consequences due to specific amounts of human exposure to PBBs through diet, the following problems have been reported and seem to be associated with this PBB exposure:

- Musculoskeletal problems, especially joint disorders (pain, swelling, and crepitation)
- Neurological symptoms (tiredness, fatigue, headaches, dizziness, and unusually long sleep hours)
- Evidence of higher liver function
- Immunological abnormalities (decreased number of circulating lymphocytes and altered responses to tests of the functional integrity of these cells)
- Elevated levels of spontaneous abortion rates among second-generation Michigan women born after the 1973 incident

- Increased risk of cancers of the breast, the digestive system and for lymphoma
- Shorter menstrual cycle and with a longer bleed time during menstruation.

Since the late 1970's, the Michigan Department of Community Health has been keeping tabs on approximately 4,000 people, mainly families and neighbors on farms who consumed the most contaminated products, and their offspring.

Incidentally, milk products (pasteurized) and beef (cooked) were not the only products affected. Feed for other animals was contaminated when it was mixed using the same machinery; carcasses of cattle not fit for sale were rendered to yield protein supplements in other animal feed. By the end of 1975, as a result of the PBB contamination, about 28,900 cattle, 5,920 pigs, and 1.5 million chickens had been destroyed. Eight hundred and sixty-five tons of contaminated animal feed were buried around the state. In addition, 17,940 lb of cheese, 2,630 lb of butter, 34,000 lb of dry milk products, and nearly five million eggs were also destroyed.

The moral of this story: In addition to the inherent disadvantages that pasteurization causes, it also does not guarantee that the final product will be free of harmful additives.

Pasteurization is not the only problem...

Proud family-run dairy farms are quickly becoming a thing of the past. Once upon a time, dairy cows would roam the pastures, eating fresh grass to their hearts' content. Many dairy cows today are confined to small, contained areas with no grass, no sunshine, no roaming around. There were over 3.7 million dairy farms in the U.S. in 1950. By the year 2000 the number had dwindled to slightly over 105,000.[113] Some of the larger confinement farms contain thousands of cows. More than half of all the milk production today in the U.S. comes from operations containing over 500 cows.

The cows themselves have become high-production milk machines. In 1950 the average output per dairy cow was slightly less than two gallons of milk per day. Cows fed a diet high in grains and growth hormones yield over six gallons per day.[114] The high incidence of disease in cows kept in confinement facilities also results in the widespread use of antibiotics, many which are resistant to prolonged heating.[115] Nutritionally, who cares? It makes sense economically -- even to the extent that the average lifespan of today's confinement dairy cow is only 42 months; cows on pasture live 12 to 15 years.

No, cows are not cats. Also, people are not cats. However, the observations made by Dr. Pottenger (chapter 20) regarding the milk from grass-fed cows as opposed to grain-fed cows on his cats should be of great concern to us humans. Grain-fed cattle also tend to have a more acidic intestine which is more conducive to harboring pathogenic bacteria than cattle fed mostly grass and hay. Grain-fed cattle were found to have a one million-fold more acid-resistant E.coli than cattle fed hay.[116] In the previous chart, you will notice E.coli contamination was found in pasteurized milk in 1994 in California.

It is almost ironic that because many cows kept in confinement conditions are overly sick and produce inferior milk, the way to insure that this inferior milk is 'safe' for human consumption is to pasteurize it![117]

Today there is a solution for the big city dweller wanting to drink healthy raw milk. It is called certified raw milk. The term 'certified' means that the milk is inspected by a board of physicians and is certified by them to meet rigid standards of cleanliness. The cows are regularly checked and must be in PERFECT health. Before milking, they are meticulously cleaned. The workers themselves with access to a certified raw milk facility must also be in perfect health and keep themselves meticulously clean. Personal habits are under constant supervision. Frequent and regular bacterial testing insures that the milk is of the highest quality.[118]

Whole books could be written on the history and all the other aspects of raw vs. pasteurized milk in our daily diet, including politics and government meddling. In fact, they already have been! My favorites are

The Untold Story of Milk by Dr. Ron Schmid, New Trends Publishing

And

The Milk Book by Dr. William Campbell Douglass II, Rhino Publishing

Both are recommended, and no, they are by no means identical. For example, they take opposite sides on the 'homogenization' issue; i.e. is homogenization of milk a cause of heart disease?[119]

To keep abreast of what is relevant and important regarding 'real milk', visit the Real Milk Campaign of the Weston A. Price Foundation at http://www.realmilk.com.

24

Two Postulates

A postulate is a hypothesis advanced as an essential
presupposition, condition, or premise
of a train of reasoning.
Merriam-Webster Dictionary

Wikipedia defines a postulate as "a statement or assumption that is agreed by everyone to be so obvious or self-evident that no proof is necessary, and which can be used to prove other statements or theorems." Simply stated, a postulate is G-d given. Period.

In junior high geometry class, we memorized geometry Postulate #1: For any two points, there is exactly one line containing them. From this postulate, we could then prove the following theorem: Two lines intersect in at most one point.

Many things in our lives are governed by this same analogy. There is the self-evident base, on which further statements or 'theorems' are derived.

Under author's notes at the beginning of this book, I stated

"This book starts out under the premise that cholesterol and saturated fat are not the causes of heart disease. Period. End of story."

I began believing this premise when writing SASHA and since its publication, I accept it lock, stock and barrel. Stated in different terminology:

Postulate

Saturated Fat and Cholesterol do
not cause heart disease.

On this assumption, I can substantiate a theorem that foods containing saturated fat and cholesterol are not harmful to my cardiovascular system. According to this argument, I could eat anything without regard to saturated fat and cholesterol content, and I would not be harming my health. This would include of course, among other things, the whole spectrum of dairy products available in any supermarket, right? What then is logically wrong with this argument as stated?

A postulate cannot be wrong by definition. It is, after all, a postulate, an axiom. I am convinced that pasteurized dairy products with the natural nutriments and enzymes missing do have a definite place in the myriad of health problems plaguing the Western world today, heart disease among them. Something is wrong with the theorem; therefore there must be something lacking in the postulate.

The type and form of the saturated fat/cholesterol that most people consume does not fit the postulate! Dr. Howell stated that when commercial fat deprived of its lipase companion confronts hydrochloric acid in the stomach, it faces a harsh experience and may be improperly metabolized when it reaches body tissues later.[120]

Conclusion: the theorem 'foods containing saturated fat and cholesterol are not harmful to my cardiovascular system' is not entirely valid so therefore cannot be automatically derived from Postulate #1 as stated. We will need to use an additional postulate and modify the first postulate to be correct in all cases.

Postulate 2

Saturated fat and cholesterol from processed/heated foods **can** cause heart disease.

Modification of Postulate 1:

Postulate 1

Saturated fat and cholesterol from raw unprocessed foods **do not** cause heart disease.

The irony of it all is that my cardiologist and all the other doctors still advocating the validity of the lipid hypothesis have been saying all along that saturated fat and cholesterol cause heart disease. Two very similar sounding postulates. Two very different consequences. So similar, but so different.

25

A Very Thin Chapter on Fats

The first law of dietetics seems to be:
if it tastes good, it's bad for you.
Isaac Asimov

The polyunsaturated fats paradox, or is it?

For decades the anti-saturated fat and anti-cholesterol campaign has been accompanied by the pro-polyunsaturated fat agenda. As recently as August 2003, the USDA was still carrying the polyunsaturated heart healthy banner 'polyunsaturated fatty acids have been linked to lower incidences of heart disease'.[121] This particular article did later mention the dark sides of polyunsaturated fats, i.e. lacking strong stability traits and being prone to oxidation, however, it did seem to stress the positive 'lower incidences of heart disease'.

Here in Israel, we have the dubious distinction of having one of the highest dietary polyunsaturated/saturated fat ratios in the world. We consume 8% more omega-6 polyunsaturated fatty acids than in the USA, and 10-12% higher than in most European countries. According to USDA guidelines we should be heart disease free. Instead we suffer from a high prevalence of cardiovascular diseases and hypertension. This was published in an article entitled *Diet and disease--the Israeli paradox: possible dangers of a high omega-6 polyunsaturated fatty acid diet.*[122]

What drew my attention to this article was a key word in the title 'paradox'. Merriam-Webster gives several definitions for the word 'paradox':

> *a statement that is seemingly contradictory or opposed to common sense and yet is perhaps true*

and also

> *an argument that apparently derives self-contradictory conclusions by valid deduction from acceptable premises*

Wikipedia states:

> *A paradox is an apparently true statement or group of statements that leads to a contradiction or a situation which defies intuition.*

The bottom line: there is no paradox here. As we shall see, the quantity and quality of the polyunsaturated fats in the Western diet is neither heart friendly or healthy.

Plaque rupture

Plaque rupture (rupture of scar tissue covering an atheroma – chapter 26) is a major trigger of acute coronary events. Sixty to seventy percent of acute coronary syndromes evolve from mildly to moderately obstructive atherosclerotic plaques.[123] The promoters of the prevalent lipid hypothesis would have us believe that aortic plaque formation is caused by eating cholesterol and saturated fat.

Atherosclerotic plaques contain a disproportionately high concentration of the omega-6 fatty acid linoleic acid; plaque content of linoleic acid correlates with dietary intake, in particular **polyunsaturated vegetable oils**. Higher plaque concentrations of linoleic acid are also associated with an increased likelihood of plaque rupture.[124]

What is the connection between saturated fats, poly-unsaturated fat and plaque formation? In 1994, Dr. Carl V. Felton et al summarized this quite nicely:

> *No associations were found with saturated fatty acids. These findings imply a direct influence of dietary polyunsaturated fatty acids on aortic plaque formation and suggest that **current trends favouring increased intake of polyunsaturated fatty acids should be reconsidered**.*[125] (Bold emphasis is mine.)

These findings were confirmed again in 2001 in a later study.[126]

Essential Fatty Acids

In SASHA I discussed the importance of steering clear of all partially hydrogenated oils and the resulting trans-fat. This is only the beginning.

Essential Fatty Acids (EFAs) are fats the body absolutely needs but does not have the ability to produce; hence the term 'essential'. Therefore, they must be obtained from the diet. The body needs only **small quantities** of EFAs for normal functioning.[127]

EFAs allow the entry into cells of important nutrients as well as the removal of toxins from the cells. In addition, EFAs are converted to substances that affect cell growth, platelet aggregation (blood clotting ability) and blood pressure, subjects of prime importance to cardiovascular health.

We have all heard of omega-3 and omega-6 fats. These are both EFAs and belong to the polyunsaturated family of fats. EFAs are used to make two classes of hormone like substances known as the prostaglandins. Prostaglandins derived from omega-6 EFAs (prostaglandin-1) typically stimulate the immune system (coagulation) and help form blood clots. Prostaglandins derived from omega-3 (prostaglandin-3) EFAs typically down regulate the immune response to maintain blood fluidity.

Our ancestors consumed a diet with a 1:1 – 3:1 balance[128] between the omega-6 and omega-3 essential fatty acids. It is speculated that in today's Western society the ratio of omega-6/omega-3 fatty acids may be as high as 20:1 - 30:1.[129] Excessive amounts of omega-6 polyunsaturated fatty acids and a very high omega-6/omega-3 ratio promotes the pathogenesis of many diseases, including cardiovascular and inflammatory disease; a lower omega-6/omega-3 ratio exerts suppressive effects.[130]

EFAs, which are polyunsaturated fats, are vitally essential for human health; on the other hand, we see that accumulated plaque in our arteries and the resulting heart disease is polyunsaturated fat intensive.

Is it only a wrong balance of omega-6/omega-3 that is causing the accumulation of the polyunsaturated junk in our arteries? Modern medicine has found a simple solution for today's omega-6/omega-3 imbalance – we should all consume more omega-3 rich foods, such as fish oil supplements. History has taught us that easy one-sided solutions can often be counterproductive, if not outright dangerous.

The last two generations were weaned on the theory that HDL is 'good' cholesterol and LDL is 'bad' cholesterol; basically we were taught that fat in general is bad. Two decades of statins to lower LDL and fats in the blood to prevent heart disease did indeed lower LDL levels, but did not curb the heart disease epidemic.

A Very Thin Chapter on Fats

The last two generations were taught that salt is 'unnecessary' – it causes high blood pressure. Supermarkets today even sell salt-free salt substitutes. It wasn't until professional athletes started suffering (even dying) from hyponatremia (low concentration of sodium in the blood) that the importance of proper salt intake was accepted.

We all 'know' that as far as breathing is concerned, oxygen is 'good' and carbon dioxide (CO_2) is 'bad'. We inhale the good and exhale the bad. Dr. Konstantin Buteyko has demonstrated that there must be enough carbon dioxide in our systems for the oxygen to circulate effectively; long term over-breathing (hyperventilation) ultimately leads to organ damage and the development of illnesses.[131]

And now the latest fad, unmonitored omega-3 supplementation to correct our imbalance.

Basic View of Polyunsaturated Fatty Acids (PUFA)

Omega-3	Omega-6
Alpha-Linolenic Acid (ALA) *	Linoleic Acid (LA) *
Eicosapentaenoic acid (EPA) **	Arachidonic Acid (AA) **
Docosahexaenoicacid (DHA) **	Gamma Linolenic Acid (GLA)**
* Essential Fatty Acid ** Conditional Fatty Acid	

There are three major forms of omega-3 EFAs that are contained in the foods we eat that are used by the body: alpha-linolenic acid (ALA), eicosapentaenoic acid (EPA), and docosahexaenoic acid (DHA). Once eaten, the body can convert some of the ALA to EPA and DHA, although in small quantities (DHA in very small quantities). Higher omega-6 to omega-3 ratios in the diet reduces this conversion further.[132] Not everyone is capable of converting some ALA to EPA and DHA.

For this reason, EPA and DHA are known as conditional essential fatty acids.

Fatty fishes supply EPA and DHA. The human brain has a high requirement for DHA. Low DHA levels have been linked to low brain serotonin levels.[133]

No doubt, obtaining enough omega-3 is important.

The main omega-6 fatty acids are linoleic acid (LA) and arachadonic Acid (AA). The body normally makes AA from LA. It is also found in animal foods (animal fats and dairy). The body can also produce GLA from LA; however, trans-fatty acids and over consumption of sugar and alcohol inhibit the production of GLA.[134]

Stating that omega-6 causes blood coagulation while omega-3 maintains blood fluidity is oversimplifying the way our body works, and the interaction between processes. AA just happens to be the precursor to prostacyclin, the most potent anti-aggretory agent[135] (a natural blood thinner). Omega-3 and omega-6 eicosanoids* work together in a complementary manner. There is a synergistic effect of omega-3 and omega-6 at low doses which is greater than the effect of high dose of omega-3 alone.[136]

Yes, adequate omega-3 intake is important, but to what extent?

The brain and nervous system, comprising 3% of the total body weight, contains a 1:1 ratio of omega-6 to omega-3 tissue composition.[137] Skin, comprising of 4% of total body weight, contains virtually no omega-3.[138] All the fatty acids in skin tissue are composed of omega-6. Organs and other tissues with 9% of total body weight are made up of a 4:1 omega-6 to omega-3 ratio. Body fat accounts for 15-35% (usually) of total body weight and is comprised of a 22:1 omega-6 to omega-3 ratio. Muscle accounting for approximately 50% of body weight

---

* Derived from omega-3 or omega-6 fats. They exert complex control over many bodily systems, including inflammatory and blood-thinning functions.

contains from 5.5 to 7.5 times more omega-6 than omega-3, depending on the degree of physical condition.[139]

The problem with most of the omega-6 fatty acids that we consume is that they are already harmful even before we consume them! One of the forms of omega-6 (linoleic acid aka LA) is found in the primary oil added to most processed foods. It is also contained in significant amounts in many of the commonly used home cooking oils such as corn oil, safflower oil, soybean oil, and sunflower oil. The modern processing of the major sources of omega-6 in our diets involves high temperatures and pressure (most vegetable oils) which has hydrogenated them into trans-fats or adulterated them with chemicals and preservatives.

This does extend the shelf life which may be great for all the middlemen along the way; however it is very harmful to the final consumer.

Here we get to the crux of the problem. By simply supplementing our diets with important omega-3 rich fish oil, we are not solving the problem of ingesting defective quantities of omega-6!

Polyunsaturated fats are susceptible to oxidation; it is the oxidation of LDL which gives LDL its bad reputation. Oxidized LDL is a predictor of atherosclerosis and cardiovascular disease.[140] LDL cholesterol by itself is not.

The LDL serves as a mode of transportation; it is the natural transporter of omega-6 and omega-3 into the cells. Consider the case of jet planes (carrier, mode of transportation) and hijackers. A plane itself carries all passengers; it does not differentiate between law-abiding citizens and murderous hijackers. Sure, we could ban all flights in order to fight the threat of hijacking. Does that sound like a logical solution? I think not.

If the EFAs we consume (polyunsaturated fats in vegetable oils) are already damaged and/or become oxidized, then simply lowering the 'mode of transportation' (LDL) to carry less EFAs and supplementing our diets with healthy omega-3 is not really solving the problem. Without elaborating on all the factors that contribute to the oxygenation of LDL, I want to emphasize again that **oxidized** LDL, and not regular LDL is a predictor of atherosclerosis and cardiovascular disease.[141]

Our creator did a magnificent job in creating us -- so many intertwined and interdependent systems. Our bodies are programmed to regulate levels of sodium, calcium and glucose to within certain limits. There must be a very good reason why our bodies were not equipped with any mechanism whatsoever to also regulate levels of cholesterol.

I will finish this chapter with a final word regarding ratios and total amounts. Olive oil, for example, is not polyunsaturated oil; it is monounsaturated oil. It is considered to be healthy oil, and is the basis of the 'Mediterranean diet'.

On the following chart[142] we see that the omega-6 to omega-3 ratio is still considered to be high – even higher than soybean oil.

Oil	Omega-6/Omega-3 Ratio
Sunflower oil	No Omega-3
Safflower oil	202:1
Corn oil	71:1
Olive oil	11:1
Soybean oil	7:1

I want to distinguish between high omega-6 to omega-3 *ratio*, and actual *amount*. In the following charts, the total amount of omega-6 and omega-3 is listed as grams per teaspoon:

Oil	Grams per teaspoon	
	Omega-6	Omega-3
Safflower oil,	10.1	0.05
Corn oil	7.9	0.11
Sunflower oil	8.95	
Soybean oil,	6.95	0.93
Olive oil	1.12	0.1

You may notice that a big advantage to olive oil is that is does not contribute to the overall total body unfavorable omega-6 to omega-3 ratio; its ratio is indeed unfavorable, however, the absolute quantities of both are low. Without getting into a discussion over the virtues of olive oil, it could also be said that olive oil is simply not as bad as the other oils.

We will return to polyunsaturated fats and Essential Fatty Acids in Chapter 34.

26

What's New Since SASHA?

You do not really understand something unless you can
explain it to your grandmother.
Albert Einstein

We all know what arteries are. I have mentioned them throughout this book. We visualize them as very small garden hoses; hoses transport water, arteries transport blood. Here the similarity ends. Whereas a garden hose is one thick layer of a single material, an artery is comprised of several different layers and cell types. Of particular importance to us are the cells that line the interior surface of blood vessels, known as 'endothelial cells'. Endothelial cells line the entire circulatory system, from the heart to the smallest capillary. This layer comprised of endothelial cells is known as the 'endothelium'.

Endothelial cells are involved in many aspects of cardiovascular health, such as atherosclerosis, formation of new blood vessels, blood clotting and blood pressure control.

Plaque that accumulates within arteries forms between the endothelium and the outer layers. It does not form on the inner surface of the artery.[143] When the plaque accumulates to

284

the point where it causes a bulge protruding the inner wall into the bloodstream, this bulge is known as an atheroma.

We will encounter endothelial cells/function extensively throughout the rest of this book.

The NIH Golomb Study

It was the NIH study[144] chaired by Prof. Beatrice Golomb regarding the negative side effects caused by statins that alerted me to the source of my dysfunction during my two statin-taking years. Among the complaints she was researching that affected me personally were memory loss, personality changes, irritability, and cognitive problems.

Today, recognition of the adverse effects caused by statins has emerged from underground and is well documented. What I do want to stress are her findings regarding a separate and serious problem suffered by the statin victims. The ignorance and/or denial of the medical community regarding adverse side effects which simply compounds the personal distress and frustration of the statin victim:

Patients perceived that physicians failed to appreciate the impact of the statin adverse effects on their quality of life. Statements attributed to physicians by many patients included: denial of existence of any statin adverse effects, denial of specific statin adverse effects (muscle, memory, neuropathy), attribution of symptoms to age, attribution of symptoms to "imagination", and dismissal of the importance of symptoms. ..... Subjects' responses suggest that many physicians may be unfamiliar with the spectrum of adverse events even for widely used preventive agents; and that physicians may be perceived to convey a lack of appreciation of the impact of symptoms on patients.[145]

EDTA Chelating Therapy

EDTA Chelating Therapy is not something new; I discussed it briefly in SASHA in 2004. Chelating therapy is very effective for people suffering from heavy metal poisoning; the process removes the excess heavy metals from the body. Its application utilizing the synthetic compound EDTA (ethylenediaminetetraacitic acid) can be utilized to improve the condition of patients suffering from clogged arteries. EDTA therapy itself consists of least 20 (generally) intravenous injections, each injection lasting several hours once or twice per week, given over the course of months. The purpose of the therapy is to 'chelate out' part of the accumulated plaque built up in arteries.

Mainstream cardiology has not embraced EDTA Chelating Therapy as a way to improve patients suffering from a variety of cardiovascular ailments. Cardiologists who are at least familiar with the procedure dismiss the process as not proven, ineffective, and dangerous. As such, it is performed at private, 'alternative' clinics. Mainstream cardiology still prefers angioplasty, PCI (stents) and bypass operations as solutions to arteries suffering from impaired flow.

Is EDTA ineffective and dangerous? "Not so," states Dr. Joel Kauffman. He evaluated dozens of clinical trials and concluded that over 87% of patients who have undergone EDTA Chelating Therapy improved.[148] In addition, no ill effects occurred when the procedure was performed correctly.

Will EDTA Chelating Therapy someday be accepted by mainstream cardiology and not remain underground? The future does look encouraging. In 2003, the National Center for Complementary and Alternative Medicine (NCCAM), a part of NIH, initiated a placebo-controlled, double-blind five-year study involving about 2,000 participants.[148] This study, which will cost approximately $30 million, is over 20 times larger than any previous study of EDTA Chelating Therapy. It is designed to be large enough to detect if there are indeed benefits or risks associated with the therapy.

Aspirin inhibits production of GLA

In the previous chapter I discussed the importance of the Essential Fatty Acids. Aspirin inhibits the enzyme Delta-6 Desaturase,[148] needed for the production of Gamma-Linoleic Acid (GLA) and important anti-inflammatory prostaglandins. GLA is of particular importance to people suffering from heart disease. It is metabolized to Dihomogamma Linlenic Acid (DGLA) which ultimately produces anti-inflammatory eicosanoids.[149] A study published in 1998 concluded that a combination of GLA and EPA polyunsaturated essential fatty acids produced a statistically significant reduction in systolic blood pressure.[150]

GLA is beneficial not only to heart patients. A deficiency in essential fatty acids, including GLA and EPA, can lead to severe bone loss and osteoporosis. Clinical studies have reported that supplements of GLA and EPA help maintain or increase bone mass.[151]

Many women suffer from Premenstrual Syndrome (PMS). PMS is characterized by breast tenderness, feelings of depression, irritability and swelling and bloating due to fluid retention. GLA supplementation proved to be highly effective in the treatment of women suffering from PMS.[152]

Millions of people take aspirin as a preventative measure against having a first heart attack or preventing a second one. I wonder how many of them have been advised to reinforce their diets with GLA. For this large population, GLA is no longer a conditional EFA; it has become an unconditional essential fatty acid, and must be consumed in the diet.

LDL levels and Statins

In 2001, I was advised to make sure my LDL levels stayed below 100. This was the reason why my Pravastatin (statin) dosage was increased from 10mg/day to 20mg/day; my LDL blood levels had surpassed the 100 threshold. For many years, high LDL cholesterol has been the accepted yardstick by family doctors and cardiologists for the off the cuff evaluation that we are in the high-risk category for heart problems.

Statins are *extremely* effective in reducing the blood level of LDL. The standard opening line when sitting across from a cardiologist is 'Let's see those cholesterol stats', and in particular, 'What about the LDL level?'

In 2005, the American Heart Association (AHA) along with the National Heart, Lung, and Blood Institute (NHLBI) published new guidelines[153] regarding recommended acceptable LDL Cholesterol Levels. For people diagnosed as moderate risk, the maximum level of LDL was set at 130mg/dL.

High-risk patients were defined as having established atherosclerotic CVD, diabetes, or ten-year risk for CHD > 20%. The recommended maximum level of LDL for high-risk people was set at 100mg/dL. Very high-risk patients were defined as likely to have major CVD events during the next few years or already had recent acute coronary syndromes or have established CHD in addition to other multiple major risk factors. The recommended maximum level of LDL for very high-risk people was set at 70mg/dL.

Until fairly recently, the cardiology world attributed cardiovascular benefits of statins to their LDL lowering abilities. This in turn strengthened the proponents of the lipid hypothesis. Recent (mid-2006, 2007) research papers appearing in peer reviewed scientific journals are finally acknowledging and stating emphatically that **beneficial cardiovascular effects of statins are independent of their LDL lowering properties**.

Medicine is a science, and changes to prevailing scientific consensus apparently never come easy. Galileo

Galilei, known today simply as Galileo, is often referred to as the 'father of modern astronomy', as the 'father of modern physics', and even as the 'father of science'. His support of the Copernican astronomy concept (sun-centered solar system) was considered to be on the border of heresy by the all-powerful Catholic Church during his time. The possible consequences of such actions are obvious.

Sure, you must be thinking -- we are more civilized today then our predecessors of 400 years ago. But are we really? In SASHA I discussed Dr. Kilmer McCully's research, which was not in line with the medical consensus. He concluded that cholesterol, particularly LDL cholesterol, was not a cause of heart disease. His research centered on homocysteine levels and ultimately resulted in his banishment from Harvard University and Massachusetts General Hospital. He was denied a new position for more than two years because of his research.[154]

This change of direction on the part of medical researchers regarding the cholesterol-independent benefits of statins is of such major importance that I will list a number of the works here. Bold emphasis is mine.

- *The benefits observed with statin treatment appear to be greater than what might be expected from reduction in lipid levels alone, suggesting effects beyond cholesterol lowering.* ***These cholesterol-independent effects have been called "pleiotropic".*** *The cholesterol-independent or "pleiotropic" effects of statins involve improvement of endothelial function, stability of atherosclerotic plaques, decrease of oxidative stress and inflammation, and inhibition of thrombogenic response. These pleiotropic effects of statins have been proposed as key properties of these drugs to reduce cardiovascular morbidity and mortality*[155]

- *..... statins, have been reported to exert actions independent of their lipid-lowering effects....*

289

*...Cerivastatin reduces monocyte adhesion to vascular endothelium under physiological flow conditions via down regulation of integrin adhesion molecules and inhibition of actin polymerization via RhoA inactivation. Our findings have **important implications for the lipid-independent effects of statins**.*[156]

- *With an increase in use and popularity, a number of beneficial actions of the statins unrelated to their cholesterol-lowering ability have been reported. .... Of central focus in this paper is the **cholesterol-independent benefit** of this group of agents on the cardiovascular system, particularly on the lowering of systemic blood pressure.*[157]

- *Acute coronary syndromes involve a complex interplay between the vessel wall, inflammatory cells, and the coagulation cascade. **Statins possess beneficial effects that are independent of low-density lipoprotein cholesterol lowering** and that have favorable effects on inflammation, the endothelium, and the coagulation cascade. There is now accumulating evidence that these lipid-independent pleiotropic effects are clinically relevant in the management of acute coronary syndromes.*[158]

- *Inflammation contributes importantly to all stages of atherosclerosis, including the onset of acute thrombotic complications. ...... Moreover, **statins have been shown to possess several pleiotropic properties independent of cholesterol lowering** in experimental settings.*[159]

- *Statins decrease mortality in patients with coronary artery disease. However, chronic heart failure (CHF) patients were often excluded in such trials. Statins possess pharmacologic properties (independent of cholesterol lowering) that may be* **beneficial on ventricular remodeling** *in such patients.* [160]

- *Macrophage cyclooxygenase-2 (COX-2) plays an important role in prostaglandin E2 and thromboxane A2 production. Statins are inhibitors of HMG CoA (3-Hydroxy-3-methylglutaryl coenzyme A) reductases and cholesterol synthesis, which block the expression of several inflammatory proteins* **independent of their capacity to lower endogenous cholesterol.** [161]

- *Accelerated coronary arteriosclerosis remains a major problem for the long-term survival of cardiac transplant recipients....... HMG-CoA reductase inhibitors, or statins, are widely prescribed to lower plasma cholesterol level. Accumulating evidence indicates* **that statins have various effects on vascular cells which are independent of their lipid-lowering effect.** [162]

- *Statins, the most widely prescribed cholesterol-lowering drugs, are considered to be first-line therapeutics for the prevention of coronary heart disease and atherosclerosis.........This article summarizes these* **cholesterol-lowering-independent effects of statins**, *termed "pleiotropic effects", and the underlying mechanisms, as well as the preclinical experimental approaches that would be useful to evaluate the effects of statins.* [163]

- *3-Hydroxy-3-methylglutaryl coenzyme A (HMG-CoA) reductase inhibitors* **(statins) exhibit a wide variety of anti-atherogenic* effects that may be independent of their property to lower plasma cholesterol.** ....

---

* Fatty degeneration of the inner coat of the arteries, an abnormal fatty deposit in an artery

The present findings suggest that statin-mediated immunomodulation by inhibiting MIP-1alpha could contribute to the beneficial effects of statin therapy independent of lowering plasma cholesterol. [164]

- *Statins are effective drugs in the prevention of cardiovascular disease. Recent studies suggested that* **statins have additional beneficial effects on the vascular wall independent of their cholesterol-lowering effects**. *......... The finding that atorvastatin inhibited ACE upregulation may represent a novel pleiotropic action and an additional beneficial effect of statins in treatment of cardiovascular disease.* [165]

- *Support for pleiotropic effects of statins in these trials has been provided not only by these acute effects but also by apparent differences in efficacy between various statin regimens that seem unrelated to their effects on serum cholesterol levels....... This article reviews some of the key statin trials in ACS and assesses the evidence for benefits of these* **drugs independent of their effects on LDL cholesterol.** [166]

- *Statins are the 3-hydroxy-3-methylglutaryl coenzyme A reductase inhibitors that function as potent inhibitors of cholesterol biosynthesis and have been used for many years for the treatment of hypercholesterolemia. However, accumulating experimental and clinical studies have revealed that the* **health benefits associated with statins treatment, particularly those conferred on the cardiovascular system, were the cholesterol-independent** [167]

- *Inflammation plays a key role in progression and destabilization of atherosclerotic plaque. 18F-fluorodeoxyglucose PET is a promising tool for visualizing inflammation of atherosclerotic plaque. Antiinflammatory action is one of* **the pleiotropic** *effects of statins. .... 18F-fluorodeoxyglucose PET visualized plaque inflammation and simvastatin attenuated it. The* **LDL-C-independent effects** *of simvastatin may participate in the beneficial effect.*[168]

- *Recently, it has been reported that 3-hydroxy-3-methylglutaryl coenzyme A (HMG-CoA) reductase* **inhibitors (statins) exhibit vasoprotective effects, which are independent of their cholesterol-lowering effects.**[169]

- *Statins inhibit cholesterol synthesis and produce pleiotropic,* **cholesterol-independent effects including endothelial NO synthase** *(eNOS) stimulation and increased expression.*[170]

- ***Statins produce cholesterol-independent, anti-inflammatory effects,*** *which result at least in part from increased endothelial nitric oxide production*[171]

- *The 3-hydroxy-3-methyl-glutaryl coenzyme A (HMG-CoA) reductase inhibitors are widely prescribed for hyperlipidemia, but they also* **exhibit anti-inflammatory actions that appear to be independent of their suppressive actions on plasma cholesterol levels.**[172]

- *Besides the action on plasma lipid levels, statins show a series of ancillary effects defined as all of their* **vascular and nonvascular effects independent from the cholesterol reduction.**[173]

- *Subgroup analyses of large clinical trials, however, have suggested that the beneficial effects of statins may extend to mechanisms beyond cholesterol reduction. Indeed, recent experimental and clinical evidence indicates that some of the* **cholesterol-independent or "pleiotropic" effects of statins** *may be mediated through improving or restoring* *endothelial function, enhancing the stability of atherosclerotic plaques, and decreasing oxidative stress and vascular inflammation.*[174]

In the beginning of this section I discussed the AHA and NHLBI recommendation for maximum LDL level of 130mg/dL for people at only 'moderate risk' and 70mg/dL for 'very high risk'.

- *Recent national recommendations have proposed that physicians should titrate lipid therapy to achieve low-density lipoprotein (LDL) cholesterol levels less than 1.81 mmol/L (<70mg/dL) for patients at very high cardiovascular risk and less than 2.59 mmol/L (<100mg/dL) for patients at high cardiovascular risk. .... For those with LDL cholesterol levels less than 3.36 mmol/L (<130mg/dL), the authors found no clinical trial subgroup analyses or valid cohort or case-control analyses suggesting that the degree to which LDL cholesterol responds to a statin independently predicts the degree of cardiovascular risk reduction. .... Clear, compelling evidence supports near-universal empirical statin therapy in patients at high cardiovascular risk (regardless of their natural LDL cholesterol values***), but current clinical evidence does not demonstrate that titrating lipid therapy to achieve proposed low LDL cholesterol levels is beneficial or safe.***[175]

- *Therefore, we could find no experimental evidence suggesting that the degree of LDL cholesterol reduction is an independent predictor of cardiovascular risk if LDL cholesterol level is less than 3.36 mmol/L (<130 mg/dL).......In this review, we found no high-quality clinical evidence to support currently proposed treatment goals for LDL cholesterol...... **We could find no published high-quality clinical evidence supporting*** *titration of lipid therapy based on proposed LDL cholesterol targets.*[176]

Statins do indeed reduce LDL levels. So what? LDL levels do not cause heart disease. I adapted this agenda as a way of life when writing SASHA. Statins do have beneficial effects for people with heart disease. Does this mean I am like many mainstream cardiologists who ponder 'Should statins, like fluoride, be added to our drinking water?'[177] Anyone who has read SASHA can guess what my answer to that would be. We will return to the statin discussion shortly.

Torcetrapib

Since Dr. Ancel Keys' 1953 so-called proof[178] that fat intake was the cause of death from coronary heart disease in his infamous 'six-country study', the cardiologic world has been searching for ways to lower fat and blood cholesterol, particularly the 'bad' LDL. Why did I label his study as 'infamous'? Dr. Keys actually had access to, and ignored, the data from an additional 16 countries; tabulation of data from all 22 countries would have confirmed that his six-country study proved nothing.[179]

Statins, which have been with us for two decades are extremely effective in reducing the level of 'bad' LDL; yet cardiovascular disease, remains the biggest cause of death in the United States. According to the American Heart Association, in every year since 1900 except 1918, CVD accounted for more deaths than any other single cause or group of causes of death in the United States.[180]

Why is mainstream cardiology unsuccessful in preventing so many deaths due to cardiovascular causes? Apparently, another 'trick' was necessary in addition to simply lowering the 'bad' LDL. Pfizer, the maker of Lipitor (LDL lowering statin), the world's best selling medication, came up with an idea of pulling an additional magic rabbit out of the pharmaceutical hat. This new rabbit -- a drug intended to increase levels of the 'good' HDL.

Pfizer was destined to become the savior of all those worried about cardiovascular diseases by supplying us with Lipitor to reduce the LDL, and a new drug which it started developing in the early 1990's named torcetrapib to raise the HDL. We would all become cardiovascular supermen!

The cardiology world was excited about the potential of this latest development. In February 2006, a leading Spanish pharmaceutical journal jumped on the bandwagon and had this to say about torcetrapib.

> *Torcetrapib, a CETP inhibitor, has been shown to be effective, safe and well tolerated when used in combination with atorvastatin therapy. Torcetrapib has been shown to increase HDL cholesterol levels by 46% when given alone and by 61% when given in combination with atorvastatin, as well as to decrease LDL cholesterol levels by more than that achieved by atorvastatin alone. When the dosage of torcetrapib was doubled (at maximum tolerated dose), HDL increased by over 100%. Combination therapy appeared safe and well tolerated.* [181]
> (Atorvastatin is the generic name for Lipitor)

And then the bubble burst!

"Doctors leading a global war on heart disease say they are *devastated* by the loss of a new drug they had expected to be an important weapon in the fight against high cholesterol."[182] This is how USA TODAY conveyed the feeling of mainstream cardiologists upon Pfizer's discontinuation of its new HDL increasing wonder drug torcetrapib. Pfizer had hoped to receive final FDA approval to market torcetrapib in the second half of 2007. MSNBC news used similar terms in its description, 'The news is *devastating* to Pfizer...'[183]

Merriam-Webster gives two main definitions for the word 'devastate':

- as to bring to ruin or desolation by violent action
- to reduce to chaos, disorder, or helplessness

According to USA TODAY one might think that doctors are no longer capable of functioning after the Pfizer announcement; according to MSNBC, one might think that Pfizer was forced into bankruptcy. Although Pfizer's stocks may have taken a bit of a beating, Pfizer, which has over 100,000 employees, annual sales of $50 billion and a $7 billion annual research budget,[184] is far from going under.

Pfizer's decision to scrap the torcetrapib project was not a pleasant decision. Since the early 1990's, it had invested close to $1,000,000,000 in torcetrapib's development. That is one billion dollars down the drain! One billion dollars can buy 50,000 brand new Ford Mustangs or over 330 million gallons of gasoline. That is one huge investment to scrap.

A late phase of a large-scale clinical trial that Pfizer hoped would prove the effectiveness and safety of the new drug was not yielding the results Pfizer hoped for. An independent board monitoring the torcetrapib trial counted 82 deaths among the patients who took the drug and 51 deaths in the group who did not take the drug.

The board called on Pfizer to halt the trial. Pfizer agreed and promptly notified the FDA and doctors who had been giving their patients the drug.[185] In addition to the 31 more deaths among the people taking torcetrapib, other discrepancies were seen in a number of patients suffering heart failure and other problems.

Two studies published during the first months of 2007 had this to say about torcetrapib:

- *In patients with familial hypercholesterolemia, the use of torcetrapib with atorvastatin, as compared with atorvastatin alone, did not result in further reduction of progression of atherosclerosis, as assessed by a combined measure of carotid arterial-wall thickness, and was associated with progression of disease in the common carotid segment. These effects occurred despite a large increase in HDL cholesterol levels and a substantial decrease in levels of LDL cholesterol and triglycerides.*[186]

- *The CETP inhibitor torcetrapib was associated with a substantial increase in HDL cholesterol and decrease in LDL cholesterol. It was also associated with an increase in blood pressure, and there was no significant decrease in the progression of coronary atherosclerosis.*[187]

Doctors are **devastated**, Pfizer is **devastated**, but what about those 82 families who hoped that torcetrapib would be the redeemer of their loved ones? These are the people who have the right to feel **devastated**.

Undoubtedly they all signed waivers before the trial confirming that they understood the risks they faced when taking experimental medicines in clinical trials. It is not easy to refuse when being asked by a doctor, who likely saved your life, to participate in a study of this type.

In 2001, while still hospitalized, I also 'agreed' to participate in the now defunct Princess study. The drug that was on trial at the time was a statin called 'Baycol' (cerivastatin). Very shortly after I started taking my daily dosage (at the time I had no way of knowing if I was taking the actual Baycol or a placebo), the project was halted worldwide because of similar reasons -- too many deaths.

Regarding those unfortunate 82 who died while taking torcetrapib, it is of little condolence that due to their low LDL and high HDL levels, they died 'healthy'.

Stents

The implantation of the stent is known medically as PCI (Percutaneous Coronary Intervention). The development of this process was an incredible achievement of technology. Just think about it. Someone arrives to the emergency room in the midst of a heart attack. After stabilizing the condition with proper medication, blood thinners, clot dissolvers, blood vessel expanding medication and the like, a blockage is identified by an angiogram, angioplasty (ballooning) is performed, and a stent is implanted (PCI) in the problem area. Next morning, the patient is on his feet; and within another day or two back to a normal routine.

The nightmare of cardiologists performing stent insertion is the eventual blockage of the stent, a process known as 'restenosis'. Restenosis literally means the reoccurrence of stenosis, which is an abnormal narrowing in a blood vessel.

After the insertion of the standard bare-metal stent, the lining layer of the blood artery starts covering the exposed metal of the stent. This natural procedure takes about a month or so to occur. This is also the reason that I was prescribed the prescription drug Plavix for the first month after my stent insertion in 2001. Together with the aspirin, Plavix is a blood thinner that helps prevent the sticking of foreign objects to the exposed bare-metal stent during that first month.

Classic restenosis is caused by a blood clot (thrombosis), at the sight of treatment or by the gradual growth of abnormal cells within the stent. In many cases, stenting is not a permanent solution, having to be done over in one to four years.[188] Medical science did find a solution for the problem of restenosis occurring in the first months after stenting caused by the growth of abnormal cells within the stent. The solution: a coated drug-eluding stent that indeed lowered the incidence of restenosis during the months following angioplasty.

A drug-eluding stent is a bare-metal stent coated with a special drug that is released from the stent over a period of time. The two leading suppliers of the newer drug-eluding stents are Johnson & Johnson and Boston Scientific. Johnson & Johnson's CYPHER® sirolimus-eluding stent received FDA approval to market in 2003. Boston Scientific's TAXUS® Express2™ paclitaxel-eluding stent entered the market in 2004.

It had seemed that medical technology had found the next generation heir to the bypass operation. The excitement, as history will show, was short-lived. Barely a year had gone by since the introduction of the drug-eluding stents and The Lancet published an article regarding the consequences of discontinuation of blood thinning medications to four stent recipients about a year after their angioplasty. The four, in a very short period of time, suffered a recurring MI (heart attack).[189]

The drug-eluding (coated) stents initially prevent restenosis by inhibiting abnormal cell growth within the stent. However, as it turns out, the drugs used to coat these stents also inhibited the growth of endothelial cells that would prevent the bare metal of the stent from being exposed to the blood.

As a result, when anti-platelet[*] medications are stopped, platelets in the bloodstream may be more likely to 'stick' to the stent, and to begin forming a clot that could block blood flow within a very short time.

In September 2006, Boston Scientific acknowledged that they found a statistically significant difference in the rates of late stent thrombosis (blood clots) when comparing its drug-eluding Taxus model with the earlier generation bare-metal stents.[190]

---

[*] Platelets (thrombocytes) are the cell fragments circulating in the blood that are involved in the formation of blood clots. Dysfunction or low levels of platelets can lead to excessive (uncontrollable) bleeding, while high levels increase the risk of thrombosis.

Johnson & Johnson was not in any hurry to jump on the guilt bandwagon. However, two papers submitted the same month at the World Congress of Cardiology in Barcelona by Drs. Eduardo Camenzind and A. Nordmann showed that Johnson & Johnson had nothing to gloat about. Dr. Nordmann observed not only an increased risk of late mortality and non-fatal myocardial infarction with the sirolimus-eluding stents, but also an apparent increase in all cause mortality after two and three years of follow-up.[191]

A 'simple' solution was found to prevent the sudden occurrence of restenosis for those walking around with the drug-coated stents. The solution is to continue taking blood thinning/anti-clotting/anti-platelet medications like Plavix for the rest of your life. Is there a downside to taking Plavix? Possibly. Plavix is a long-lasting drug that does not have a readily available antidote. Once you start taking it, your platelets are basically out of commission for about seven to ten days, the time it takes for your body to get rid of the old platelets and make new ones.

This could be critical if one is seriously injured in an accident, or needs an urgent operation, etc.

An interesting phenomenon occurred in the stock prices for both Johnson & Johnson and Boston Scientific in the beginning of February, 2007. They both took off south bound. The reason: the long-awaited American College of Cardiology convention to be held in New Orleans at the end of March. At the convention Dr. W. Boden reported that many heart patients routinely implanted with stents to open arteries gain no lasting benefit compared with those treated with drugs only.[192]

Dr. Michael Maeng released the results of a study he conducted involving 12,400 patients in Denmark who were randomly given bare metal or drug-coated stents. He found that the rates of blood clots and heart attacks were similar over 15 months; however, over the last three months of that period, an increased risk of blood clotting and heart attack was seen with drug-coated stents.[193]

Due to the concerns over blood clots, the market saturation of the drug-coated variety of stents dropped to approximately 70% of the market, down from 95% a year earlier. It is no wonder that Boston Scientific's and Johnson & Johnson's stock prices reacted as they did.

What does the future hold for stents? At the March 2007 convention, newer technology stents were presented. Abbott presented a totally bioabsorbable drug-eluding stent made of polylactic acid, which is designed to be fully absorbed and slowly metabolized by the coronary artery. Their everolimus-coated stent will release the drug into the artery and then be slowly absorbed over time. The goal is to leave a healed natural vessel behind.

OrbusNeich's innovation for preventing thrombosis and minimizing restenosis is a stent coated with a substance designed to attract stem cell-like cells from the bloodstream to help the artery heal.

Cordis' experimental stent contains an anti-clotting drug that is contained in tiny wells designed to dissolve over time so that after six months or so the device turns into a plain bare-metal stent.

Will these new stents decrease the occurrence of stent restenosis? Only time will tell. For now, Dr. Camenzind, whose September 2006 presentation at the Barcelona World Congress of Cardiology sparked the current controversy over drug-eluding stents, has his own idea. He finds that the original simple balloon angioplasty device that is currently used as a way to inflate stents may now provide a less invasive way of preventing restenosis.[194]

All in all, a stent is not a natural phenomenon that occurs in the body. Lifestyle habits that are beneficial to people without stents could be harmful to people with them. In SASHA I discussed the importance of keeping homocysteine levels within reasonable limits. One of the ways of accomplishing this is increasing folic acid and vitamins B_6 and B_{12} in the diet. However, for those with stent implantations, it is not recommended to take a B_6/B_{12}/Folate supplement. A conflicting study showed that this vitamin combination caused an increased risk of in-stent restenosis. [195]

To stent or not to stent – that is the question. There are basically two situations when stenting (PCI) is performed. The first is the situation when a patient arrives in the hospital in the midst of a heart attack occurring in real time. The stent is implanted to immediately save the life, or at least minimize imminent permanent damage that may be caused by any other delay. This is NOT the scenario that occurs in most situations.

Most people who have a stent implanted are in a state known as 'stable ischemia'. Something somewhere is blocked up to some degree; however, it is not life threatening in the foreseeable future. Stenting in this case is one of possibly alternatives available to improve or correct the existing problem. In this scenario, it is my opinion that implanting or not implanting a stent is one of the more crucial decisions that one may face in a lifetime. It is no less critical than deciding to marry or not, and to whom; to bring children into this world, or not to; to leave an established stable place of work for whatever reason; and any other major personal/family decision.

The procedure itself has become routine. It might not be the most pleasant procedure in the world; however, it certainly is not all that terrible. As previously mentioned, the recovery and return to normal routine happens within a day or two.

The downside of receiving a stent is long term. Restenosis occurring suddenly at any stage has claimed fatalities, or in a more fortunate situation, a bypass operation. One of the tools doctors still use to try to keep the stent open and free flowing at all costs is to artificially lower blood cholesterol levels. This naturally leads to increased dosages of the famed statins -- the more statins, the lower the LDL. Your cardiologist may be happy with the numbers, but how will you still be functioning? In the case of stable ischemia, in my opinion, the use of stents should be considered as a last resort, and not as a standard practice.

Shock Wave Therapy

A new shock wave therapy for the heart has been found to improve the condition of people with heart blockages/damage by increasing blood flow in the affected region. The method, known as Extracorporeal Cardiac Shock Wave Therapy (CSWT) is based upon the 1980's noninvasive therapy to break up kidney stones (Extracorporeal Shock Wave Lithotripsy). The cardiac shock wave generated is a low-level shock wave as compared to the wave generated to break up kidney stones; it is approximately 10% of that used for lithotripsy treatment.

In 2004, pigs treated with shock wave therapy grew more blood vessels than a control group after only four weeks. There was an increase in the regional myocardial blood flow without any adverse effects.[196] A paper presented to the 12th World Congress on Heart Disease in 2005 stated that:

> *We conclude that CSWT is a new, safe and efficient non-invasive therapy for treating chronic ischemia in CAD patents with refractory angina which are ineligible for other interventions.* [197]

An additional study reported the results regarding nine patients with end-stage coronary artery disease. During a typical session they were hit in 20 to 40 different areas of the heart with 200 pulses each. The hits were focused on areas as small as a two-square-millimeter area. In all patients, blood flow increased and symptoms were alleviated, suggesting the growth of new blood vessels.

> *Myocardial perfusion was improved only in the ischemic area treated with the therapy. These*

beneficial effects persisted for 12 months. No procedural complications or adverse effects were noted. ..... These results indicate that our extracorporeal cardiac shock wave therapy is an effective and non-invasive treatment for end-stage coronary artery disease, although further careful evaluation is needed. [198]

Yes, the researchers are meanwhile very optimistic, however, as stated, 'further careful evaluation is needed'.

Nearly 16 million Americans are living with coronary heart disease.[199] Despite progress over the past two decades in treating cardiac disease, there is basically no way to fix damaged heart muscle. During heart attacks, tissue is destroyed when blood is temporarily cut off to a section of the heart, and this tissue can never be repaired.

Close to home here at the Technion University in Haifa, beating cardiac tissue has been created in a lab from human embryonic stem cells, leading to the creation of tiny blood vessels within the tissue.[200] The creation of a vascular system in the tissue is critical for its acceptance by the body.

The technique is aimed at helping patients who have cardiac insufficiency due to heart attacks, making possible tissue implantation into a human heart to repair the damage caused by the attack.

27

Green Gold

*$a^2 + b^2 = c^2$ where c is the hypotenuse of a
right-angle triangle.*
The Pythagorean Theorem

This theorem is of fundamental importance in Euclidean
Geometry. It serves as a basis for the definition of
distance between two points. Decades ago in high school
I knew at least one proof of this theorem, as did all the other kids
in my math class. Little did I know then that almost 40 years
later, Mr. Pythagoras's personal eating doctrines would have
such a profound effect on my own eating habits.

Most of us today associate Pythagoras with mathematics.
He was also a preacher of mystic doctrines and the founder of
the mystic, religious and scientific society called Pythagoreans.
It is ironic that Pythagoras received his culinary inspiration here
in what is modern day Israel, at a site located a short two-hour
drive from where I now live.

The famous historian Flavius Josephus claimed Judaism
and/or Hebrew religious thought influenced Pythagoras's
thinking.[201] This concurred with other reliable sources, among

306

them Hermippus, an Athenian writer, and Porphyry, a Neoplatonist philosopher.[202]

Pythagoras studied with the Essenes* on Mount Carmel, located on the outskirts of modern day Haifa.[203] The Essenes were one of three leading Jewish sects mentioned by Josephus as flourishing in the second century B.C.E., the others being the Pharisees and the Sadducees. The Essenes was a mystic, messianic, even apocalyptic sect of Judaism. They led a very humble existence; they wore very simple clothing, were very pacifistic, and possessions were collectively owned. Members of the northern Essene sect were also known as 'Nazarenes'; Jesus, who was raised in Nazareth (located in the upper Galilee – less than a half-hour drive from modern day Mount Carmel), was known as Jesus the Nazarene.

It was at Mount Carmel with the Essenes that Pythagoras learned about live foods. He took this knowledge with him upon his return to Greece. Pythagoras then became a fruitarian (diet consists of raw fruit and seeds only). He used raw food to cure people with poor digestion. This knowledge was later passed down to Socrates and Plato.[204]

Adapting an eating habit from an ancient practice from a part of the world so steeped in Jewish and early Christian history is definitely very inspirational. Certainly more inspirational than being influenced by some new processed junk food advertised on TV -- don't you think so?

Nearly 2500 years after Pythagoras, a Swiss physician Maximilian Oskar Bircher-Benner, founder of the famed Bircher-Benner Clinic in Zurich, Switzerland, discovered the

---

* There was also a southern Essene sect located closer to Jerusalem. The Dead Sea scrolls comprising more than 800 documents were discovered between 1947 and 1956 in eleven caves in and around the ruins of the ancient settlement of Khirbet Qumran, on the northwest shore of the Dead Sea. Scholars believe that most of the Dead Sea Scrolls were produced by the Essenes.

writings of Pythagoras and began experimenting with live foods. Around the turn of the previous century (1900) he used a balanced diet of raw vegetables and fruit as a means to heal patients at his sanatorium in Zürich. He was enchanted with chlorophyll (a product of photosynthesis in which plants convert sunlight into carbohydrates), and labeled it 'concentrated sun power'.

> *These plant-units contain everything which the human organism requires, and in the right proportions: enough of the various proteids, a wealth of the best energy givers, the carbohydrates, from which fats can at any time be formed in the organism or the fats themselves; the minerals necessary for life in the excited state and in the right proportion, and accordingly also the vitamins.....No one therefore need wonder any longer that man can amply nourish himself, grow and keep well with these alone, that ox, horse, stag, roe and even the elephant can build up their proteid-rich bodies from grasses, herbs, leaves and blossoms[205]*

Dr. Bircher stated that nature uses chlorophyll as a body cleanser, rebuilder, and neutralizer of toxins.

In 1930, Dr. Hans Fischer won the Nobel Prize for Chemistry[206] for research on red blood cells. During his research he noticed that hemin, a component of the hemoglobin in blood that carries oxygen, is nearly identical to chlorophyll on the molecular level. The significance of chlorophyll being similar to human hemin is great. A study done 80 years ago showed that the animal body is capable of converting chlorophyll to hemoglobin.[207] It is no wonder that one Steve Meyerowitz labeled chlorophyll as the blood of plants.[208] We will return to Steve very shortly.

Hemin is a web of carbon, hydrogen, oxygen and nitrogen atoms grouped around a single atom of iron.

Chlorophyll is a similar web of the same atoms, except that its centerpiece is a single atom of magnesium. This should be of special interest to people worried about heart disease, as magnesium deficiency has been shown to correlate with a number of chronic cardiovascular diseases.[209] It was also found that oral magnesium supplementation in patients with Coronary Artery Disease results in a significant improvement in exercise tolerance, quality of life and possibly beneficially alters outcomes in patients with CAD.[210]

Presenting Dr. Ann

For many people already familiar with the health benefits of chlorophyll, Dr. Ann needs no further introduction; stating her family name would be a redundancy. For those less informed, Dr. Ann is Dr. Ann Wigmore. Dr. Ann was not the only person within the last 100 years to actively promote chlorophyll and wheatgrass for health benefits. Charles Schnabel and later V. Earl Irons made significant strives in promoting wheatgrass/chlorophyll products in America in the early and mid-1900's; however, wheatgrass today is overwhelmingly equated with Ann Wigmore.

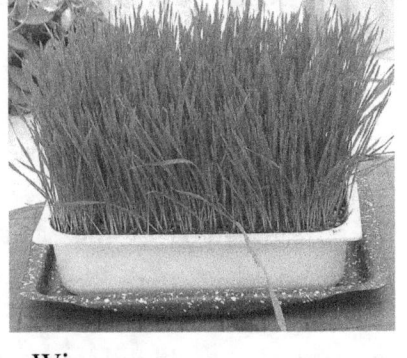

By the age of 50, Dr. Ann was battling colon cancer, arthritis, and depression. Like most other 50-year-olds, she also had normal gray hair, a sign of the natural aging process. It was then that she developed her Living Foods Lifestyle® and within several years returned to excellent health. She essentially abandoned her American-style eating habits, to which she attributed her deteriorating health. One of the principle aspects of her raw-food lifestyle was adapting the daily habit of drinking fresh liquid chlorophyll. The source of her chlorophyll: fresh wheatgrass juice.

Dr. Ann helped people recover from chronic disorders for 30 years using wheatgrass. She tragically perished in a fire at the age of 83 in 1993. Up until her premature death, she was limber, energetic, and intellectually sharp. Her hair color had even returned to its natural brown.

Indeed, of the many books that she wrote, the one that she is most famous for is *The Wheatgrass Book*.[211] She stated that starting the day with a shot/glass of fresh chlorophyll containing wheatgrass juice is starting the day with a storehouse of vitamins, minerals, hundreds of enzymes, amino acids and oxygen in liquid form.

There are many other benefits of drinking fresh wheatgrass. The following is a very partial list:[212]

- Normal metabolism causes the constant production of body acids. An excess of acidity in the body weakens bones and teeth, and reduces our immunity from colds and other illnesses. The abundance of alkaline minerals in wheatgrass juice helps to reduce over acidity in the blood.

- Amino acids are the basic structural building units of proteins. Wheatgrass contains 17 amino acids including the eight essentials.

- Speeds up blood circulation and metabolic rate – helping to control weight, thus enhance digestive powers melting the excess fat in the body.

- Protects us from free radicals

- Stimulation and regeneration of the liver

- Destroys harmful germs and microbes

- Contains selenium – (see Chapter 23 – Post Pasteur)

- Requires little energy to digest

- Increases antioxidant levels
- Inhibition of Carcinogens

According to Dr. Theodore M. Rudolph, the daily use of chlorophyll is very beneficial for people suffering from hardening of the arteries (arteriosclerosis). He believes that chlorophyll's ability to combine with oxygen, and its cleansing ability, contributes much to the removal of foreign matter from the walls of the blood vessels.[213]

Grow your own wheatgrass

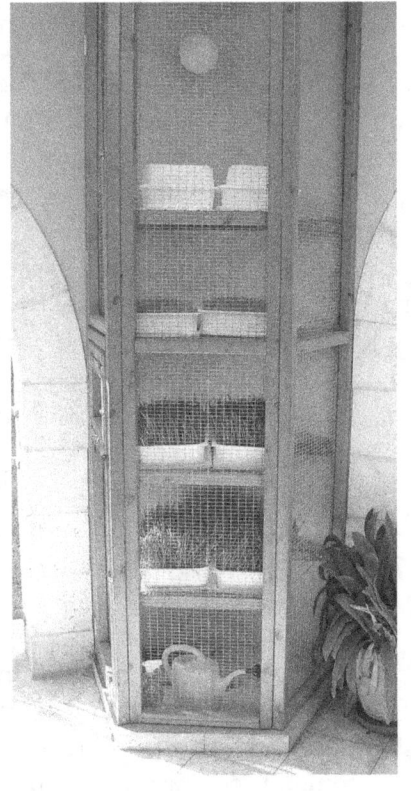

I was not content to simply stop my poor eating habits that contributed to my heart attack in 2001. The elimination of trans-fats and partially hydrogenated oils undoubtedly slowed down further deterioration of my personal health. I wanted to make a conscious effort to improve my health, and not only maintain the existing status quo.

Today I start my day with a shot of wheatgrass, and my purpose for describing here how I grow it is to emphasize that wheatgrass can be grown and enjoyed by anyone; it is not a privilege enjoyed only by the die-hard naturalists and those eating 100% or close to 100% raw and natural food. Growing wheatgrass is something that is doable by anyone. It is also an important step in ingesting a greater percentage of healthy food in our daily diets. While wheatgrass can be (and usually is) grown indoors by many people, I grow it outdoors in an old birdcage that I converted for this endeavor. Interested parties are strongly encouraged to obtain further information from the sources listed at the end of this chapter.

The type of wheatgrass seeds usually used are those known as 'hard' or 'winter' wheat berries. Like other natural seeds and nuts, their own enzyme inhibitors protect them. This allows them to survive until growing time. Therefore, before planting, the wheatgrass seeds must be sprouted.

Sprouting

The amount of seeds to be prepared depends on the size of the growing trays you will be using. The trays I use are 12½" x 10½" (32cm x 27cm). Fill a wide-mouth jar with one cup of seeds. Secure a piece of nylon screen over the jar and secure it with a rubber band. Rinse the seeds by filling up the jar and spilling out the water several times. Fill the jar with water, and place it in a dark area for approximately 12 hours. After the 12-hour soak, rinse the seeds several times (through the secured nylon screen), and let the jar drain at a 45-degree angle for another 12 hours.

Depending on the season, you may have to modify sprouting procedures; there is no absolute right and wrong. Dr. Ann recommended the 12-hour soak and 12-hour drain time. Dr. Bernard Jensen, well versed in a wide variety of holistic healthcare disciplines, favors planting immediately after the initial 12-hour soak.[214] Steve Meyerowitz, the 'sproutman' and current wheatgrass guru recommends an initial soak of 9-12 hours, rinsing well, then germinating the seeds in a sprouter bag for two days, making sure to rinse at least twice a day.[215] The instruction CD that I received with my wheatgrass juicer recommends soaking for 12 hours and draining for another 12. I seem to obtain best results when soaking for 9 - 12 hours, and draining (with rinsing) for about another 24 hours.

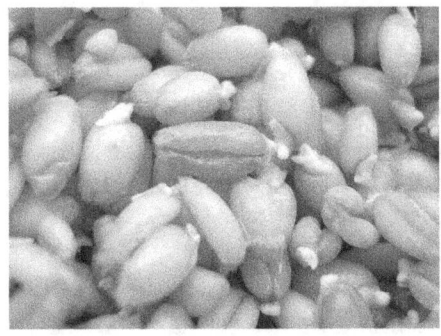 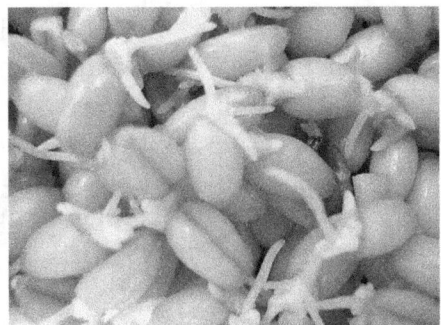

Wheatgrass seeds after 12-hour draining

Wheatgrass seeds after 24-hour draining

Planting

Once sprouted the wheat berries are ready for planting. The seeds are ready to plant when they have doubled in size and the tips of the roots are visible. The tips will be longer if the seeds are drained for 24 and not 12 hours. Fill the tray with an even layer of soil and gently spread the wheat berries over the soil. I favor Dr. Ann's method of not piling up the wheat berry seeds on top of one another. The instruction CD that I mentioned earlier recommends spreading the seeds two or three deep. This is done to promote a thicker harvest. My growing trays have adequate draining holes drilled out of the bottom. Water the seeds (the dirt should be moist and not soaked) and cover the tray with another empty tray

Remove the upper tray when the wheatgrass reaches a height of about one inch and leave in indirect sunlight. Water as necessary in accordance with the weather, humidity and temperature. If the trays are sitting on a flat tray to catch excess water, elevate the upper tray slightly; a couple of pebbles in the corners are adequate. This will allow for all the excess water to drain out of the seeded tray and not be trapped within. The biggest problem I encounter is a greenish blue mold just above soil level, which seems to happen because of over-watering and/or overly hot weather. When the wheatgrass reaches seven to ten inches (18-25 cm) in height, it is ready for harvesting. Use a pair of large scissors to cut it as low as possible.

I cut and juice the wheatgrass first thing in the morning. Once juiced, it should be drunk immediately. Cut wheatgrass can be kept under refrigeration for up to a week. I prepare and plant a new batch every two to two and a half days. You may, if you decide to, harvest your tray a second time. From my experience, this depends on the quality of the first harvest. If it was basically mold free, then I may wait to see how the second batch develops.

Dr. Ann goes into detail on how to recycle the used wheatgrass mats. Here you have a choice on deciding to which doctrine you want to adhere. Dr. Ann's doctrine is organic. She goes with the natural composting to improve and maintain the fertility of soil. For this you must be prepared to wait upwards of three months for this natural process to occur, including the physical place to hold three or so barrels/large trash cans. It helps to obtain earthworms to help 'process' the recycled mats. See references at the end of this chapter.

Changing of the wheatgrass guard

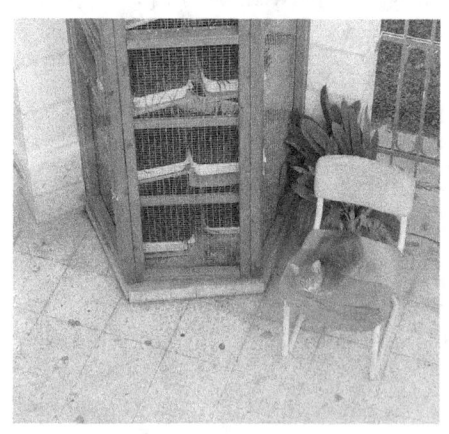 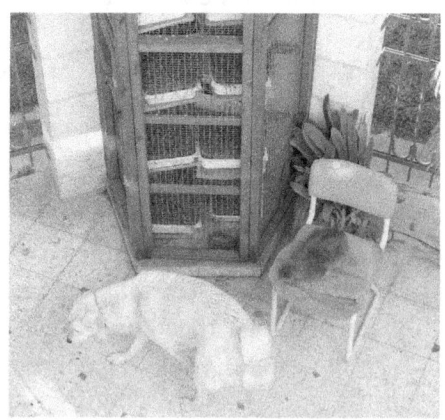

Where's Lambchop? Late as usual!   Nice you decided to show up!

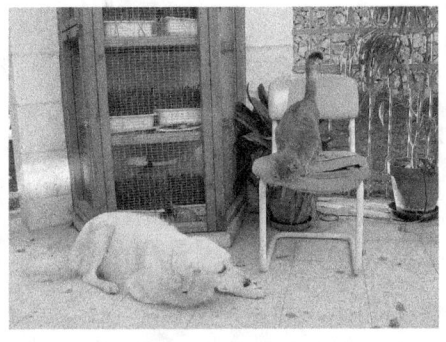
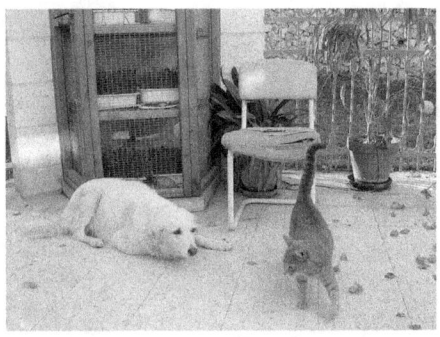

OK, Lambchop, if you're in place, I'm gonna take off.

Have a nice night off, Gray. See ya tomorrow, Lambchop.

Another use for wheatgrass seeds

Wheatgrass seeds can also be used to make a healthy, tart and slightly carbonated drink called rejuvelac.[216] After the wheatgrass seeds have sprouted for several days (rinsing twice a day), instead of planting them, place them in a large glass container, and rinse well. Add one quart of water per every cup of wheatgrass seeds, again cover with the nylon screen mesh and let stand for two days (less in summer). When ready, filter through the screen mesh. It should be cloudy, tart but not too sour; if too sour, it may be spoiled. I also pour it through a clean cloth diaper as an additional filtering method. (Diaper? We will encounter diapers again in the next chapter.) Refrigerate and consume within a couple of days.

Return the sprouted seeds back into the large glass container, fill again with water, and the next batch will be ready in another 24 hours. The process can be repeated a third time.

Make very sure that the seeds you are using to make rejuvelac are organic and have not been sprayed with pesticides. Don't forget, the wheatgrass seeds are soaking in what you ultimately will be drinking.

Before filtering the ready rejuvelac, if whitish foam is floating at the top, it can be easily sifted off with a spoon.

I am also a Victoria fan

The name 'Victoria' may not yet be as universal as 'Dr. Ann' so I will present her by her full name, Victoria Boutenko – the same Boutenko mentioned in chapter 20. The Boutenko family arrived to the U.S. from the former Soviet Union. They adapted quite well to American life, which included succumbing to a wide range of 'normal' diseases resulting from eating 'normal' foods. Victoria herself had arrhythmia and edema. She was also obese and depressed. Her husband suffered from painful rheumatoid arthritis and had severe hyperthyroid. Their kids rounded out the list with juvenile diabetes and asthma.

In 1994, the Boutenkos embarked on a diet of entirely raw foods, returned to perfect health, and have since been known as the Raw Family.

Victoria points out in *Green for Life*[217] the anatomical resemblance between chimpanzees and us humans. In fact we both share an approximate 99.4% of the same DNA sequence.[218] There is a good reason for this. Many anthropologists tend to believe that the modern human being evolved from a chimpanzee-like ancestor.[219]

Victoria observed that there is a huge difference in the chimpanzees' eating habits and our own. Chimpanzees do not eat most of the foods that we humans eat. These include all the cooked foods, the starchy carbohydrates, oils and junk food in general. The small amounts of the vegetables we do eat are mostly roots. The chimps on the other hand consume close to 50% of their diet as fruit, and the majority of the remaining 50% as greens.

Modern chimpanzees, however, are not herbivores; they are actually omnivores, like us.[220] Although chimpanzees generally subsist on fruits and greens, they will hunt monkeys on occasion, even when fruits are plentiful.[221] This is not characteristic behavior of a true herbivore.

In direct contrast to the roots (of the greens) that we consume, the chimps eat the leafy part of the vegetable. They eat roots only when there is a shortage of the usual fruits and greens.

The invention of the Victoria Smoothie

Nature has its unique way of protecting its treasures and allowing their survival. The primary structural component of green plants is cellulose. Its strength is what keeps the plant cells rigid and protects the valuable nutrients that are stored inside the cells. For all her motivation and heath awareness, Victoria knew that having to chew the greens to a creamy consistency adequately enough to release the nutrients from their protective cells was not practical for us humans. Enter the high-speed food blender; rupturing the strong cell walls was now accomplished. In addition to the greens, add some fruit into the blender, and the resulting drink is both healthy and tasty.

Blending the greens to a drinkable pulp has advantages over juicing and throwing away the solid byproduct. The cellulose of plants is not digestible by humans. It is an insoluble dietary fiber, in contrast to the soluble fiber which is found in the fruit. Fiber plays an important role in our digestive system. The main purpose of fiber is elimination. If we do not consume enough fiber, the toxic wastes of various sources and dead body cells accumulate in our bodies.

The soluble fiber improves bowel movements by increasing the volume of bulk in the colon. The insoluble fiber acts as a sponge, absorbing toxins. Both types of fiber are necessary for elimination. According to the American Heart Association both types of fiber are associated with a decreased risk of cardiovascular disease.[222]

Varying the greens in our diet also insures the digestion all of the essential amino acids that are vital for protein production.

Introducing the Mike Shlush

What is a Mike Shlush? Basically, it would contain the same or similar ingredients as a Victoria smoothie. In *Green for Life* Victoria supplies a comprehensive choice of what ingredients and in what amounts to prepare a smoothie. I generally use whatever greens (usually lettuce, coriander, spinach, parsley, etc) that happen to be in the house.

The big difference is in the hardware. Victoria uses a powerful high-speed Vitamix Blender. Its blade spinning at 240 miles per hour will liquefy practically anything she happens to blend; hence the name of her creation – the liquid Victoria smoothie. I am using a 25-year-old Magi mix Food Processor – maybe the only one of its kind still left in the Middle East. The result is not a pure smoothie; it's more like a shlush that still has to be somewhat munched before swallowing – hence the semi-liquid Mike Shlush.

Recommended reading:

The Wheatgrass Book, Ann Wigmore, Avery/Penguin Putnam

Wheatgrass Nature's Finest Medicine, Steve Meyerowitz, Book Publishing Co.

Green For Life, Victoria Boutenko, Raw Family Publishing.

28

Fermenting

Often, the less there is to justify a traditional custom,
the harder it is to get rid of it.
Mark Twain

There are many things that are passed down from generation to generation. This is known as tradition. There are things that exist generation after generation, and eventually peter out. My maternal grandmother could never understand how it was possible for me to grow up not learning/knowing Yiddish. My folks of course understand it, they can still converse in it to some extent.

My siblings and I are totally Yiddish illiterate. Am I sorry that as a tot I was not exposed to Yiddish? Of course I am because during early years, foreign languages seem to be absorbed easily and naturally. Do I really have the need for Yiddish in my daily life? Not really, but the idea of having been able to learn it painlessly and effortlessly seems to be an unexploited opportunity.

Do I blame my folks for this unutilized opportunity? Not really. I committed a much greater blooper. When Esty and I were married, seven years after my immigration to Israel, my

Hebrew was already better than her English. It naturally followed that Hebrew became the daily spoken language in our home.

Nevertheless, I proclaimed that when we will be blessed with children, I would speak with them in English only. With Naamah, the plan got off to a promising start. For the first year of her life, I spoke to her only in English. Then we moved to a different city due to a job change, I started working longer and longer hours, and the rest is well known. I decided to improve this endeavor when Sagi was born, and again when Rakefet was born and of course when Tuval came along.

We have a video movie of baby Tuval correctly answering questions like 'Where is your diaper?' and 'Where is your elbow?' Several years later, diaper and elbow were no longer any part of his vocabulary. That was my blooper, my responsibility. The kids today of course do speak English. This, however, is more to the credit of the school system here and the Simpsons, but they definitely do not speak it with a North American accent.

Tradition is also not necessarily based solely on historical fact. It is also based on how we remember the past, which is not always identical to how the past really was. My folks grew up eating traditionally prepared foods from the traditional kosher kitchen. I have no doubt that in my earliest years this tradition was still in effect. However, like most people, I have very little recollection from those very early years. If you would ask my mom, she would tell you that I was crazy about her lamb chops. The fact that I really don't remember the lamb chops doesn't mean there weren't really lamb chops!

I was born in 1950, but for me, the food tradition at home dates only as far back as I can remember -- 1956? 1960? 1965? And what do I remember about traditional American food as I approached my teen years? It was the hotdogs, hamburgers, fries, pizza, and submarine sandwiches.

Foods known as authentic traditional foods were of course in existence well before the start of my own personal memory or existence. How far back does this tradition go? Not hundreds, but thousands of years. One of the ancient methods of preparing and preserving foods was utilizing natural fermentation. We all know the term fermentation as a process used to produce wine, beer and vinegar. Wine jars dating back more than 7000 years ago have been excavated at Hajji Firuz located in modern day Iran.[223]

In the more general sense, fermentation refers to the conversion of sugar to alcohol using yeast, or the chemical conversion of carbohydrates into alcohols or acids. Fermentation also has some uses exclusive to foods. Fermentation can produce important nutrients which are elements or compounds necessary for contributing to an organism's metabolism, growth, or other functioning. Fermentation also eliminates anti-nutrients (also known as enzyme inhibitors), which are substances that interfere directly with the absorption of vitamins, minerals and other nutrients.

Lacto-fermentation is the process whereby friendly bacteria transform sugars and starches into beneficial lactic acid. Lactic acid acts as a preservative that inhibits pathogenic bacteria (undesirable microorganisms) in the food or drink undergoing fermentation. Recommended sources for additional and technical information regarding fermentation can be found at the website of the Weston A. Price Foundation.

One does not have to be a die-hard naturalist living on a farm somewhere out in the boondocks in order to begin receiving the benefits of fermentation. It is the purpose of this chapter to show you that anyone, in any kitchen, can easily supplement any diet with healthy naturally fermented foods.

Kefir

The culturing of dairy products, found almost universally among pre-industrialized peoples, enhanced the enzyme content of those products. Kefir is a drink prepared by inoculating milk with the grains of previous kefir batches. Kefir grains are a combination of bacteria and yeasts in a matrix of proteins, lipids and sugars. They contain over 30 probiotic bacteria proven highly beneficial to humans. The term probiotic refers to live microorganisms which when administered in adequate amounts, confer a health benefit on the host.[224]

As the term itself implies, probiotic is the opposite of antibiotic. Probiotic: 'pro' refers to 'for'; 'biotic' refers to 'life' -- the result, 'life promoting'. Antibiotic: 'anti' refers to 'against'; 'biotic' refers to 'life' -- the result, 'against life'. The protein contained in cultured (lacto-fermented) dairy products is the very highest quality available for human consumption. And as a bonus for those still worried about their cholesterol levels, an anti-cholesteremic milk factor (lowering of blood levels of cholesterol) has been discovered in fermented milk and fermented milk products.[225]

Homemade kefir is very easy to make. You do need to start with a small handful of kefir grains. The Internet provides a good source for finding kefir grains; there are a number of worldwide forums dedicated to kefir, kefir making and how and where to obtain grains. I prepare kefir using a small wide-mouth Mason jar. Simply put the kefir grains in the jar, add a glass of milk, and gently stir or agitate. The jar should not be more than 2/3 full. Initially, the fresh milk will thicken until it obtains a consistency much like smooth yogurt. With longer fermentation, it separates into a layer of thick curd floating on top of greenish whey. The mixture should be shaken or stirred two or three times per day.

I like the Mason jars because they can be closed hermetically for shaking/agitating without having the mixture splash out. Esty is still very unused to sharing the kitchen with me -- even when I don't mess up! I usually leave the lid on the Mason jar loose enough to allow carbon dioxide produced in the fermentation process to escape from the jar. Leaving the jar closed tightly will give the kefir more of a sour taste.

Fermentation is dependent on temperature, time and the activity of the specific grains. The longer it ferments, the tarter the taste. As a general guide kefir will ferment twice as fast at 86°F (30°C) as at 68°F (20°C), but remember, as you approach 100°F (37°C) degrees, the grains lose their potency. Fermentation time takes between 24 to 48 hours. Once the kefir has cultured to your liking, strain it through a sieve using a spoon to gently separate the kefir drink from the grains. If you prefer to drink it cold, refrigerate as necessary before drinking. Return the Kefir grains into the Mason jar with fresh milk and repeat the process.

Most any type of milk can be used -- even dead pasteurized homogenized cow milk. At the end of chapter 23 (Post-Pasteur), I did mention without going into any detail the existence of pro and con camps regarding homogenization and heart disease.[226]

The ultimate solution -- use goat's milk! First, if you are not sure where you stand on the homogenization issue, there is no need to homogenize goat's milk. Fat molecules of goat's milk are one-fifth the size of cow's milk.[227] You can verify this yourself. The next time you are in the dairy section of your local supermarket, check out the commercially sold goat's milk. It is pasteurized; however, it is not homogenized.

There are a number of health advantages to using goat's milk, especially raw (unpasteurized) goat's milk.

- Goats are among the healthiest and hardiest of domestic animals.[228] They are naturally immune to diseases, such as tuberculosis.[229]

- Goats are clean by nature.[230] Cows are not. A cow's 'personal hygiene would embarrass a pig'.[231]

- The molecules of goat's milk are closer in size and composition to human milk, making it easier to digest. Goat's milk protein is also substantially less

- allergenic than cow's milk protein in susceptible individuals.[232]

- Our bodies can digest goat's milk in about 20 minutes; it takes two to three hours to digest cow's milk.[233]

- Goat's milk contains a unique essential balance of vitamins, minerals, proteins, carbohydrates, enzymes and fats; it is one of the few whole foods that are able to sustain life. [234]

- Goat's milk is the highest source of selenium (Chapter 23) of any of the milks.[235]

- Fresh goat's milk (like mother's milk) is alkaline and has a tendency to neutralize acids in the body.[236] Cow's milk has an acid reaction. [237]

- Goat's milk differs from cow's milk in that it contains more of the essential fatty acids (linoleic and arachidonic) and it has a greater percentage of medium and short-chain saturated fatty acids. These differences suggest that the fat of goat's milk may be more readily digested than that of cow's milk.[238]

- Crohn's disease is caused by the microorganism Mycobaterium avium subspecies paratuberculosis, or MAP which is common in U.S. dairy herds. The MAP in cow's milk fails to be killed by conventional pasteurization. Transmission of MAP is passed from infected cattle to humans through cow's milk. No disease like MAP affects goats.[239]

- A controversial drug called rBGH (Recombinant Bovine Growth Hormone) is used quite extensively by most dairies in the U.S. It causes cows to produce more milk. rBGH is a product of genetic engineering. A higher rate of cattle disease is reported among cattle being given rBHG which results in a greater use of antibiotics. These antibiotics are passed down to the milk.[240] Incidentally, rBGH use was approved by the FDA in 1993.

♥ ♥ ♥

The milk I use (when I can obtain it) is fresh raw goat's (or sheep's) milk. I will have to clarify somewhat what I mean by fresh. Raw milk of any type, as in many states in the U.S.A., is not marketed over the counter for human consumption. Finding sources is by word of mouth, friend brings friend. The problem is that my present source is a couple of hours drive away. It is also not available all year around -- depending on the parturition season. This means that most of the milk that I buy at one time winds up in the freezer, so technically it's not really fresh by the time I use it. After thawing out though, it still makes great kefir.

Over time, the Mason jar becomes 'not very aesthetic'. I have a couple of spare Mason jars on hand so that when one enters the dishwasher, there is a spare ready. Make very sure that the kefir is not exposed to chlorinated water! This means that all jars, utensils etc. must be bone dry before using them. There are those who will use only non-chlorinated water for cleaning all utensils being exposure to kefir. Following are other tips for taking care of your kefir grains:

Severe cold (freezing temperatures) or heat (over 100°F/40°C) can damage the grains. Last summer's heat almost killed off my grains altogether. I do not believe that summer daytime temperatures in my kitchen went over 100°F, however, the grains stopped growing, and they shrank down in size. Keeping the kefir in the fridge during the hottest part of the day seemed to help the grains to recuperate. Another option – during the cooler winter months, the grains grow and multiply rapidly. I accumulate the excessive grains and refrigerate them in a 'milk bath' and use them to reinforce the kefir grains in the hot summer months. Every couple of weeks I replace the milk.

I do not let the grains come in contact with metal, although there are those who claim this is not important. The spoon I use to separate the grains from the kefir is actually a plastic won-ton soup spoon. The mesh of the strainer sieve is plastic/nylon. Do not keep your kefir/grains in direct sunlight. When stirring or filtering the grains, do not squeeze them. Be gentle!

Keep in mind that the grains are living entities. As you would not want to do without food, neither would they. The only exception to this if you need to store the grains. There are proper methods for dehydrating them and preparation for freezing. Check out the forums or other relevant articles on the net.

The living grains are constantly growing, which allows one to share them with friends every couple of weeks. If it isn't already obvious, the grains are also edible.

Fresh Cream Cheese

Usually one of the first things I do after obtaining fresh raw goat's or sheep's milk directly from the farm is to use the first couple of liters to make a couple of small tubs of cream cheese (14-17.5 oz / 400-500 grams).

When I first started making my own cream cheese, I followed standard popular recipes which involved slowly heating the fresh milk to 180°F (82°C), and then adding vinegar or lemon juice. This caused the milk to curdle and separate from the liquid whey; the cheese curds were then separated from the whey by straining. While this did supply me with homemade cheese and homemade whey, I did realize eventually that this was partially self-defeating. Although I did produce a product without any artificial preservatives, the heating was still killing off the beneficial enzymes in the process, so what was I ultimately gaining?

My present method of making cream cheese is based on a simple recipe by the Weston A. Price Foundation head Ms.

Sally Fallon Morell.[241] Raw milk, with all of its natural enzymes intact, separates into milk curds and whey when left unrefrigerated for several days (longer in winter, shorter in summer – it's a function of temperature).

Cheese making – summer months

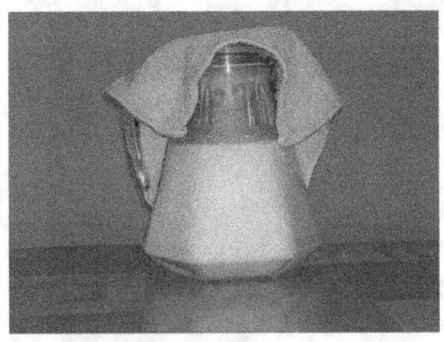

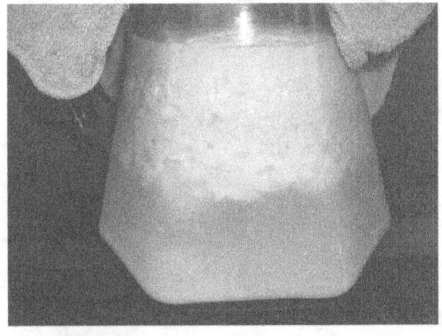

Day 1: Pour raw milk into a large glass container.

Within a day or two (or three, depending upon the temperature), the whey separates from the cheese curds.

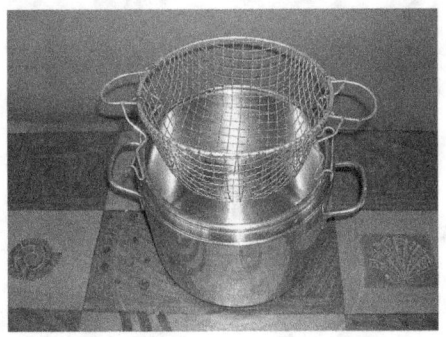

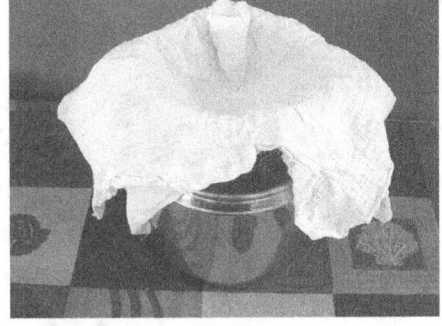

Prepare a large pot (stainless steel). On top of it, place a drain screen (same as used for draining the oil from deep frying).

Place a cloth diaper (or cheese cloth) into the strainer.

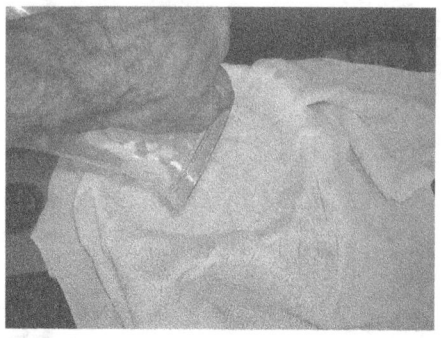

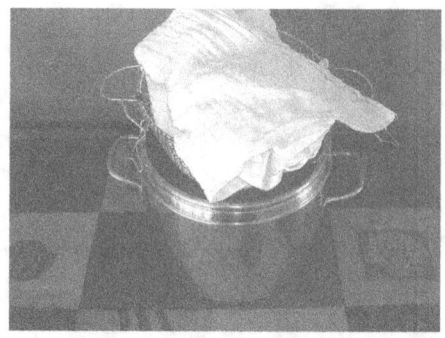

Empty the contents of the container (whey and cheese curds).

Drain, and place as is in refrigerator for several more hours.

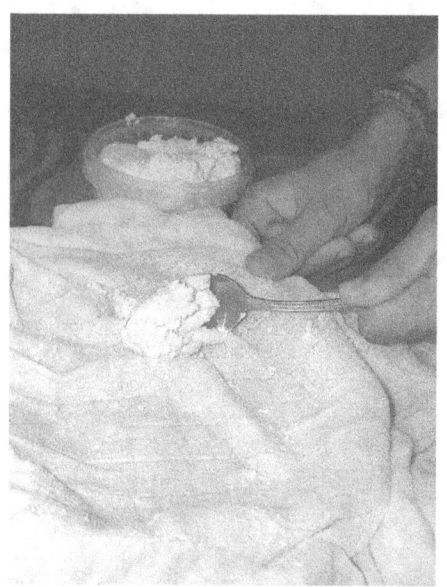

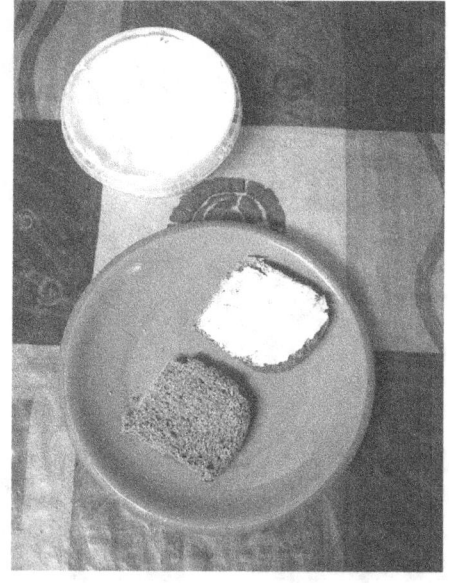

Store the cheese in containers -- use a spoon to scrape off the diaper.

With some fresh homemade whole wheat bread straight out of the oven – Bon Appetit!

I learned at the beginning of last winter that leaving milk out in a cold kitchen is basically leaving it in a 'not very cold refrigerator'. It simply doesn't want to separate! I found a novel way to speed up the separation. Use a simple yogurt maker; the heat is very mild. If you remember the test for enzyme tolerance from Chapter 20, the heated yogurt maker does not approach being uncomfortable when handling. It does not damage the enzymes and separates the milk within two days. The major difference is using a number of regular-sized glasses that fit into the yogurt maker instead of one single large vessel to house the milk while waiting for it to separate into curds and whey.

Cheese making – winter months

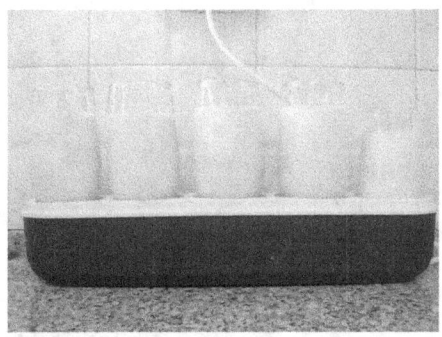 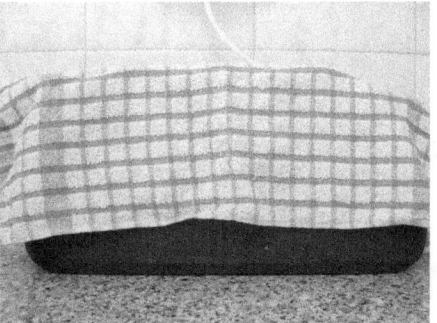

Day 1: Pour raw milk into separate glasses and put in low heat yogurt maker.

Cover glasses completely to keep them heated evenly.

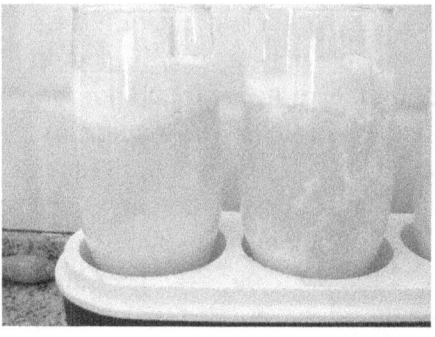

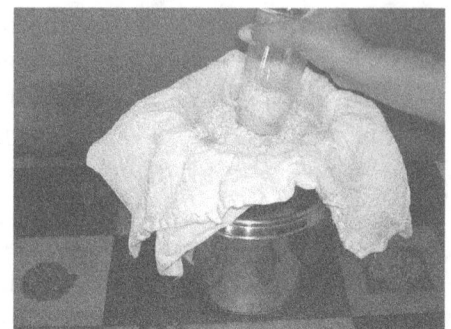

Within a day or two (or three, depending upon the temperature), the whey separates from the cheese curds.

Pour into diaper-lined strainer and continue as above.

Making the cheese dryer

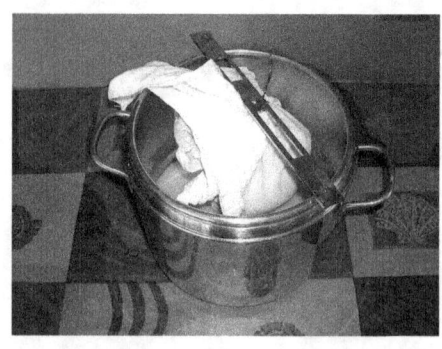

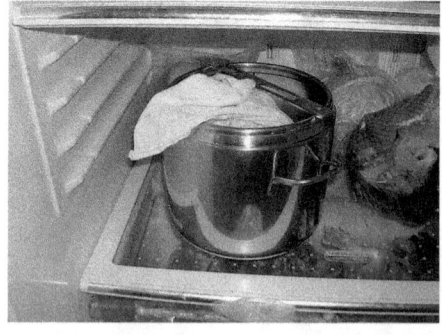

After initial draining, tie the diaper/cheese cloth into a bundle and suspend it so it does not touch the whey.

Place as is into the refrigerator for another eight hours.

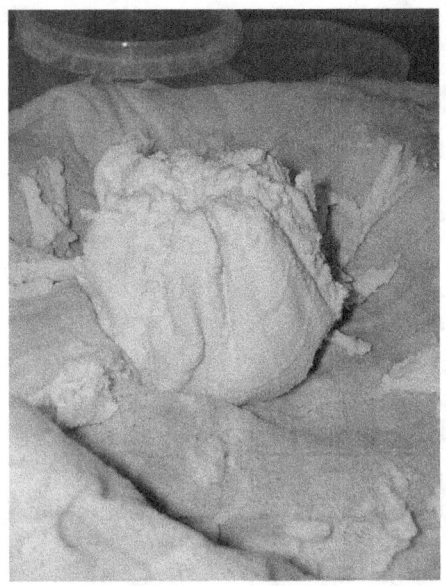 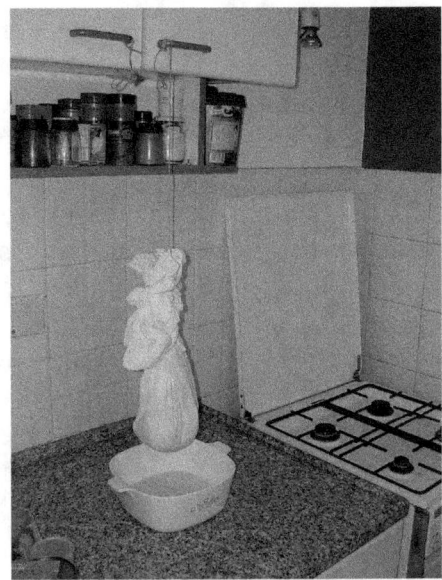

Voila! Open the diaper. The cheese is less creamy and more solid.

This is another way to hang the cheese to dry, however, not especially recommended if your wife has things to do in the kitchen….....

Whey

Does it seem strange that I make my own cheese? After all, I can, and usually do bring back some homemade goat's cheese from my milk supplier. The reason why I make my own cream cheese is because I am not only interested in the cheese itself, but interested in the byproduct that is produced in the process.

I am referring to the yellowish colored liquid that separates from the cheese known as 'whey'. Whey is an excellent source of protein, vitamins, minerals and lactose. Historically, the cheese industry viewed whey as the waste material in cheese production and either discarded it or used it as a fertilizer. Recently, its worth as both an animal feed and a food ingredient has been recognized. Its price has soared to about 79 cents a pound[242] -- a good cash item for cheese diaries. The founding fathers of medicine, Hippocrates, and later Galen, recommended whey to their patients to cure a variety of diseases.[243]

It is also indispensable for making homemade fermented vegetables, grains and beverages. Whey is rich in lactic acid, which speeds up the process of fermentation. It was through this process of lacto-fermentation that our forefathers were able to preserve vegetables before the invention of freezers and canning methods.[244]

My first homemade fermented dish made with whey was sauerkraut. The recipe and directions come from, where else, again Ms. Sally Fallon Morell.[245] Even a lifelong non-kitchen person such as me can follow her easy to understand recipes.

How do I discard excess whey that I have no foreseeable use for? I pour it over the recycled soil mats before replanting new wheatgrass seeds. It may not have the same effect as using Dr. Maynard Murray's method of using diluted ocean water for its rich balanced mineral content as a natural fertilizer;[246] however, it is a way of natural recycling.

29

Aw Nuts……..

You are as old as your arteries.
Hanna Kroeger[247]

There are a number of expressions that one uses to express great dissatisfaction at any given moment, such as 'oh sh--' and other four-letter words. People who are more cultured and who do not want to swear in public but still need to verbalize current dismay can safely say 'Aw nuts!' instead, and still retain their civilized identities.

Another usage of nuts: Esty at times (if not most of the time) thinks that I'm nuts. And this was even before some of the eating habits I have acquired since my heart attack, which she still has trouble adjusting to. But I have a license to be nuts. James Bond, 007, has a license to kill. I survived my heart attack. I later survived the statins; I earned the license to be nuts.

Seriously though, what made me start adding various types of nuts to my diet? It came about with my changing lifestyle, specifically leaving my last job and starting a job involving shift work. Basically I was interested in increasing my knowledge regarding health pitfalls to watch out for now that I was leaving the normal day/night schedule. There was a necessity to alter my sleep habits according to my new work schedule. This involved both the afternoon/evening shift (arriving home after one a.m.) and later, the graveyard shift -- starting either ten or eleven p.m. and arriving home in the morning when most people have already had breakfast and on their way to work.

Published information was not especially encouraging:

- *Heart problems also have been noted more often among shift workers than day workers.....Researchers found that the longer people worked shifts, the more likely they were to develop heart disease....*[248]

- *These results suggest that shiftwork has direct and unfavourable effects on cardiac autonomic activity and that this might be one mechanism via which shiftwork increases the risk of cardiovascular disease. It is postulated that sleep loss could be one mediator of the association between shiftwork and cardiovascular health.*[249]

What are the possible consequences of altering my natural circadian rhythm, and what can I do to minimize the resulting health hazards?

Circadian rhythms are important in determining our sleeping and feeding patterns. There are clear patterns within our 24-hour normal day/night schedule of hormone production, brain wave activity, cell regeneration and other biological functions. Anyone who has ever experienced jetlag knows firsthand what happens when his/her circadian rhythms are interfered with. Common symptoms are fatigue during the daytime, disorientation and insomnia at nighttime and possible mood disorders. This circadian clock is normally timed to the

Earth's natural light and dark cycles, which is perfect for the regular daytime job.

Most circadian rhythms are controlled by the SupraChiasmatic Nucleus or SCN, which acts as the body's clock. The SCN rests in a part of the brain just above the point where the optic nerves cross. Light that reaches photoreceptors in the eye retina creates signals that travel along the optic nerve to the SCN. Signals from the SCN travel to several brain regions, including the pineal gland. This gland responds to light-induced signals by switching off production of the hormone melatonin.

For people maintaining the normal day/night schedule, melatonin level rises during nighttime sleep. It reaches a peak between eleven p.m. and two a.m., and then drops significantly during sunrise. One of the major problems of working shift work is not getting enough high-quality sleep. This in turn results in a vicious cycle of sorts; the lack of nighttime sleep causes a reduction in melatonin production and the shortage of adequate levels of melatonin prevent us from getting enough sleep! Adequate melatonin levels are also associated with assisting us in dealing with stress, and lowering blood pressure and the risk of heart rhythm problems.[250]

An interesting study involving the seeds of plants may shed some light on the importance of melatonin to cardio health in us Homo sapiens:

> *This level of melatonin is much higher than the known physiological concentrations in the blood of many vertebrates. Since the seed, particularly its germ tissue, is highly vulnerable to oxidative stress and damage, we surmise that melatonin, a free radical scavenger, might be present as an important component of its antioxidant defense system.*[251]

How then is it possible to raise melatonin levels, besides trying to simulate night conditions during the daytime by sleeping in a totally dark room or at least covering the eyes? The answer is via our diet. More specifically, a handful of nuts helps raise our melatonin level, which ultimately helps us sleep better. Nuts contain important nutrients and beneficial phytonutrients and also have many characteristics vital for keeping our cardio systems running smoothly.

♥ ♥ ♥

Walnuts contain melatonin and also contribute to the antioxidative capacity of the blood.[252] Walnuts are relatively high in arginine, an essential amino acid. Essential amino acids cannot be synthesized by the organism and therefore must be obtained via food diet. Amino acids function as building blocks in protein biosynthesis. In the body, arginine is converted into nitric oxide (NO), a chemical that helps keep the inner walls of blood vessels smooth and allows blood vessels to relax. Both atherosclerosis and acute coronary events increase when NO levels decline.[253] Foods high in arginine help the body produce its own nitric oxide.

Almonds are an excellent source of the amino acid tryptophan. Tryptophan is a precursor (forerunner or predecessor) of melatonin. The building blocks for natural melatonin production in the body include sufficient amounts of vitamin B6, vitamin B3 and most importantly, tryptophan.

In SASHA I discussed the serious consequences of reduced levels of brain serotonin levels resulting from the use of statins. Tryptophan is also a precursor for serotonin, which is an additional reason to eat almonds. Serotonin is the neurotransmitter responsible for feelings of well-being, mood, self-confidence and concentration. The only source for serotonin in the brain is tryptophan. It cannot be converted from any other substance. Some serotonin is converted in the pineal gland to melatonin. Melatonin production is inversely proportional to that of serotonin, a chemical.[254] Generally during the night, when the mind is less active, less serotonin and more melatonin is produced.

Almonds contain much more vitamin E than all other nuts, and most other foods in general.[255] Vitamin E, a fat-soluble vitamin, is an antioxidant vitamin involved in the metabolism of all cells. It protects essential fatty acids from oxidation in the body cells, helps deactivate free radicals and prevents breakdown of body tissues. Almond skins contain flavonoids which act synergistically (combined effect greater than separate individual effects) with vitamins C and E to enhance LDL resistance to oxidation.[256] Hanna Kroeger, a staunch advocate of natural healing methods recommends an almond drink spanning the course of 30 days to be done once a year.[257]

Peanut lovers (peanuts are technically legumes, and not nuts) will be happy to hear that they contain significant amounts of both tryptophan and arginine.

Do nuts have a downside? They may if proper precautions are not taken. First of all, nuts, like grains, contain numerous enzyme inhibitors that can put a real strain on the digestive mechanism if consumed in excess. In SASHA I mentioned that I soaked my homemade granola (incidentally oats are also a good source of tryptophan) to neutralize the phytates (enzyme inhibitors).[258] Nuts are easier to digest and their nutrients are more readily available if they are first soaked[259] in water and then dried. Besides neutralizing the enzyme inhibitors, this can increase the vitamin and mineral content. Before the food revolution of the last century, traditional people always soaked or partially sprouted their seeds and nuts before they were eaten. You can of course make the nuts crunchy again by roasting; however, extended roasting at high temperature kills the enzymes and damages the nuts' delicate fats.

Is there a downside to peanuts? First of all, peanuts contain an especially high amount of enzyme inhibitors. They must never be eaten raw. Secondly, a study performed in 1988 showed peanut oil to be unexpectedly atherogenic for monkeys, rabbits, and rats.[260]

Keep in mind that walnuts, as opposed to many other types of nuts, are extremely susceptible to rancidity.[261] In warm conditions they quickly go rancid particularly after shelling. Heat, light and humidity will speed spoilage. The best way to preserve them is to buy them in the shell, or keep them in an airtight container in the refrigerator or even in the freezer.

Neutralizing the enzyme inhibitors in nuts is not enough. It is important to understand the connection between nuts and Essential Fatty Acids omega-3 and omega-6 -- and the infamous O6/O3 ratio (chapter 25). I will discuss this further in Chapter 34.

30

The Next 20,000

Life is like riding a bicycle. To keep your
balance you must keep moving.
Albert Einstein

The next 20,000? The next 20,000 what? 20,000 Leagues Under the Sea?* I mentioned in the preface that anyone who has read SASHA would probably be able to guess what the 20,000 stands for; and indeed it is the next 20,000 kilometers (12,427 miles) of bicycle riding. It will be a bit difficult to explain this significance in only a paragraph or two; it relates to my post heart attack period when the side effects of the statins I was prescribed started taking their toll.

The effects totally disrupted my profession and personal life. What had started as being simply a tool to maintain physical conditioning in post heart attack life, the bike riding slowly became a total obsession. It was how I started my day every morning; it was the only thing I enjoyed doing during the day. The daily riding improved my stamina, which allowed me

---

* Sorry Jules

to take very long bike rides over the weekend. After a few months of riding, I set my annual goal to 4,000 kilometers (2,485mi) which was eventually revised to 5,000 kilometers (3,107mi), and finally to 5,215 (an exact 100 kilometers a week average for the entire year).

In fact, an entire chapter in SASHA was devoted to my personal race to get to that 5,215th kilometer by year's end. Does this obsession sound a little strange? It should; welcome to the world of statin side effects. That is basically what prompted me to write SASHA in the first place.

At the end of that first riding year, I picked my goal for the new riding year based upon my improved stamina over the previous couple of months. The new goal: a 140km (87-mile) average per week for the entire year. This is basically how SASHA ended, reaching the 12,570km (7,810mi) goal by the end that second riding year. The goal I set for myself for the third riding year was to reach a cumulative total of 20,000km (12,427mi). A goal is a goal is a goal. Towards the end of that third year I was averaging 180km (112mi) per week for the last month and a half in order to obtain this goal. And I did reach it.

I mentioned earlier that one of the benefits of writing a book is the personal research one does when working on the project. Yes, writing a book like this is definitely a project. I discovered when writing SASHA that sometimes a single article or even a single sentence is enough to kindle an urge to dig up more information regarding a new idea.

Grisanti? Who is Dr. Grisanti?

Dr. Ronald Grisanti authors one of the newsletters I subscribe to. Why is Dr. Grisanti an authority to me? Basically, I share his views on the real causes of heart disease. He is not a believer in the conventional lipid hypothesis. I share his visions of the non-role of cholesterol and saturated fat with regards to the real cause of heart disease.

One newsletter was headlined with 'Do you want to prevent having a heart attack?' That certainly is a headline that talks my language. After all, I did have one. The gist of the newsletter was that long-duration, low-intensity aerobics do not offer us protection against suddenly experiencing a fatal heart attack; in fact they 'can actually speed up your trip to the grave' as he put it.

That particular line rang a bell for me as I was reading it. Then it rang a gong!

The Bell

What was it that rang the bell? Dr. Grisanti mentioned that Jim Fixx, author of *Complete Book of Running*, had a fatal heart attack… while running.

The Gong

Dr. Grisanti specifically mentioned marathon runners as common fatal heart attack victims. It is said that a picture is worth a thousand words. In this case, I think that this direct quote from SASHA will drive the point home.

> *Do I plan to continue bike riding? Definitely! And while on the subject of bike riding and physical exercise in general, I would like to point out that exercising alone does not provide any guarantee against heart attacks and/or an even worse scenario - not surviving a heart attack.*
>
> *A recent event provided good proof of that. Brian Maxwell, the creator of Power Bars (convenient energy bars used by athletes to give them an energy boost while competing), died this week (April 2004) of a heart attack at the age of 51. What is significant here is that he was a former world-class marathon runner. In 1977, Maxwell was ranked as*

the third best marathon runner in the world by Track and Field News.

While on the subject of runners, it was 20 years ago (1984) that Jim Fixx had a massive heart attack while jogging and died immediately. He was 52 at the time. It was Fixx's best-selling book "Complete Book of Running" that started the big jogging craze in the seventies.[262]

Was I partially barking up the wrong tree? It was my intention at the time that Fixx's great personal endurance was not enough to keep him healthy. The implication was that if his eating habits were poor then even his fantastic fitness would not guarantee his good health. I am not personally familiar with Maxwell's specific 'Power Bars'. I do know, however, that many health stores sell convenient power/energy bar type snacks for athletes that contain partially hydrogenated fat. I repeat, partially hydrogenated fat ingredients being sold by 'health stores'!

Dr. Grisanti likens the effects of long-duration, low-intensity aerobics on the heart to an old VW Beetle engine. The VW engine, small and economical, runs all day on a single tank of gas. What happens if that same VW with the small economic engine with four full-sized adults sitting in it suddenly has to go up a big hill full speed and needs the power of a Ferrari? Simply put, it cannot handle the load.

How many times have you heard about someone having a heart attack after lifting something heavy, or suddenly after receiving very bad news? Sound familiar? Not being able to temporarily handle the sudden load?

Dr. Grisanti promotes the use of high-intensity 'Grizzly Bear Intervals' several times a week instead of the basic daily aerobic exercising that is prevalent today.[263] Why the name Grizzly Bear? It is based on the simple principle that during aerobic exercise sessions, one should do several sets of exercise at a pace as if a hungry grizzly bear was chasing you. Dr.

Grisanti himself states that he didn't invent Grizzly Bear Interval training. However, he has fine-tuned it into a very precise way of exercising.

A check through the medical literature shows that this trend of thought is by no means a new idea. There have been quite of few studies conducted on this subject through the years.

As early as 1990 a study was done on subjects that had already undergone coronary bypass surgery. It concluded that interval type exercise was preferable over constant exercise:

> *Exercise training according to the I (exertion and recovery phases alternate each minute) method involves both the aerobic and anaerobic capacity of the organism, whereas exercise training according to the C method (constant exertion) involves only oxidative capacity. After coronary bypass surgery, the I method is better suited to increase physical performance and is more effective in economizing the cardiac function.* [264]

This particular study mentioned both aerobic and anaerobic capacities. A person utilizes his/her muscles to perform physical work. This is accomplished through muscle contraction. Contraction can be performed only when biochemical energy is converted into mechanical energy. Two types of biochemical energy are involved.

- Aerobic: energy is supplied to the muscles in the presence of oxygen.

- Anaerobic: energy is supplied to the muscles in the absence of oxygen

Aerobic activities are typically of a low to moderate-intensity and can be continued over a considerable amount of time. Walking and jogging would be examples of aerobic activities. Anaerobic activities are very intense and for that reason can only be continued for a very limited time. Running a 100-meter sprint at full speed would be an example of an anaerobic activity. While aerobic fitness is a characteristic of the person as a whole, anaerobic fitness is a local characteristic of the muscle or local muscle group because of its independence on blood and oxygen supply to the area.

A popular worldwide test for measuring anaerobic fitness is the Wingate Anaerobic Test (WAnT). It was developed at the Department of Research and Sport Medicine of the Wingate Institute for Physical Education and Sport in Israel in the seventies.

> *It is used as a standard in accessing muscle power, muscle endurance and fatigability. It has also been used as a reproducible, standardized task that can help analyze physiologic and cognitive responses to supramaximal exercise.*[265]

In 1998 a study showed that skeletal muscle fatigue develops in both high-intensity and also low-intensity exercise; however, it was demonstrated that these are two totally separate fatigue mechanisms. What is interesting is that the low-intensity exercises caused the same pathological intracellular chemical imbalances that are found in heart failure patients.

> *We conclude that with high-intensity exercise perturbations of Na+ and K+ in muscle cells may contribute to fatigue, whereas with endurance type of exercise and in heart failure patients the skeletal muscle fatigue is more likely to reside in the intracellular control of Ca2+ release and reuptake.*[266]

Basically, there has been a substantial amount of research done proving the advantages of short duration high-intensity exercise, over long-duration low-intensity workouts – a few more examples:

- *There is an inverse association between relative intensity of physical activity (an individual's perceived level of exertion) and risk of CHD, even among men not satisfying current activity recommendations.*[267]

- *It was concluded that relatively brief but intense sprint training can result in an increase in both glycolytic and oxidative enzyme activity, maximum short-term power output, and VO2 max.*[268]

- *We conclude that short sprint interval training (approximately 15 min of intense exercise over 2 wk) increased muscle oxidative potential and doubled endurance capacity during intense aerobic cycling in recreationally active individuals.*[269]

- *High-intensity aerobic interval exercise is superior to moderate exercise for increasing VO2peak (peak oxygen uptake) in stable CAD-patients. As VO2peak seems to reflect a continuum between health and cardiovascular disease and death, the present data may be useful in designing effective training programmes for improved health in the future.*[270]

- *These results indicate that high-intensity cycling training in 14 sessions improves enzyme activities of anaerobic and aerobic metabolism.*[271]

And finally, the importance of adequate rest periods and *not* working out every day:

However, performance did not improve in a short training programme that did not include days for recovery, which suggests that muscle fibres suffer fatigue or injury.[272]

The fact that I am learning about this now when the facts have been known for quite some time is actually not surprising. I wonder how many people in the Western world suffering from heart disease have ever heard of Dr. Uffe Ravnskov. It is the Western world that is suffering from heart disease today. He is undoubtedly the spiritual father of the ANTI 'saturated fat and cholesterol cause heart disease' movement that is today gaining momentum. The first edition of Dr. Ravnskov's classic book *The Cholesterol Myths* was first published 16 years ago. How many new cases of heart disease cropped up in the last 16 years during the present reigning lipid hypothesis era?

In SASHA, I went into detail regarding the accepted way and widely publicized method of calculating resting and maximum heart rate for exercise workouts. The maximum rate calculations given were based on starting with a pulse calculation of 220, and subtracting various amounts according to variables of the exerciser (age, etc).

Actually, this widely published formula for maximum heart rate has no scientific merit for use in exercise physiology and related fields.[273] Dr. Grisanti also claims that this calculation will be missing the boat for most people. It will be adequate for about one third of the people using it, but the calculations will be high for one third of others, and low for the other third.

Dr. Grisanti calculates what resting, basic training level and maximum aerobic heart rate should be; however, his calculations are entirely different, and not based upon the 220 starting point.

He instructs the exerciser to perform an exact number of sets tailored personally for anyone using them, which takes into consideration the present fitness of the exerciser. This allows the exerciser to stop the daily exercise before entering the over-training stage, which is counterproductive to maintaining good health. Dr. Grisanti puts a great deal of emphasis on making sure not to over exercise. There are inherent dangers in strenuous exercise, which can, and do, result in the death of supposedly very fit people who are in excellent health.[274]

He recommends walking, stationary bike riding or similar methods as the best way to implement the Grizzly Bear Interval workout. These types of exercise lend themselves well to the accurate adherence to exercising according to the calculated pulse rates.

What attracts me to Grisanti's approach to exercising is that I am an analytic type of person. I often go by numbers when doing something. In SASHA, I had the goal to reach 5,000km, and then revised it to exceed 5215. The next year I chose the 140km weekly average for the year. Numbers are something that can be measured. If they are in any way related to a personal goal to obtain something, it makes the whole mission measurable and accountable.

That said, I personally do not like stationary bikes. I like the real bike, fresh air, sunshine, even if the sunshine is in the middle of the hot summer, or the fresh air is in the middle of the cold winter. I simply enjoy the outside bike riding.

Fresh air vs. inside air -- is there really a difference? The home/apartment/office is a source of a myriad of dangerous materials that influence the air quality.[275] The list includes, but is not limited to: combustion sources such as oil, gas, kerosene, coal, wood, and tobacco products; building materials; asbestos-containing insulation; wet or damp carpet; formaldehyde from cabinetry or furniture made of certain pressed wood products; products for household cleaning and maintenance; products for personal care, or hobbies; central heating and cooling systems and humidification devices; air fresheners; the use of solvents in cleaning and hobby activities; cleaning products and pesticides in housekeeping, etc. High-pollutant concentrations can remain in the air for long periods after some of these activities.

The question is: Is my bike riding more like long-duration aerobatic stationary bike riding, or closer to the Grizzly Bear Interval workout? It's probably a combination of both. After reading about his calculations, I did my next ride in the neighborhood with a pulse meter in order to get the feel of where my resting, maximum and duration laps are according to his calculations. Does this mean that every time I take a ride I am always monitoring my pulse? The answer is no. However, it has changed my awareness of how I ride if it is for exercise purposes only.

I choose my daily route according to how I want to exercise for the day. I now separate my easy bike stroll days from days when I go for the grizzly bear style workout. It is also a good solution for those days when I happen to be in a big hurry and want to finish a good workout in a minimum amount of time.

Grizzly bear intervals comprise only the first half of Dr. Grisanti's exercise workout. The second part involves strength training and its importance to overall muscle tone. Dr. Grisanti advocates the Grunt and Growl Strength Training method, in which the exerciser reaches his own personal momentary muscular failure point following only one set of each specific exercise at a predetermined weight/resistance. Similar to his grizzly bear workouts, Dr. Grisanti spells out a very detailed way of working out in the gym. This includes how the exerciser can determine his/her own exercise workout weights to be used.

Another source of information, one that I consider to be most reliable and informative, also advocates working out in a gym in addition to doing some type of aerobatic workouts. The source: Mr. Anthony Colpo.

Who is Anthony Colpo?

Anthony Colpo is not a university professor, nor associate professor. He is not a medical doctor; he is not a doctor of any sort. He is a certified fitness professional. I guess in my college days we would have called him a physical trainer or 'jock' for short. I don't know if the term is still used today, but you remember the jock stereotype: a 250lb illiterate running back that runs the 100 meters in 11 seconds; or the scholarship to the 6'6" guard that hits 70% of his three pointers. Not only that, but Colpo is from............... oh my gosh......Australia!......... I admit that we native born and educated Americans were taught very little about all those 'other' countries out there. In school we did learn that Australia is full of kangaroos and aborigines; however, it wasn't until that specific episode of *The Simpsons* when Homer et al. traveled to Australia that I got to see Aussies in action in their parliament firsthand.

Does this last paragraph seem to be overly cynical and ridiculous? It should. Could there be some correlation between the lackadaisical approach to teaching world geography at the grade school level and the lackadaisical approach of many research professionals in interpreting the actual results of sooooo many studies involving the lipid hypothesis? Although the previous paragraph was written in jest, the thought is frightening.

What is even more frightening regarding that previous paragraph is that it follows the same unwritten guidelines that many of the medical research studies follow, especially if sponsored by an interest group. I am referring to 'consensus' and 'source'. First, an American 'consensus' that all natives of any faraway country inhabited by aborigines and kangaroos are primitive, confirmed by the 'source' -- Lisa Simpson, the rational genius of the Simpson clan. It is insignificant that Lisa Simpson is animated. She is a 'source' and represents a 'consensus'.

Why then would I blindly follow health advice of a non-doctor like Anthony Colpo? The reason is simple. If I had to choose one book, and one book only regarding what causes heart disease, and more importantly, what does NOT cause heart disease, it would be his *The Great Cholesterol Con*. Although Mr. Colpo is not a doctor, perhaps someday a broadminded university will indeed bestow on him an honorary doctorate degree for his superb independent research in such an important field.

Both Dr. Grisanti and Mr. Colpo take their physical training very seriously. With Dr. Grisanti, it's a family thing. In one of his newsletters, he published a picture of both he and his wife in bathing suits. If there is such a thing as a Mr. and Mrs. America (married) contest, they would be very serious contenders. Mr. Colpo is more modest, and I do not recall seeing a picture of him in a bathing suit; however, according to his neck circumference, it definitely appears that he takes his personal physical training VERY seriously. As a certified fitness professional, he personally pumps the iron big time. The bottom line -- both Dr. Grisanti and Mr. Colpo are diehard advocates of purposeful physical activity for maintaining good health.

I personally have never cared for the gym surroundings for working out -- the loud music, the 'stench' despite the air conditioners working full force.

Esty does like working out at the gym. She also has an interesting observation regarding the difference between the men and women that come to the gym to work out. Men come already stinky to the gym because they will be showering after the workout anyway. Women come to the gym already after a shower and smelling nice......

No, I prefer strength workouts that I can do at home. I don't exercise because I expect to compete in some Olympic strength event. I simply want to stay fit. My preference is isometric or isometric/isotobic type exercises. Isometric workouts are based on exerting a maximum force against an immovable object. This is in contrast to an isotonic type exercise, such as lifting barbells. Isotobic exercise is similar to isometric, only the immovable object is pressing back.

Isometric exercises have been with us for quite a while, even before the name isometric was actually coined. The inventor of modern-day isometric exercise was someone born in 1893 named Angelo Siciliano. Never heard of him? You probably know him by the name of Charles Atlas, crowned the world's most perfectly developed man in the years 1922 and

1923; his isometric exercise method was registered as dynamic tension®.

Anyone growing up in the fifties and sixties who read comic books like I did always saw his advertisements appearing before or after the ads 'Learn to be a locksmith' on the front or back inside covers. Charles Atlas indeed was a 97-pound weakling; the episode where the skinny guy gets sand kicked in his face was based on his real life story.[276]

Charles Atlas rose to fame well before sports, all sports, including bodybuilding, were tainted by anabolic steroid usage. Charles Atlas was natural; he was pure. Testosterone was not synthesized until the 1930's; it was not introduced into the sporting arena until the 1940's and 1950's. Today with the wide use of anabolic steroids, there are no doubt bodybuilders who are bigger and stronger than Charles Atlas; however, none will ever reach his immortality.

It's almost like comparing Barry Bonds to Babe Ruth. Bonds has already surpassed Ruth's total homerun tally; as this is being submitted for printing, he is now very, very close to catching Hank Aaron. Bonds' name has been tainted by possible forbidden drugs usage. Ruth, however, would sign autographs; he visited kids in the hospital; he played ball with kids in the street. Babe Ruth remains a legend. Charles Atlas also remains a legend.

2007

A study published in the April edition of Medicine & Science in Sports & Exercise[277] confirms all the previous conclusions regarding HIIT. Maximum oxygen uptake is considered to be the most important factor determining success in aerobic endurance sports. In this study, subjects were split up into four groups.

1. Long slow distance running (LSD) – 70% of maximum heart rate (HR)

2. Lactate threshold running (LT) – 85% of maximum HR
3. 15/15 interval running – 47 repetitions of 15 seconds intervals, 90-95% of maximum HR with 15 seconds of rest of 70% max HR
4. 4 X 4 min interval running – 4 intervals of 4 minutes at 90-95% HRmax with 3 min of rest at 70%

The results:

The high-aerobic intensity training performed by the 15/15 and 4x4 min groups increased absolute VO_{2max} significantly compared with the LSD and LT training. Between the 15/15 and the 4 X 4 min groups, no significant difference in training response was observed.

31

What Really are Degenerative Diseases?

*The illiterate of the 21st century will not be those who cannot
read and write, but those who cannot learn,
unlearn, and relearn.*
Alvin Toffler

Cardiovascular diseases account for more than half of total mortality before the age of 75 in industrialized countries.[278] Merriam-Webster defines disease as 'a condition of the living animal or plant body or of one of its parts that impairs normal functioning and is typically manifested by distinguishing signs and symptoms'. Most of us equate the term 'disease' with what is properly known as 'infectious disease'.

Infectious diseases result from the activities of microorganisms (living creatures) such as viruses, bacteria, and fungi that invade the body. Influenza, Tuberculosis, Malaria, Measles, Syphilis, Rabies, Smallpox and Polio are examples of infectious diseases. Vaccines and other medications are the tools of the trade in combating infectious diseases.

Heart disease is not an infectious disease. It is defined as a 'degenerative disease'. It is not caused by live microorganisms invading our bodies. I have yet to hear of someone receiving a 'vaccination' against heart disease.

What then is the definition of degenerative disease? The National Cancer Institute defines degenerative disease as 'a disease in which the function or structure of the affected tissues or organs changes for the worse over time'. Simple, right?

Melinda Meade and Robert Earickson in *Medical Geography* define degenerative disease not as a point-blank definition, but rather in terms of its **characteristics**; 'degenerative diseases are *characterized* by the deterioration or impairment of an organ or the structure of cells and the tissues of which they are a part'.

I will concentrate on two particular definitions that I feel zero in on what degenerative diseases really signify. The first is a superb non-technical definition coined by Dr. Ruza Bogdanovich in *The Cure is the Cause*.

> *Degenerative disease occurs when the body does not get what it needs. When it doesn't, it degenerates.*

Another definition appears in Wikipedia:

> *A degenerative disease is a disease in which the function or structure of the affected tissues or organs will progressively deteriorate over time, whether due to normal bodily wear or **lifestyle choices** such as **exercise** or **eating habits**.* (Bold emphasis is mine.)

Lifestyle choices! Exercise and eating habits! Eating habits entail, of course, food choices. And what is food exactly? According Merriam-Webster, food is 'material consisting essentially of protein, carbohydrate, and fat used in the body of an organism to sustain growth, repair, and vital processes and to furnish energy'.

There is nothing negative regarding this definition of food. Sure, we eat food to supply us with energy, but if what we eat impairs growth, repair and vital processes, why then do we still call it 'food'? It should be called 'anti-food'. Food does not cause degenerative diseases, anti-food does. The mass of anti-food that you can buy in most supermarkets is mind-boggling!

Modern medical technology has indeed found medical solutions to keep us going when we develop 'degenerative diseases'.

I arrived that one Friday afternoon to Hadassah Hospital in the midst of a heart attack, had an additional two attacks that night while still hooked up to all of the intravenous infusions. Sunday morning I had a stent implanted and first thing Monday morning I was already back on my feet, planning my recovery and return to normal routine. That is fantastic medical technology. Future side effects and additional medications aside, it is still a very impressive feat of technology.

The bypass operation is another favorite tool used by cardiology surgeons. Executed for the first time by Dr. René G. Favaloro at the Cleveland Clinic in 1967,[279] bypass operations are now very commonplace the world over. The term itself also brings back fond memories, but not related in any way to heart surgery.

A month before my 17th birthday, I passed my driving test. The routine was receiving a learner's permit, and having an adult family member teach you how to drive in the family car. Our family car at the time was an old 1956 Ford Station Wagon sporting a 292 cubic inch engine. This was the same engine used in the new small two-seater sports car, the Ford Thunderbird. In that big station wagon, it was a powerful engine; those early sporty T-birds must have really flown! Yep, that Ford was big, blue and..... rusty. (I bet you thought I was about to say big, blue and beautiful.)

This was a time when my fellow students would arrive to do their driving test in the new smaller compact cars -- the Chevy Corvair, Ford Falcon and the like. Truthfully, doing parallel parking or the three-point turn-around with a small, and possibly automatic transmission car was a big plus. Looking back, I guess the DMV tester gave me some extra points for showing up to do the test in an 11-year-old huge blue tank with the three-speed manual transmission on the column. I passed the test on my first try.

Sometime after the test, when the old engine was all gummed up on the inside, the oil wasn't circulating from the bottom crankcase to the top of the engine. This caused the car to overheat and lose even more oil. Mechanics then were creative; possibly they received inspiration from their medical colleagues.

The solution: a set of copper 'bypass' pipes connecting the bottom crankcase to the head of the engine. At the time we were so impressed with the recent heart bypass process that whenever anyone asked us what those strange copper pipes were on our engine, we proudly answered that the car had a bypass operation, just like they do now on real people.

Cars are mechanical and made out of metal. There is a natural non-renewable deterioration of the materials and moving parts over time. It is natural for a car to develop a 'degenerative disease'. It is not necessarily natural for us humans, especially before old age.

Cancer is another example of a 'degenerative' disease. Like heart disease, cancer also has its technological solutions. The cardiologist has angioplasty, stent implantation and bypass operations in his bag of tricks. The oncologist has at his disposal chemotherapy, radiotherapy and surgery. These are all 'fixes'. We hear all the time about all the efforts being made to find the 'cure' for cancer.

Well over a half a century ago, Nobel Prize Laureate Otto Heinrich Warburg[*] discovered that cancer is caused by

---

[*] Otto Warburg was awarded the 1931 Nobel Prize in Physiology or Medicine. It is believed he was selected for a second Nobel Prize in 1944, but as a Jew was not allowed to accept the prize due to the policies of the German Nazi

impaired cell respiration due to a lack of oxygen at the cellular level. This in turn results in hyper-acidity at the same cellular level. Dr. Wigmore cured her own cancer by lifestyle changes, which included a diet more alkaline that acidic. In the 1980's, Dr. Keith Brewer[280] successfully treated patients with various cancers using Cesium, nature's most alkaline mineral, not with radiotherapy and chemotherapy.

What do heart disease and cancer, two degenerative diseases, have in common? Cardiology and oncology researchers spend tremendous resources on improving the 'fixes'; the direction should instead be on 'prevention'. Prevention for both in many cases is feeding the body foods as nature intended, and eliminating the junk that overly taxes the body's ability to digest it. Dr. Maynard Murray was quoted in M.D. Magazine as saying:

> ... *the human race is very much what it eats, and if we would pay a bit more attention to the quality of what goes into our mouths, we might be able to find some solutions to two of mankind's more pressing health problems – cancer and arteriosclerosis*

I humbly submit my own supplement to Dr. Bogdanovich's definition of degenerative disease.

Degenerative disease occurs when the body gets what it doesn't need. When it does, it degenerates.

---

government at the time. This has never been confirmed by The Nobel Foundation.

32

Angiogram #2

February 2007

Chronologically, this is the natural continuation following Chapter 19, which ended with 'to be continued...'. This is the continuation. I did want to review some basic knowledge before reverting back to my personal story. It has been over five and a half years since my heart attack in July 2001. The angiogram performed at that time determined that my main LAD artery (Left Anterior Descending coronary artery) suffered from a blockage of 90%. A blood clot that was unable to navigate the blocked artery was basically the essence of my heart attack. Angioplasty (ballooning) was performed and a stent was installed in the blocked area to keep the artery open.

Two days before my scheduled second angiogram, I arrived at the hospital for the pre-angiogram blood tests and checkup. The doctor performing the checkup asked me the usual questions. Has there been chest discomfort? Do I exercise? She also asked me a question that really took me by surprise. "How many angiograms have you already gone through in the past?"

What bothered me at the time was the intonation in the doctor's voice that this was a typical routine question. It has always been my impression that angiograms are not procedures that people would do routinely many times -- silly me! I answered, "This will be my second time." She recorded the answer and continued with the next question.

Two days after that pre-checkup, I was back on the angiogram table in order to discover and correct the cause of the marginal results of my latest stress test and the subsequent positive results of the thallium heart scan. I had not been experiencing any chest discomfort. Even my professor of cardiology said the angiogram may show the need for a quick, minor correction only, and possibly not even that.

After all, I was feeling great. I had been slowly but surely making vast improvements in my eating habits, and was still considered to be very physically active (bike riding) for my age group. I was well past the initial period when most cases of restenosis (stent blockage) with the standard non-coated stents occur (or so I thought).

The results of the angiogram not only totally surprised me, but my professor of cardiology as well. The stent was totally blocked up -- not a 90% artery blockage like in 2001, however, a full 100%. For two and a half hours, the doctors performing the angiogram tried without success to perform an angioplasty and open up the blockage.

This entire episode raised a number of perplexing questions and uncertainties regarding future action to be taken.

Aren't there usually warning signs of some type when this occurs -- chest pains? fatigue? something? Interestingly, the literature shows that 40% of patients with restenosis may be free of chest pain.[281] According to my cardiologist, the discontinuation of the statins played a critical role. A stent is nevertheless not naturally found in human arteries. Is its closing up somehow concerned with a possible natural body defense mechanism? Didn't my improving eating habits and serious approach to exercising influence this process at all? Did the rest of my arteries suffer similar advancing blockages, or was the problem localized to the stent area only?

How was it I was 'still alive' and fully functioning with a 100% blockage in this critical artery? Will I now need an emergency bypass operation? Medical terminology has another way of referring to a totally blocked artery. It is known as Chronic Total Occlusion (CTO). It was explained to me that while the stent was slowly closing up (probably over the last couple of years) my cardiovascular system was developing new alternative blood vessels (collaterals) to circumvent the constantly narrowing main artery.

Amazing -- my own in-house bypass operation! Many people, the lucky ones not experiencing sudden death, require immediate emergency bypass surgery when this occurs. An immediate ultrasound performed while still on the angiogram table showed that this was unnecessary for me. Why was I one of the lucky ones? Was this due to all the bike riding I do? Improved eating habits? NOT taking statin medication?

And exactly how well are *my* new collaterals functioning. When Chronic Total Occlusion occurs, well-developed collaterals may provide flow equivalent to a 90-95% stenosis[282] (equivalent to a 90-95% blockage of the original occluded artery). Is this sufficient?

As far as my doctors are concerned this is even more reason to take statins, to protect these new delicate blood vessels. Am I being naive or in self-denial, telling myself that in a sense my own cardiovascular system has performed a sort of internal bypass operation and that I can continue worry free with the status quo? What about the rest of my arteries; are they progressively blocking up also?

I mentioned in SASHA that I was verbally informed back in 2001 that there were additional blockages in my arteries; however, only that one specific blockage in the critical LAD artery required medical intervention. I never received the 2001 angiogram report. My official hospitalization then was at the Mount Scopus branch of Hadassah Hospital; angiograms, angioplasty and such are performed at Hadassah Hospital's Ein Kerem branch.

My present angiogram was done on a Thursday. I was discharged from the hospital Friday morning, a day most offices are already closed for the weekend. First thing Sunday morning, the first day of the normal work week in Israel, I went back to the hospital to see if I could get a copy of that 2001 angiogram report for comparative reasons. I did find the appropriate department, my personal identity information was typed into the terminal, and I could see the report being printed out on the office printer.

This was an exciting moment for me. Besides the 100% blocked stent, has the overall cardiovascular condition of my arteries deteriorated since 2001? Have I been on a 'good path' these last couple of years or simply have I been very, very foolish? In a few seconds I would know.

33

Vindication

*We can't solve problems by using the same kind of
thinking we used when we created them.*
Albert Einstein

This chapter is actually a natural part of the previous
chapter, however, for me it is of prime importance. It
may be a very short chapter, but the personal significance
of this chapter for me is overwhelming, and therefore it stands as
a separate independent entity.

I compared the 2001 angiogram report with the fresh
2007 one. With the exception of the total restenosis in 2007
(100% stent blockage), **the same partially blocked locations
and the percentage of those blockages in 2001 were identical
to the present blockages -- my overall condition had not
worsened.**

Vindication

2001 Angiogram report

.51 גיל החולה

צינתור שמאלי נערך ביום 15/07/2001 עם שימוש בצנתרים Judkins right 6F , Judkins left 6F .

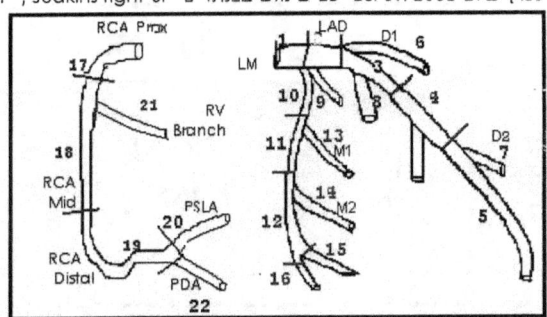

המימצאים בעורקים הכליליים

העורק השמאלי הראשי תקין, מערכת LAD ראה פירוט, מערכת CIRC ראה פירוט, מערכת RCA ראה פירוט.

שם ומספר הסגמנט	דרגת היצרות מ"מ 3 - 0	זרימה קולטרלית	קוטר ואזי מ"מ	מיקום	אפיונים למיקטע	מתאים לבלון לניתוח	
1- LEFT MAIN	תקין					○	○
4-LAD mid	> 90%					⦿	○
12-CIRC distal	קל					○	○
14-Second Marginal	50-70%					○	○
18-RCA mid	קל					○	○

2001 -Translation:

Name and Segment No.	Degree of Blockage
4 – LAD mid	>90% (angioplasty necessary)
12 – CIRC distal	Light
14 – Second Marginal	50-70%
18 – RCA mid	Light

2007 Angiogram report

גיל החולה 57.

צינתור שמאלי נערך ביום 01/02/07 עם שימוש בצנתרים Judkins right 6F , Judkins left 6F .

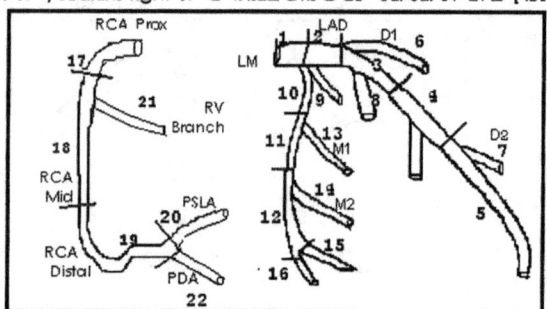

המימצאים בעורקים הכליליים

העורק השמאלי הראשי תקין, מערכת LAD ראה פירוט, מערכת CIRC ראה פירוט, מערכת RCA ראה פירוט. העורק הימני דומיננטי.

שם ומספר הסגמנט	מיקום היצרות מ"מ 0-3	דרגת TIMI	קוטר	זרימה קולטרלית		אפיונים למיקטע	מתאים לבלון לניתוח	
				מאין	איכות			
4-LAD mid	100%					prox to stent	◯	⦿
14-Second Marginal	50-70%						◯	◯
18-RCA mid	קל						◯	◯

2007 - Translation:

Name and Segment No.	Degree of Blockage
4 – LAD mid – prox to stent	100% (angioplasty necessary)
14 – Second Marginal	50-70%
18 – RCA mid	Light

After three and a half years without the statins and not being on a low-fat low-cholesterol agenda, the angiograms did not indicate any significant deterioration in my artery condition. There was even a light blockage (12–CIRC distal) that showed up in 2001 that was deemed insignificant enough not to state in 2007.

This was a tremendous relief to me -- a vindication that my eating/exercising habits were indeed keeping the condition of my arteries from deteriorating further. I brought this up with my professor of cardiology who said that really doesn't really confirm anything; the angiogram looks at the inside of the arteries only and certainly doesn't measure possible hardening or thickening of the arteries. This may be a valid point; however, it doesn't negate the fact that I have succeeded in maintaining the status quo -- and without the statins!

I also wonder how many of his patients that come in for the '15-minute' tune up to balloon stents from time to time also take statins, and still need the ballooning. After all, the stent still remains a foreign metal object implanted in a very critical area. One of the functions of cholesterol is to 'bandage' inflamed/damaged arteries. This is a natural defensive action that our bodies perform. The body's natural tendency to insulate the stent from its surroundings is a defensive mechanism.

Chronic total occlusions are found in approximately one-third of the patients with significant coronary disease who undergo angiography.[283] There are three accepted options for dealing with the options available to anyone suffering from Chronic Total Occlusion (CTO).[284]

One option is Percutaneous Intervention, or as more commonly known, angioplasty treatment. Recanalization of a CTO is attempted in only 8-15% of patients undergoing angioplasty.[285] As stated before, this attempt was not successful on me.

The presence of a CTO is a common reason for referral to a second option[286] - coronary artery bypass surgery (CABG). But even a successful bypass operation does not promise a lasting solution. Sections of blood vessels used to create detours around the original blockages tend to develop clogs five to ten years after a bypass.[287] While I realize that a bypass operation is a potential reality for me, I hope to be able to avoid one. In addition, nearly a quarter of the million patients a year who need stents have had bypass surgery in the past.[288] I already have one stent. I really do not want another one.

A third option is described simply as 'medical management'. Bring on the Beta-blockers, ACE-inhibitors, and in particular, the statins. I've gone that route before also. That is basically what SASHA was all about.

In my particular situation, it is imperative to encourage the development of additional blood vessel generation and promote adequate blood flow in my existing cardiovascular system; this is especially true due to the fact that test results show that I am not functioning 100% at the higher heart stress rates. The bottom line, and an agonizing question for me, do I now have to consider the statins in the terms of personal profit and loss?

Dr. Uffe Ravnskov in his pioneering epic *The Cholesterol Myths* acknowledged the cardio health benefits of statins[289] and explained why they are independent of their cholesterol-lowering properties. The statins inhibit the production of a substance called mevalonate, which is a precursor of cholesterol. As mevalonate production decreases, so does cholesterol production. However, mevalonate is also a precursor of other substances in the body that control other important biological functions, some which influence arterial health.

Today there is no doubt that statins do have a beneficial effect on the cardiovascular system. Statins can impair or reverse atherosclerotic plaque formation; improve arterial function; has anti-clotting, anti-inflammatory and antioxidant effects; and prevents atherosclerotic plaque rupture.[290] Cost vs. benefit. I remember all too well my personal costs of the low cholesterol levels caused by the statins.

I respectfully submit my own variation to this third option of 'medical management'. In place of the medications (ESPECIALLY statins), a change in food choices and adequate exercise, the subject of the next chapter.

34

Bottom Line

Off the shelf may be great for software,
but not for your stomach[*]

Food

Anyone from my generation remembers the Watergate scandal during President Nixon's administration and the list of the stars involved. One of the stars was G. Gordon Liddy. He was one tough cookie. It was Liddy's refusal to talk about his role in the Watergate scandal that sent him to prison for a longer term than any other Watergate figure. Time Magazine, in its April 21, 1980 issue, printed some excerpts from his then recent autobiography *Will*.

> *Then I got the idea for a test to destroy forever any dread I might still harbor for rats. For the next hour, I roasted the dead rat. With a scout knife I skinned, then cut off and ate the roasted haunches of the rat.*

---

[*] I made that up

For some strange reason, I had always remembered a response that appeared in the Letters to the Editor from a reader who stated:

> *To G. Gordon Liddy's self-imposed requirement to eat a roasted rat and his activities as an adult, I can only remark,* **"You are what you eat.**"[291] (Bold emphasis is mine.)

Yes, we are what we eat. Not only is this a literal expression, but it also now used figuratively as well. The point I am making is both literally and figuratively, *live* people should make an effort to eat more *live* food. Eating only dead food should be seen as expediting the trip to the next whatever-it-is that awaits us all, whether it be a shorter lifespan due to 'natural causes' or an abrupt exit due to some degenerative disease.

My standard breakfast

My basic 'appetizer' is a shot/half a glass of freshly squeezed wheatgrass juice. However on a non everyday schedule which I will discuss shortly, I precede this by dissolving a teaspoon of freshly ground turmeric root in a glass of water. Turmeric has been used for thousands of years to treat a variety of diseases. The active substance in turmeric is curcumin. Curcumin reduces inflammation (a major cause of atherosclerosis) and is also a powerful antioxidant[292] (reduces free radicals).

I follow that with a 'Mike Shlush' (modified Victoria smoothie from chapter 27). I also grind in one clove of garlic (high sulfur content) and ginger (strong free radical scavenging property and known for its anti-inflammatory properties[293]).

I then have my own variation of the Budwig drink. Dr. Johanna Budwig, a German biochemist and multiple Nobel award nominee did extensive research on the properties and benefits of Essential Fatty Acids (EFA's) combined with sulfurated proteins in the diet. Sulfur is a mineral that has the ability to carry oxygen in the body.

Her basic Budwig tonic is based on blending low-fat cottage cheese (or yogurt) with flax seed oil and/or freshly ground flax seeds. When flax seed oil and sulfur-rich protein are combined, the EFA's in the flax seed oil become water-soluble and electron-rich. This increases the stability of the cell membrane and facilitates the transfer of materials and energy between the inner and outer cell membrane.[294] It was her contention that such oils should be consumed together with foods containing the appropriate proteins; otherwise the oils will cause more harm than good.

We saw in Chapter 25 that most of the plaque clogging our arteries is composed of polyunsaturated fats that we consume in our diet. Essential Fatty Acids are polyunsaturated fatty acids that our bodies cannot produce and must be consumed in our diets as polyunsaturated fats.

Nutritionists will come up with different, if not outright conflicting recommendations regarding absolute minimum and maximum requirements. I too have my sources which I choose to accept.

Anthony Colpo mentions that polyunsaturated fats should comprise no more than 4.5% of our total daily calorie intake.[295] Dr. Mary Enig, a world-renowned biochemist specializing in the nutritional aspects of fats and oils, has coauthored many articles with Weston A. Price Foundation head Ms. Sally Fallon Morell. Dr. Enig recommends that we take in at least 2 to 3% of our calories as fat in the form of omega-6 fatty acids and at least 1 to 1.5% in the form of omega-3 fatty acids.[296]

My variation of the Budwig drink:

Instead of yogurt, I use my homemade kefir. I should point out that Dr. Budwig did not specifically mention kefir; it is my own substitute. I mentioned in Chapter 12, when making kefir, the jar must be shaken one to two times per day. This combines the separating whey back into the mixture. Whey proteins contain sulfur, which in turn contains the amino acids cysteine and methionine. The basis for the Budwig drink is sulfur-rich protein.

The kefir I usually make ferments for 48 hours, however only 24 hours during the hot summer months. The extra fermentation time burns off more of the natural milk sugar.

To the kefir I add several tablespoons of freshly ground flax seeds, which is rich in Omega-3. I prefer to use freshly ground flax seeds and not flax seed oil, because the oils become rancid very easily if not properly cared for. Flax seed oil is found in the refrigerated section of your health store; it should be cold-pressed and packaged in an opaque container.[297] At home it must also be kept refrigerated. Flax seed oil should never be heated[298] (as in cooking and frying). Omega-3 is important; however, if you start developing skin rashes, you may be overdoing it with the flax/oil.

I mix in several drops of borage oil. This is my compensation for the aspirin effect of neutralizing the D6D enzyme that promotes production of the conditional fatty acid GLA. It was also found that administration of relatively small amounts of GLA, (up to 360 mg/day) raises the blood levels of arachidonic acid (AA), which is also an important conditional essential fatty acid.[299] Do not overdose on Essential Fatty Acids. Stay within set maximum limits. It was shown that a very high dose of borage oil over a span of a month and a half enhances platelet aggregation;[300] this is something heart patients should be particularly aware of.

I also add a tablespoon of cocoa. Cocoa flavanols may lower inflammation, keep blood pressure in check and prevent platelets from clotting.[301] Cocoa is also a good source of copper. Remember Dr. Klevay and copper deficiency from SASHA?

One third to one half of a teaspoon of fish oil meets requirements for the daily intake of EPA and DHA.[302]

I also add several almonds and walnuts that have been pre-soaked and rinsed.[303] I then add several tablespoons of raw (non-toasted) oat flakes that have also been pre-soaked[304] in whey (phytates and anti-nutrients, remember?). Keep in mind that whole grains are acidic in nature.[305] Slightly aged whey is considered to be a weak acid. Germinating/soaking the grains in an acid medium[306] makes them more alkaline.[307] This reaction is termed 'alkaline-forming' foods.

For 'dessert', I usually have a soft-boiled egg. I buy only organic 'free range' eggs. The nutritional quality of eggs is a function of the food the hens eat. Organic 'free range' eggs have a more balanced healthier omega-3 to omega-6 fatty acid ratio (chapter 25) than commercially grown indoor caged hens. In addition, the eggs of outdoor free range hens are rich in Vitamin D.

My lunch or supper is typically a big salad with meat, fish, or chicken.

My third meal is generally another glass of kefir, and one or more cream cheese (Chapter 28) sandwiches. I no longer make my own baked whole wheat–rye bread as I used to. I now opt for unbaked 'flat bread' made in a food dehydrator. For a great introduction on the use of food dehydrators and illustrated (non wheat) bread recipe, check out 'Igor's Live Flat Bread' by Igor Boutenko - that's right, Victoria's (raw-food) husband. I also use Igor's recipe as the basis of my own variations, such as oat bread/crackers.

During the day I will also 'snack'. Snacks include having another egg or some fruit ('sour' fruits such as apple/grapefruit, and later a sweet fruit such as a banana). I will also drink a glass or two of rejuvelac (chapter 27) if I have some on hand.

Good rules to live by: stay off of sweets, sugars (ESPECIALLY fructose) and white flour as much as possible! Canola oil still does NOT enter my household. I realize that it is still a favorite with 'heart' dieticians because it is a monounsaturated oil like olive oil. Anything you need to know about Canola oil can be found on the Weston A. Price website.

I have said it before, but I will say it again -- eliminate totally all partially hydrogenated ingredients from your diet. *THE* Internet site on partially hydrogenated oils and trans-fats is Stephen Joseph's www.bantransfats.com[*].

Statins (HMG CoA reductase inhibitors)

Immediately following my two-and-a-half-hour angiogram, I took another look at the short-term benefits vs. costs of taking statins. I did decide to resume a hydrophilic statin[**] temporarily -- for four weeks and taper off by the sixth week. This was not to lower my cholesterol levels, but rather for other short-term effects which may be specifically beneficial for me after getting 'poked at from within' on the angiogram table, i.e. anti-inflammatory effects, anti-clotting, prevention of plaque rupture[308] etc. Statin therapy does appear to reduce the incidence of stroke, myocardial infarction, and death within 30 days after angioplasty and stent placement.[309] However, this time I also took coenzymeQ$_{10}$ with it - not because my doctor told me, but because of all the evidence that statins deplete the body of coenzymeQ$_{10}$.

Warning:
HMG CoA reductase inhibitors block the endogenous biosynthesis of an essential cofactor, coenzymeQ$_{10}$, required for energy production. A deficiency of

---

[*] See how you can get your own 'Don't partially hydrogenate me' T-shirt and bumper sticker!

[**]as opposed to a lipophilic statin – for the most up-to-date and complete guide to statin medication, visit Dr. Duane Graveline's website http://www.spacedoc.net

coenzymeQ$_{10}$ is associated with impairment of myocardial function, with liver dysfunction and with myopathies (including cardiomyopathy and congestive heart failure). **All patients taking HMG CoA reductase inhibitors should therefore be advised to take 100 to 200mg per day of supplemental coenzymeQ$_{10}$.**[310] (Bold emphasis is mine.)

It may have been prudent to also take selenium supplements during this period, but for the limited period I didn't.

We noted that the pattern of side effects associated with statins resembles the pathology of selenium deficiency…… A negative effect of statins on selenoprotein synthesis does seem to explain many of the enigmatic effects and side effects of statins, in particular, statin-induced myopathy (muscular weakness)[311]

I stated previously that I am functioning normally in spite of the blocked main artery due to the generation of new blood vessels which circumvented my blocked stent. Let's take a closer look at what I referred up until now as simply 'new blood vessels'.

Angiogenesis

Angiogenesis is a process by which new capillary blood vessels sprout from a preexisting blood vessels. Stated more scientifically, it is a process in which endothelial cells proliferate and differentiate to form a fine capillary tree.

Capillaries are designed to provide maximum nutrient delivery efficiency. A greater number of capillaries also allows for greater oxygen exchange in our bodies. The driving force for angiogenesis is ischemia[312] (restriction in blood supply, generally due to factors in the smaller blood vessels). Angiogenesis is also induced by hypoxia[313] (shortage of oxygen). Hypoxia would be a natural consequence resulting from ischemia.

Angiogenesis, however, has not been shown to be correlated with increased blood flow,[314] (angiogenesis is not compensation for an occluded artery) which brings us to our next term:

Arteriogenesis

Arteriogenesis is the rapid proliferation of preexisting standby collateral arteries known as arterioles; it refers to an increase in the diameter of existing arterial vessels. Newly generated arteries can expand up to 20 times the diameter of the original arteriole.[315] In principle this mechanism resembles a deflated bicycle inner tube that stays flat until needed. When pumping it up with physical force, the once flat, airless inner tube becomes an expanding diameter air-filled tube.

Mechanically, arteriogenesis is linked to elevated pressure (physical force). This in turn increases radial wall stress, and fluid shear stress (elevated flow), which increases endothelial surface stress. Chronically elevated fluid shear stress was found to be the strongest trigger of arteriogenesis under experimental conditions.[316]

As I have personally experienced, it is possible to functionally replace an occluded (blocked) artery completely by collaterals.[317]

The most basic differences between angiogenesis and arteriogenesis are summarized on the following chart: [318]

	Angiogenesis	Arteriogenesis
Initiated by	Ischemia (blockage)	Shear Stress
Substrate	Preexisting capillaries	Preexisting arterioles
Result	Increased capillary density	New arteries
Time	Days	Days to weeks

Obviously, angiogenesis and arteriogenesis are terms that have taken on a new significance for me. In this regard, will statins be beneficial for me? Studies indicate that statins have a biphasic potential either to promote or inhibit angiogenesis. Low statin doses induce a pro-angiogenic effect, and high statin doses cause an anti-angiogenic effect.[319]

Studies are great for the researchers, but for us patients what does this really mean? Are the current doses in clinical use that we humans take pro-angiogenic or anti-angiogenic? This was a question I put to a number of researchers. An answer that I received is 'current doses in clinical use are probably pro-angiogenic, however, this remains an educated guess.' As I learned from my two-year, 20mg Pravastatin period, not all patients have the same tolerance to medication as others. What may be a low dose for someone could very well be a high dose for someone else. Let's assume for the argument that it is indeed pro-angiogenic in most cases. Is that a good thing or a bad thing? For a damaged area of the heart, it may be a very good thing; however, does this mean that artificially stimulated angiogenesis is good for the body as a whole? The National Cancer Institute states[320] that:

> *Cancer spreads by metastasis, the ability of cancer cells to penetrate into lymphatic and blood vessels, circulate through the bloodstream, and then invade*

and grow in normal tissues elsewhere.... Cancer researchers studying the conditions necessary for cancer metastasis have discovered that one of the critical events required is the growth of a new network of blood vessels. This process of forming new blood vessels is called **angiogenesis.** (Bold emphasis is mine.)

Dr. Judah Folkman stated as early as 1971 that cancer tumors were angiogenesis-dependent.[321] Dr. Napoleone Ferrara stated straight to the point and very bluntly:

Abnormal regulation of angiogenesis has been implicated in the pathogenesis of several disorders, including cancer.[322]

Angiogenesis? I prefer to depend on my own body chemistry to regulate my angiogenesis rate by natural means. Am I being overly panicky? With regards to statins and their relationship to cancer:

- *Use of cholesterol-lowering drugs should be restricted to those at high risk of short-term CHD death, such as those with prior CHD.*[323]

- *A disturbing increased incidence of cancers has been reported in two randomized controlled trials of the hydrophilic 3- hydroxy-3-methylglutaryl CoA (HMG-CoA) reductase inhibitor pravastatin—Prospective Study of Pravastatin in the Elderly at Risk (PROSPER;ref.1) and Cholesterol and Recurrent Events (CARE;ref.2). In the PROSPER[*] trial, the*

---

[*] CARE and PROSPER were two studies researching the effects of statins on heart disease – the cancer findings were an added surprise.

*reduction in deaths from vascular events was completely negated by the increase in deaths from cancer. In the CARE trial, breast cancer occurred in a significantly greater number of women treated with pravastatin.......**There is clearly an urgent need for further controlled trials of the individual statins with inclusion of cancer mortality as a clinical end point.**[324]* (Bold emphasis is mine.)

- *Squalene, the immediate precursor to cholesterol, has anti-cancer effects, according to research.[325]*

I mentioned previously that I grind up a teaspoon of the spice turmeric in the morning – but not every morning. The active ingredient in turmeric is curcumin, which has been shown to be an inhibitor of angiogenesis. If my primary health concern today was fighting cancer, I probably would take turmeric every morning. Since today I am more concerned with the anti-inflammatory benefits of turmeric, I do not take it every morning in order to minimize my own interference in my natural angiogenesis process.[326]

I hope I am wrong, however, my gut feeling tells me the next decade will see a dramatic increase in research studies proving a definite positive correlation between statin usage and an increase in the incidence of cancer.

Will a cancer epidemic overtake the heart disease epidemic as the number one cause of death?

As important that angiogenesis is for small capillary generation, my main concern, due to the stent blockage, is blood flow and arteriogenesis. Do statins affect arteriogenesis positively or negatively? Tests do show that statins improve general arterial function by specifically improving endothelial function.[327]

Interestingly, the positive effects of statins on endothelial function disappear a short time after discontinuation of taking them. A test involving atorvastatin (Lipitor) showed these benefits disappeared in a mere 36 hours. Incidentally, the half-life of atorvastatin is approximately 14 hours, which is about 10 times longer than the half-life of most other statins.[328]

An important regulator of coronary collateral growth is nitric oxide.[329] The statins ability to increase nitric oxide production[330] leads to an increase in Endothelial Progenitor Cells (EPC) and improved endothelial function.[331]

Is there a relationship between the dose of the statins and development of the collaterals? Good question. One study says no[332] (and by the way also specifically states that there is no relationship between collateral development and LDL cholesterol levels). Another study found that collateral development was viable only with statin doses of at least 10mg of atorvastatin or equivalent.[333]

Again, is artificially interfering with production of progenitor cells beneficial or harmful? A 2007 study warns that:

> *caution should be used in the manipulation of circulating progenitor cells for therapeutic strategies.*[334]

A bit confused? You should be; so am I. There is a much better way to increase nitric oxide production and increase circulating Endothelial Progenitor Cells. The answer – EXERCISE! In the last years, several groups were able to show the positive effects of exercise on Endothelial Progenitor Cells.[335]

It has been shown that growth of these collateral arteries is triggered by physical forces, which increases fluid shear stress on the vessels. Fluid shear stress initiates the activation of Endothelial Cells.[336] And as a bonus, shear stress is also known to lead to the release of nitric oxide.[337]

I prefer to increase my nitric oxide production and my circulating EPC's by bike riding rather than by statin popping. Antioxidants (found in nuts and seeds), a little garlic and keeping a lid on sugar also promote nitric oxide (NO) production. [338]

Regarding NO production and arteriogenesis in particular:

Maintenance, or improvement, of NO production and signaling, such as with regular exercise, may improve endothelial cell function and thus may help preserve the arteriogenic potential of preexisting collateral networks.[339]

Statins are the ultimate invention of the twentieth/twenty-first century. For those who cannot, or simply will not exercise by choice, the statin offers a solution, a calculated risk solution. For those who choose not to eat properly the statin does offer an alternative, again, a calculated risk alternative.

What exactly is a calculated risk? When Israeli Prime Minister Ariel Sharon had a minor stroke on December 18, 2005, the cause was attributed to a clot lodged in a small 1 - 2mm hole in his heart. The hole was a minor birth defect, also found in 15-20% of the population.[340] Prime Minister Sharon was given heavy doses of blood-thinning medication, which can be associated with an increased risk of brain hemorrhage; this was the calculated risk. The purpose of this medication was to prevent another occurrence of a clot pending the heart operation. On January 4, 2006, the night before his scheduled heart operation and while still at home, he suffered a major stroke with massive internal bleeding. He has been in a vegetative state ever since.

To statin or not to statin -- that is the question. It comes down to a choice between two alternatives.

I start the day off with a shot of wheatgrass, which I have been growing and nurturing for the last seven to ten days. I make my own personal breakfast cereal which includes homemade kefir; the kefir is made from raw milk that I have to obtain from the 'underground'. It has been fermenting for the last 48 hours and has to be filtered to separate the grains from the liquid. To this I add oats that have been soaking for the last 24 hours in whey (slightly acidic), walnuts and almonds that have been soaking in a salt solution, freshly ground flax seeds, besides other ingredients. I repeat this filtering process for another glass of kefir in the evening. I make my own cheese; total processing time is measured in days. I find the time for daily deliberate physical activity that can range from half an hour to one and a half hours.

Or…….

I can simply take a statin.

For me the choice is obvious. I willingly choose the former. My gripe is that statins are now given as a first-choice method of treatment; due to their disastrous side effects I consider them to be more of a last resort. If, as I grow older and find that for reasons beyond my control I will no longer be able to exercise as much as I believe to be necessary, I will again weigh the costs vs. the benefits of taking statin medication. And even then, the dosage will be much smaller than the accepted clinical dosages prescribed today.[341] For now, I prefer the natural alternatives.

Exercise

While still on the angiogram table, my professor stated that it was probably the bike riding that helped develop my internal bypasses. Indeed, medical studies do confirm that blood vessels enlarge when chronically exposed to high flows.[342] What then would be the ultimate exercise method to maintain these new bypass arteries at an optimal level? Research also shows that once new arteries open up, they also rapidly decrease in size if overall decreased blood flow warrants it (decreased wall stress).[343]

Introducing HIIT (grizzly bear) workouts in my riding routine has allowed me to have an adequate workout, when short of time or when especially poor weather keeps me inside. With all of its benefits for cardiovascular health (chapter 30) is it, however, the best way to promote and maintain arteriogenesis? Is arteriogenesis better served by longer-term moderate exercising? Dr. Ulrich Laufs and associates demonstrated that:

> *Intensive and moderate exercising for 30 min, but not for 10 min, increased circulating levels of EPC, which may represent an important beneficial outcome of physical exercise.*[344]

EPC's (Endothelial Progenitor Cells) are made in the bone marrow, enter the bloodstream and go to areas of blood vessel injury to help repair the damage. The number of circulating Endothelial Progenitor Cells in an individual's blood may be an indicator of overall cardiovascular health.[345] Therefore, depletion and aging (senescence) of EPC's may contribute to blood vessel disease.

All exercise is beneficial, as long as not overdoing it.[346] I have adapted several different bike-riding styles to my riding routine. I try at least once a week to go out for an enjoyable off-road trail ride, which encompasses several hours of all the elements of intensity and duration according to the terrain. I use a pulse meter to regulate my efforts as necessary.

During the week when I am usually more pressed for time, I may do alternating days of HIIT (grizzly bear) workouts;

days with longer-duration lower-intensity including steady uphill riding, or simply an enjoyable easy fresh-air ride.

This way I am hopefully benefiting from the best of all worlds -- overall cardiovascular health with an emphasis on arteriogenesis.

The role of the 2-P's in long term exercise planning

The reality of functioning with an occluded artery has reinforced the importance of maintaining a structured riding schedule. As with most other aspects in life, we must work hard to achieve our goals. It takes both persistence and perseverance- the 2 P's - to reach long term goals. For this reason, I want to lump the 2 P's together for the purpose of achieving long term goals as follows:

> Persistence/perseverance is the technique utilized to obtain an ambitious long term goal. A long term goal does not necessarily have a set time deadline. In order to achieve the long term goal, it is divided into a number of short term goals. Each short term goal DOES have a deadline. Moreover, the success or failure of the short term goal must be measurable by some objective method. Persistence/perseverance is the sequence of successfully achieving short term goals over time.

My master long term goal is to maintain the status quo regarding my existing heart disease. This is a *v-e-r-y l-o-n-g t-e-r-m* goal without a set time deadline. One of the means at my disposal to obtain this master goal is to set another smaller *long term* goal WITH a deadline, that involves physical exercise in general, and my bike riding in particular. I have been riding an average 6,000km (3,730mi) per year, and this has become my yearly goal. 6,000km!?! That is further than the air space between New York and Madrid, Spain! Sounds impossible?

Even if there was a bridge connecting both sides of the Atlantic Ocean?

As per my 2-P's doctrine, I divide this ambitious long term goal into 52 short term goals, or, my weekly quota. That is more or less the distance of a weekly round-trip bike ride between Baltimore and Washington D.C.; this still sounds ambitious, but not as 'impossible' as riding the distance between New York to Madrid. In order to meet this short term goal, I keep track of the kilometers/miles that I ride each week. An hour to an hour-and-a-half of daily riding allows me to achieve my weekly goal. The sequence of successfully achieving short term weekly goals over time ultimately results in my meeting my annual goal, which is simply the means to the end of maintaining my status quo.

And it works.

The additional payoff of daily riding and keeping in shape allows me to really enjoy my weekend bike treks with family and friends. Pictures from some of my bike trips are posted on my web site (www.heartrecovery.net).

I will be very happy when a serious researcher will determine

1. if there is a greater positive correlation between 'HIIT and arteriogenesis' as compared to 'longer-duration lower / moderate exercising and arteriogenesis'.

2. if there is any (positive or negative) correlation between HIIT and the cardiovascular health of the specific areas in the arteries that are most susceptible to potential or existing heart disease (areas experiencing the greatest 'sheer stress').[347]

Important tip – when riding in the summer on hot days, be sure to supplement your water with natural salt.[348]

If you are the gym type, then definitely go to the gym. My isometric/isotobic exercise I do at home.

And finally and maybe most important…

And finally and maybe most important…

And finally and maybe most important…

In SASHA, I stated that I considered the heart attack to be a technical temporary setback; I would be back to normalcy in a minimum amount of time. Granted, the statins took me off this timetable for a number of years, but they didn't quell my innermost desire to be 'healthy' again.

Everything up until now stated in this book as been technique only. Proper eating habits and proper exercise are important; however, they are not enough. Anyone who dwells on personal setbacks 'oh I am a miserable unfortunate guy' will always be that, a miserable unfortunate guy. Despite my heart attack, the stent, the total restenosis (blockage) in my main LAD artery, **I am healthy**. No doctor can convince me otherwise!

35

Epilogue

To copy one person's work is plagiarism, to
copy many, is research

According to this definition from an unknown source, this book is certainly not plagiarism; I have quoted from many other works. Does that qualify it as research? I think not! There is nothing truly original in this book. I have invented nothing. I have collected previously published information that I believe will contribute to keeping my cardiovascular system as healthy as possible for my own personal health benefits. Some of my sources are well known, such as Ms. Sally Fallon Morell and her associates from the Weston A. Price Foundation; Dr. Anne Wigmore and others; some of the other sources are not as well known.

Anyone interested in implementing habits that I have acquired to maintain my cardiovascular health should keep in mind that I attribute my current health status to the complete package I have written about. Anyone deciding to 'simply stop taking statins like Mike did', but is not willing to make necessary changes in diet and invest the necessary effort in physical exercise is only deceiving himself.

It may very well be that only a certain few of the changes I have made are responsible for a significant improvement in health; while the effects of some of the changes may be of marginal value only. Taking the easy road out may be risky and lead to undesirable consequences.

It is also difficult to implement a decision when it contradicts the accepted way of doing things, especially if the decision involves personal health issues. The accepted way of preventing and treating heart disease is keeping cholesterol levels at 'acceptable levels'. The accepted ways of accomplishing this is by keeping to low-fat diets and supplementing the process with medications, i.e. statins. Why? Because as far back as our personal memories go, **that's the way it's always been**. End of story.

An amusing story of unknown origins illustrates this point quite well. It is presented to management training students. The story involves a 'study' of five monkeys in a cage. A banana was hung from the top of the cage and a set of stairs was placed under it. For those unfamiliar with monkeys, they naturally like bananas. Almost immediately a monkey started to climb up the stairs in order to retrieve the banana. As soon as he touched the stairs, all of the other monkeys were sprayed with cold water. After a while, another monkey made an attempt with the same results. All the other monkeys were sprayed with cold water. Ultimately, when any monkey tried to climb the stairs, all the other monkeys prevented him from doing so in order not to get the cold shower.

At this stage the cold shower mechanism was disconnected, then one of the original monkeys was removed from the cage and replaced with a new one. The new monkey saw the banana and dashed to the stairs. To his surprise, all of the other monkeys attacked him. After another attempt and attack, he knew what the consequences would be if he tried to climb the stairs.

Again, another of the original five monkeys was replaced with a new one. The newcomer went for the stairs and was attacked. The previous newcomer participated in the punishment with all the other veterans. Next, a third original monkey was replaced, then the fourth, and finally the fifth. Every time the newest monkey took to the stairs, he was attacked. The newest monkeys that were attacked had no idea why they were not permitted to climb the stairs; they also had no idea why they were participating in the beating of the newest monkey.

After all the original monkeys were replaced, none of them had ever been sprayed with cold water. Nevertheless, no monkey ever again approached the stairs to try for the banana. Why not? Because **that's the way it's always been.**

♥ ♥ ♥

Man is capable of doing marvelous things. Man has put other men on the moon. Man has built computer chips executing millions of operations per second.

Man is also capable of doing the most heinous acts, the mass murder or mutilation of other human beings. The English language has a term for this; it is called genocide. The term itself was coined by Raphael Lemkin in 1943, from the roots *genos (Greek)* for family, tribe or race) and *-cide* (Latin) - *occidere* or *cideo* - meaning to massacre.

Genocide is defined by the Convention on the Prevention and Punishment of the Crime of Genocide[349] (CPPCG) Article 2 as:

> *any of the following acts committed with intent to destroy, in whole or in part, a national, ethnic, racial or religious group, as such: Killing members of the group; Causing serious bodily or mental harm to members of the group; Deliberately inflicting on the group conditions of life calculated to bring about its physical destruction in whole or in part; Imposing measures intended to prevent births within the group; and forcibly transferring children of the group to another group.*

Unfortunately, the twentieth century alone, despite all of its technological advances, bore witness to many atrocities. To name just a few:

- 1915-1918: 1,500,000 Armenians slaughtered.
- 1932-33: 7,000,000 perished in Ukraine due to the deliberated caused famine by Joseph Stalin.
- 1938 through 1945: Despite denials by some so-called scholars, as well as several of today's world leaders, the Nazi holocaust DID happen. It was real. Six million Jews perished in the death camps.
- Cambodia: 2,000,000 deaths due to executions, deliberate starvation and overwork - Khmer Rouge leader Pol Pot.
- Rwanda: up to 800,000 Tutsis were killed by Hutu militia using clubs and machetes.
- More recently – the on-going atrocities going in the Darfur region of western Sudan against the non-Arab villagers.

And this horrific list is not all-inclusive.

No doubt, decent people the world over are appalled by these atrocities. But what does one call a non-violent systematic method that kills and maims millions every year?

Medicines to lower blood pressure and bad cholesterol are already effective and widely used, yet heart disease remains the biggest cause of death in the United States, killing 911,000 people in 2003, according to the American Heart Association.[350]

There was nothing exceptional regarding heart disease as the leading cause of death in 2003. In every year since 1900, except 1918, cardiovascular disease accounted for more deaths than any other single cause or group of causes of death in the United States.[351]

Shouldn't the millions and millions of deaths caused by CHD generate the same disgust that death by genocide creates? The data shows that over the last 100 years, with the widespread use of all types of modern manufactured food, including the pasteurized dead milk products and hydrogenated oil products, just to name a few, the rate of mortality due to CHD has almost tripled.

In 1901 in the USA, there were 140 deaths[352] per 100,000 caused by 'diseases of the heart'. This number peaked to 375.5 deaths[353] in 1963 and since then has been tapering off. The medical establishment sees this as verification that it is making headway in stopping heart disease. This is a naive outlook. Although the medical establishment should be commended for making technological advances in improving medical procedures (stents/bypass operations) for saving heart attack victims, heart disease itself is not declining.

Overwhelming evidence proves that the lipid hypothesis is based on bad science. It is not valid. Simply put, it is not the cholesterol or saturated fat that has caused the rate of deaths due to CHD to nearly triple over the last hundred years. This increase occurred in spite of a decline in the saturated fats in the American diet and improved techniques for taking care of heart attack patients over the last 40 years.

Here we get to the crux of the problem. This is no single tyrant, Adolf Hitler or Pol Pot, that can be blamed for this phenomenon of millions dying because of CHD. The industries that for many years were utilizing partially hydrogenated oil in their products, resulting in high trans-fat content, were encouraged and promoted by official U.S. agencies that were established to protect our health. Pasteurization is firmly set by law, the sale and distribution of non-pasteurized milk/products is either outright illegal in most states, or overly restricted.

With no intent to insult the feminist movement, breast-feeding is by far the healthiest and cheapest way to feed babies.

Baby formula was the natural response to the higher mortality[354] and higher sickness rate of babies fed pasteurized cow's milk instead of natural mother's milk.

In 1976, it was reported that in a particular Californian city, it cost almost three times as much to buy ready made baby formula as it did to buy food for the nursing mother.[355] Respected multinational companies actively market expensive substitute milk formulas in .... Africa... of all places. The cost of purchasing milk substitutes in many third world countries is a crippling slice of the monthly salary.[356] This also does not take into consideration the hidden costs of chronic illnesses and inferior development of the babies in the future who were denied mothers' milk.[357]

I mentioned in the beginning of SASHA that I was never an avid reader; as such I do not possess an especially rich treasury of words. I was not able to find an existing word that accurately describes this phenomenon of peaceful genocide that I want to discuss now. As a result, I am forced to coin my own term.

Troficide - *trofi (Greek)* for food and *-cide* (Latin) - *occidere* or *cideo* - meaning to massacre.

I also respectively submit a definition for this new term:

Troficide is the systematic nutritional killing or maiming of humans regardless of national, ethnic, racial or religious group, as such: Killing members of the group; Causing serious bodily or mental harm to members of the group; Deliberately inflicting on the group conditions of life calculated to bring about its physical destruction in whole or in part; and forcibly transferring children from their mothers' breasts.

Man is capable of doing marvelous things. Man has put other men on the moon. Man has built computer chips executing millions of operations per second.   Man is also capable of putting an end to 'troficide'.

.

36

Post-Epilogue

Coexistence... what the farmer does with the turkey
- until Thanksgiving.
Mike Connolly

Here is another one "The only alternative to coexistence is codestruction" - Jawaharlal Nehru. On this optimistic introduction, and with the intent of closing this book on a lighter note and not with 'troficide', I leave you with the following question. How does one half of a couple who needs significant freezer space to freeze fresh raw milk, and additional refrigerator space to cool dripping fresh cheese, bottles of whey, rejuvelac and fermenting sauerkraut, coexist in what is otherwise known as a normal kitchen/household?

Leave it to Esty to come up with a creative solution to my unconventional eating habits. Esty recently surprised me with my very own refrigerator. Yes, you read that correctly. No, it is nowhere as large as the family fridge, and I did have to clean out a corner of a storage room to fit it in; however, it has made sharing the same kitchen 'more pleasant'. No, it was not intended as a present for the 'man who already has everything'.

You can categorize the fridge as the type of present where the 'giver' benefits as much as the 'givee'. I get to buy larger quantities of fresh raw milk at a time, and Esty keeps me out of 'her' freezer!

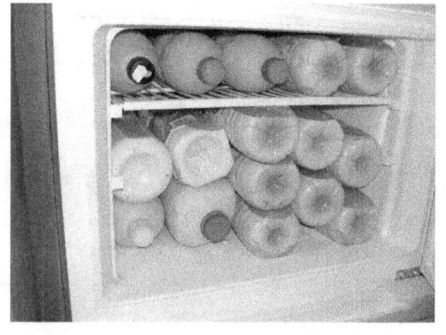

According to my spellchecker, it appears that I have created another new word, 'givee'. I probably should have used the word 'recipient'.

But then again, after the stent and the statins, I have learned to bend the existing rules a bit.

July 13, 2007 3:30 PM

Exactly six years ago today I arrived to Hadassah Hospital in Jerusalem in the midst of a heart attack. Much has occurred in the Stone household over the last six years. When I first started writing this book well over a year ago, I wrote (chapter 18):

> Within six years after a recognized heart attack (MI), 18% of men will have another heart attack, about 22% will be disabled with heart failure, 8% will have a stroke and 7% will experience sudden death.[358]

At the time I was still under the illusion that the 'six-year rule' did not apply to me. Why should it? I had extensively changed my eating and exercise habits. As destiny would have it, I discovered following routine testing that the stent inserted in my critical main artery (LAD) had become 100% clogged -- 100% restenosis.

However, I did *not* have another heart attack; I was *not* disabled with heart failure and did *not* experience sudden death.

Despite this total blockage in such a critical area, a bypass operation in the foreseeable future is not even in the cards. Except for the pinpoint blockage at the stent location (chapter 33), my overall condition has not deteriorated despite my abandoning many of the consensus-accepted rules for coping with/preventing heart disease. You are free to draw your own conclusions.

And for the record, the cats that participated in the 'cat scan' in chapter 23 are all alive, well and smiling.

37

2010

*Discovery consists in seeing what everyone else
has seen and thinking what no one else
has thought.*
Albert Szent-Gyorgyi

I s there such a thing as Post Statin Syndrome (PSS)? In 10 years time, if you google this term, this book might be the only place where the term occurs – or – it may be the most searched for illness in the first part of the 21st century.

There is a myriad of information regarding the negative side effects of statin medication, cognitive problems, memory loss, personality changes, and irritability. Regarding irritability, case studies have demonstrated that

> *Manifestations of severe irritability included homicidal impulses, threats to others, road rage, generation of fear in family members, and damage to property.*[359]

But what happens AFTER the physical effects subside after the discontinuation of the statins? As I discussed in

395

SASHA, I felt an emotional recovery very shortly after discontinuing the statins in 2003. Dr. Golomb mentioned in her research that cognitive dysfunctions return to pre-statin functioning after approximately 6 months.

What then is Post Statin Syndrome (PSS)? Time is a dynamic entity. It waits for no one. It goes back for no one. Physical, mental and emotional functioning of the individual may revert back to pre-statin levels. However, what about the effect that the statin period has on one's interactions with his/her personal surroundings? To the best of my knowledge, there are no research endeavors of the 'post' statin period. I can only relate what a post statin period looks like from my own personal perspective. I discussed in SASHA my cognitive dysfunction at work. I also mentioned a schism in my relations at home with Esty.

What I didn't delve into at the time was what had occurred with colleagues and co-workers during this period. As I am approaching some forty odd years of gainful employment, I can say that what characterized my interpersonal relationships throughout my work career, was that I truly got along with everyone - superiors, colleagues, subordinates - everyone. During my statin period, I found myself in the strange setting of NOT getting along with superiors, colleagues and subordinates.

I mentioned time is dynamic? Towards the end of 2003, when I was totally weaned off of the negative effects of the statins, my messed up relations with others at work stayed messed up. Maybe if I was of stronger character, I could have been more proactive in trying to mend impaired relations with colleagues, as I was able to accomplish with Esty. But I wonder how many people that get caught up in the statin web never really manage to escape it.

Almost two years after the physical effects of the statins had subsisted, at work I nearly found myself in a physical fight with co-worker almost young enough to be my son. Sure, the guy was an obnoxious bastard and was capable of dissecting me in a physical confrontation.

However we encounter types like this all the time - in stores, on the road, at gas stations, even neighbors. We certainly cannot go around 'slugging' people just because they are obnoxious bastards. In mid 2005, which coincided with two years after getting off the statins, I realized that there was just too much to fix in repairing strained relationships at work. I decided to resign - the final necessary step to seal off my post statin syndrome period. I left a job with a good salary and excellent benefits; I quit for the unknown.

Not fair? If you are at the age where you can list on your curriculum vitae (CV) of life that you have had a heart attack, then you can probably count the decades you have left on this planet with the fingers on one hand. No one is really born with inalienable rights. It's a great campaign slogan for politicians, but that is not how the real world works. Play the cards you are now holding, get on with the rest of your life, and move on. That works for me; I hope it works for you.

References

Chapter 2

1. Essentials of an Adequate Diet", USDA (1956), milk and milk products; meat/fish/poultry/eggs/dry beans/nuts; fruits and vegetables; grain products.

Chapter 3

2. Dean Ornish, "Dr. Dean Ornish's Program for Reversing Heart Disease", Random House, 255-256,280-281

3. Robert Atkins, "Dr. Atkins' New Diet Revolution", Avon Books,6,7,12,57-63,174

Chapter 9

4. Hans Selye, "The Stress of Life", McGraw-Hill,31-33,64-65

5. Meyer Friedman, Ray Rosenman, "Type A Behavior and Your Heart", Alfred A. Knoph,100-103

6. Conclusions of the Western Collaborative Group Study (WCGS) conducted in 1961

    Later studies led to conflicting conclusions whether or not Type A behavior was or was not a good predictor of CHD, summarized by:

    Schwalbe FC, Relationship between Type A personality and coronary heart disease. Analysis of five cohort studies.J Fla Med Assoc. 1990 Sep40;77(9):803-5

    Other studies suggest that a specific subcomponent of Type A behavior, the "Anger/Hostility dimension" does appear most predictive of CHD:

    Smith TW, Frohm KD. What's so unhealthy about hostility? Construct validity and psychosocial correlates for the Cook and Medley Ho scale. Health Psychology 1985; 4: 503-20.

    Schneiderman N, Chesney MA, Krantz, DS. Biobehavioral aspects of cardiovascular disease: progress and prospects. Health Psychology 1989; 8: 6349-76.

Chapter 10

7. Franz X. Mayr ,"Fundamente zur Diagnostik der Verdauungskrankheiten" -1921 (Foundations for the diagnostics of the digesting diseases)

Chapter 11

8. B. A. Golomb, M. H. Criqui, H. White, and J. E. Dimsdale, Conceptual Foundations of the UCSD Statin Study: A Randomized Controlled Trial Assessing the Impact of Statins on Cognition, Behavior, and Biochemistry Archives of Internal Medicine, January 26, 2004; 164(2): 153 – 162

9. D. Gaist, U. Jeppesen, M. Andersen, L. A. García Rodríguez, J. Hallas and S. H. Sindrup Statins and risk of polyneuropathy: A case control study Neurology, May 2002; 58: 1333 – 1337.

10. Bailey DG, Dresser GK, Kreeft JH, Munoz C, Freeman DJ, Bend JR. Grapefruit-felodipine interaction: effect of unprocessed fruit and probable active ingredients. Clin Pharmacol Ther. 2000 Nov;68(5):468-77.

11. Kantola T, Kivisto KT, Neuvonen PJ., Grapefruit juice greatly increases serum concentrations of lovastatin and lovastatin acid, Clin Pharmacol Ther. 1998 Apr;63(4):397-402.

12. Klotz U., Pharmacological comparison of the statins, Arzneimittelforschung. 2003;53(9):605-11

13. Becquemont L.,Interactions medicamenteuses et hypolipemiants (Drug Interactions with Lipid Lowering Drugs), Therapie. 2003 Jan-Feb;58(1):85-90

14. Lilja JJ, Kivisto KT, Neuvonen PJ.Grapefruit juice increases serum concentrations of atorvastatin and has no effect on pravastatin, Clin Pharmacol Ther. 1999 Aug;66(2):118-27

15. Fukazawa I, Uchida N, Uchida E, Yasuhara H., Effects of grapefruit juice on pharmacokinetics of atorvastatin and pravastatin in Japanese,Br J Clin Pharmacol. 2004 Apr;57(4):448-55

16. Lilja JJ, Kivisto KT, Neuvonen PJ., Duration of effect of grapefruit juice on the pharmacokinetics of the CYP3A4 substrate simvastatin, Clin Pharmacol Ther. 2000 Oct;68(4):384-90

17. New Scientist vol 180 issue 2424 - 06 December 2003, You're my wife? page 14;

    Duane Graveline, "Lipitor: Thief of Memory, Statin Drugs and the Misguided War on Cholesterol", Infinity Publishing

18. Golomb BA 1998. "Low cholesterol and violence: Is there a connection?", Annals of Internal Medicine, 128:478-487

19. DeMyer MK, Shea PA, Hendrie HC, Yoshimura NN.,Plasma tryptophan and five other amino acids in depressed and normal subjects., Arch Gen Psychiatry. 1981 Jun;38(6):642-6

20. Mann J, McBride A, Brown R, et al. Relationship between central and peripheral serotonin indexes in depressed and suicidal psychiatric inpatients. Arch Gen Psychiatry. 1992;49:442-446;

    Ozer OA, Kutanis R, Agargun MY, Besiroglu L, Bal AC, Selvi Y,Kara H.,Serum lipid levels, suicidality, and panic disorder., Compr Psychiatry.2004Mar-Apr;45(2):95-8

    Engelberg H., Low serum cholesterol and suicide.Lancet. 1992 Mar21;339(8795):727-9

21. Bliznakov E, "The Miracle Nutrient Coenzyme Q10", Bantam Books

22. Langsjoen PH, Langsjoen AM.,The clinical use of HMG CoA-reductase inhibitors and the associated depletion of coenzyme Q10., Biofactors. 2003;18(1-4):101-11

    Langsjoen H, Langsjoen P, et al., Usefulness of coenzyme Q10 in clinical cardiology: a long-term study. Mol Aspects Med. 1994;15 Suppl:s165-75

23. Davis E, Mercury the Element, Wise Traditions in Food, arming and the Healing Arts, (Weston A. Price Foundation),Summer 2003

24. Vimy MJ, Lorscheider FL.,Intra-oral air mercury released from dental amalgam., J Dent Res. 1985 Aug;64(8):1069-71.;

    Vimy MJ, Takahashi Y, Lorscheider FL.,Maternal-fetal distribution of mercury (203Hg) released from dental amalgam fillings.Am J Physiol. 1990 Apr;258(4 Pt 2):R939-45

References

25. Siblerud RL.,The relationship between mercury from dental amalgam and the cardiovascular system. Sci Total Environ. 1990 Dec 1;99(1-2):23-35

26. Salonen JT, Seppanen K, Lakka TA, Salonen R, Kaplan GA, Mercury accumulation and accelerated progression of carotid atherosclerosis: a population-based prospective 4-year follow-up study in men in eastern Finland., Atherosclerosis. 2000 Feb;148(2):265-73.

27. Fereydoon Batmanghelidj, "Your Body's Many Cries for Water", Global Health Solutions, 17,18,71-76,83-86,160-162

    USA Acres Magazine, June 99, Vol 29,No 6,p24,Water is Medicine

28. Kilmer McCully: pioneer of the homocysteine theory. Lancet 1998 352: 1364.

    McCully KS. Vascular pathology of homocysteinemia: implications for the pathogenesis of arteriosclerosis. Am J Pathol 1996;56:111-28

29. NJ Wald et al,Homocysteine and Ischemic Heart Disease,Arch Intern Med. 1998;158:862-867.;

    Clarke R, et al, Underestimation of the importance of homocysteine as a risk factor for cardiovascular disease in epidemiological studies.J Cardiovasc Risk. 2001 Dec;8(6):363-9.

30. Nygard O, Vollset SE, et al,Total plasma homocysteine and cardiovascular risk profile. The Hordaland Homocysteine Study. JAMA. 1995 Nov 15;274(19):1526-33.

31. Klevay LM. Dietary copper and risk of coronary heart disease,Am J Clin Nutr. 2000 May;71(5):1213-4

32. Klevay LM. Coronary heart disease: the zinc/copper hypothesis. Am J Clin Nutr. 7-28: 764;1975

33. Albert MA, Ridker PM., The role of C-reactive protein in cardiovascular disease risk., Curr Cardiol Rep. 1999 Jul;1(2):99-104.

34. Miller M., Raising an isolated low HDL-C level: Why, how, and when? Cleveland Clinic Journal Of Medicine Volume 70 • Number 6 June 2003

35. Gaziano, J.M., Hennekens, C.H., O'Donnell, C.J., et al., "Fasting Triglycerides, High-Density Lipoprotein, and Risk of Myocardial Infarction," Circulation, 96(8), 1997, pages 2520-2525.

Chapter 12

36. Booyens, Louwrens, Katzeff, The role of unnatural dietary trans and cis unsaturated fatty acids in the epidemiology of coronary artery disease Med Hypotheses. 1988 Mar;25(3):175-8

37. Ascherio A., Katan M. B., Zock P. L., Stampfer M. J., Willett W. C.,Trans Fatty Acids and Coronary Heart Disease, N Engl J Med 1999; 340:1994-1998, Jun 24, 1999

38. Willett WC, Ascherio A. Trans fatty acids: Are the effects only marginal? Am J Public Health 1994; 84:722-724

39. Ascherio A, Willett WC.,Health effects of trans fatty acids. Am J Clin Nutr. 1997 Oct;66(4 Suppl):1006S-1010S

40. Gofman, J W, et al. The role of lipids and lipoproteins in arteriosclerosis. Science 1950; 111: 166-181, 186

41. W F Enos, R H Holmes, J Beyer. Coronary disease among United States Soldiers killed in action in Korea. Preliminary report. Journal of the American Medical Association 1953; 152: 1090

    D Groom, "Population Studies of Atherosclerosis," Annals of Int Med, July 1961, 55:1:51-62;

    W F Enos, et al, "Pathogenesis of Coronary Disease in American Soldiers Killed in Korea," JAMA, 1955, 158:912

42. McNamara JJ, Molot MA, Stremple JF, et al. Coronary artery disease in combat casualties in Vietnam. Journal of the American Medical Association. 1971; 216: 1185–1187

43. The Bogalusa Heart Study - A study involving over 14,000 children and young adults in Bogalusa Louisianna

44. Sally Fallon, Mary G. Enig Nexus Magazine 2002 volume 9, Number 5, THE GREAT CON-OLA;

    Sally Fallon, Mary G. Enig,"Nourishing Traditions", New Trends Publishing, 19,128

References

45. Fifty years of data collected from residents of Framingham, Massachusetts to identify major risk factors associated with heart disease, stroke and other diseases

46. Kannel WB, et al ,Optimal resources for primary prevention of artherosclerotic diseases. Atherosclerosis Study Group.Circulation. 1984 Jul70(1):155A-205A

47. Castelli WP. Arch Int Med 1992; 152: 1371-1372

48. Enig M, Fallon S, The Oiling of America, Nexus Magazine, Vol 6 Num 1, 12/98-1/99

49. Nutrition Science News, July 1999, Kilmer McCully, M.D. Connects Homocysteine and Heart Disease

50. McGill Jr HC, Arias-Stella J, Carbonell LM, et al., "General Findings of the International Atherosclerosis Project," Laboratory Investigations, 1968, 18:(5):498

51. CBS News, March 8, 2004

52. New York Times, July 20, 2004, Seeking a Fuller Picture of Statins

53. Ravnskov U. Implications of 4S evidence on baseline lipid level, The Lancet 1995, 356, 102-103

54. Soma MR, Corsini A, Paoletti R., Cholesterol and mevalonic acid modulation in cell matabolism and multiplication, Toxicology Letters 1992, 64/65 1-15

    Ravnskov U.,"The Cholesterol Myths", New Trends Publishing, 207

Chapter 13

55. John G. Peterson, Michael S. Lauer, "Using Aspirin and ACE inhibitors in combination: Why the hullabaloo?" Cleveland Clinic Journal of Medicine , June 2001

56. Kilmer McCully,"The Heart Revolution",Harper Perenial,Chap1,28

57. Liu SM, Stampfer MJ, Hu FB, et al. Whole-grain consumption and risk of coronary heart disease: results from the Nurses' Health Study. Am J Clin Nutr 1999;70:412–9.

Anderson JW, Hanna TJ. Whole grains and protection against coronary heart disease: what are the active components and mechanisms? Am J Clin Nutr 1999;70:307–8.

58.   Sally Fallon "Nourishing Traditions", New Trends Publishing, 452,453

59.   Cohen AM.,Fats and carbohydrates as factors in atherosclerosis and diabetes in Yemenite Jews, American Heart Journal, 1963,65:291-293

60.   Felton CV, Crook D, Davies MJ, Oliver MF.,Dietary polyunsaturated fatty acids and composition of human aortic plaques.Lancet. 1994 Oct 29;344(8931):1195-6

Chapter 17

61.   Benjamin Franklin, Poor Richard's Quotations (1975)

Chapter 18

62.   Ignarro L., NO More Heart Disease: How Nitric Oxide Can Prevent -- Even Reverse -- Heart Disease and Stroke, St. Martin's Griffin; 2006, page 31

63.   Ravnskov U, The Cholesterol Myths: Exposing the Fallacy that Saturated Fat and Cholesterol Cause Heart Disease NewTrends Publishing, 2000, 50-52

64.   Stone M. Surviving a Successful Heart Attack second edition, Lulu, 2005, 30-39

65.   Kauffman J. Malignant Medical Myths: Why Medical Treatment Causes 200,000 Deaths in the USA each Year, and How to Protect Yourself, Infinity Publishing, 2006,165

Chapter 19

66.   Fuster V et al, Hurst's The Heart, Mcgraw-Hill 2000, 7

Chapter 204

67.   Howell E., Enzyme Nutrition, Avery, 1995, xv, 3-5,7,16,33-35,80,123,148,149,154

68.   Bairoch A, The Enzyme database in 2000, Nucleic Acids Res 28: 304-305

69.   Becker Gh, Meyer J, Necheles H. Fat absorption and atherosclerosis. Science. 1949 Nov 18;110(2864):529

      Becker Gh, Meyer J, Necheles H. Fat absorption in young and old age. Gastroenterology. 1950 Jan; 14(1):80-92

70.   Pilgeram LO, Deficiencies in the lipoprotein lipase system in atherosclerosis., J Gerontol. 1958 Jan; 13(1):32-42

71.   Pottenger FM. Pottenger's Cats: A Study in Nutrition, Price-Pottenger Nutrition Foundation, 1995

72.   Pottenger FM, 18

73.   MacDonald ML et al. Nutrition of the domestic cat, a mammalian carnivore., Annu Rev Nutr. 1984; 4:521-62

74.   Knopf K et al. Taurine: an essential nutrient for the cat., J Nutr. 1978 May; 108(5):773-8

75.   Sturman JA et al. Feline maternal taurine deficiency: effect on mother and offspring J Nutr.1986 Apr; 116(4):655-67

76.   Fallon S. Nourishing Traditions: The Cookbook that Challenges Politically Correct Nutrition and the Diet Dictocrats Sec ed., NewTrends Publishing 1999, xi xii

77.   Pottenger FM, 3

78.   Boutenko V et al., Raw Family: A True Story of Awakening, Raw Family, 2000

79.   Kroeger H. God helps those that help themselves, Privately printed, 1984, 13, 220

Chapter 22

80.   Antoine Béchamp, La Théorie du Microzyma (preface)

81.   Douglass WC. The Milk Book: The Milk of Human Kindness Is Not Pasteurized, Rhino Publishing, S.A., 2004, 121

82.   New York Times, The Doctor's World; Revisionist History Sees Pasteur As Liar Who Stole Rival's Ideas, May 16, 1995

83.   Washington Post, USA Today Reporter Resigns Over Probe Thursday, January 8, 2004; Page C01

84. Hume ED. Béchamp or Pasteur? A Lost Chapter in the History of Biology Sec ed., E.W. Daniel Company, 1932, 205

85. Id at 281

86. Lanctôt G. The Medical Mafia: How to Get Out of It Alive and Take Back Our Health & Wealth, Here's the Key 1995, 157

87. Hiestand S&D, Electrical Nutrition: A revolutionary approach to eating that awakens the body. Avery, 2001, 67

88. Pfizer Inc. 2006 Financial Report page 78, Pfizer website http://www.pfizer.com/pfizer/annualreport/2006/financial/p2006fin79.jsp - viewed May 19, 2007

89. IBID

90. IBID at 16

91. Graveline D. Lipitor Thief of Memory, Infinity, 2004

Chapter 23

92. Douglass WC. 16

93. Schmid R. The Untold Story of Milk: Green Pastures, Contented Cows and Raw Dairy Products, NewTrends Publishing, 2003, 206

94. National Nutritional Conference for Defense May 14, Federal Sea Agency, pp 176

95. Family Practice News, Sept 1, 1981

96. Schmid R. 229

97. Krauss, W.E., Erb, J.H. and Washburn, R.G. Studies on the nutritive value of milk, II. The effect of pasteurization on some of the nutritive properties of milk," Ohio Agricultural Experiment Station Bulletin 518, page 9, January, 1933

98. Schmid R 102

99. Douglass WC. 138

100. Howell E. 149

101. Schmid R. 101

102. Colpo A. The Great Cholesterol Con, Lulu, 2006, 283

103. Rodriguez EM, Sanz AM, Diaz RC, 1999 Chemometric Studies of Several Minerals in Milks, Journal of Agriculture and Food Chemistry, 47:1520-4

References

104. Consumer reports January 1974

105. Douglass WC. 62

106. Douglass WC. 18

107. Annand JC. The case against milk protein. Atherosclerosis, 1971 vol. 13, p. 137.

    Annand JC. Further evidence in the case against heated milk protein. Atherosclerosis, vol. 15, no. 1 (Jan. 1972), pp. 129-133.

108. Jernigan D&S. Beating Lyme Disease: Using alternative medicine and god-designed living, Somerleyton Press, 2004

109. Hippocrates used raw milk to cure tuberculosis. Until pasteurization became the norm, medical literature extensively praised the disease-fighting ability of raw milk.

    Potter CS. Milk Diet as a Remedy for Chronic Disease, 1908

    Dr. J.E. Crewe, from the Mayo Foundation, Minnesota, reported the therapeutic uses of raw milk in 1923. For 15 years, he employed the raw-milk-diet treatment in various diseases including tuberculosis, which is ironic considering that tuberculosis was blamed on raw milk...

110. Response to letter from Ted Elkins, Deputy Director, Office of food Protection and Consumer Health Services, Maryland Department of Health and Mental Hygiene, from Sally Fallon, President, The Weston A. Price Foundation, May 23, 2006. Downloaded at www.westonaprice.org/federalupdate/aa2006/ResponseToMDH MH.pdf

111. State of Michigan Department of Community Health, PBBs (Polybrominated Biphenyls) in Michigan Frequently Asked Questions downloaded at http://www.michigan.gov/documents/mdch_PBB_FAQ_92051_ 7.pdf

    Environmental Politics and Science: The Case of PBB Contamination in Michigan MICHAEL R. REICH, PHD Am Public Health, March 1983; 73(3) 302-312

112. Brilliant LB, Wilcox K, Van Amburg G, et al: Breast-milk monitoring to measure Michigan's contamination with polybrominated biphenyls. Lancet 1978; 2:643-646

113. Schmid R.194

114. Schmid R.194-196

115. Schmid R.222, 223

116. Diez-Gonzalez F et al, Grain feeding and the dissemination of acid-resistant Escherichia coli from cattle, Science, Sept 11, 1998 281:166-168

117. Schmid R. 205

118. Douglass WC. 259, 260

119. Based on the research of Dr. Kurt Oster, summarized in Homogenized Milk May Cause Your Heart Attack - The XO Factor by Kurt A Oster. There is dispute among researchers today regarding the validity of this premise.

120. Howell E. 149

Chapter 25

121. United States Department of Agriculture Agricultural Research Magazine, August 2003 - Vol. 51, No. 8, page 18

122. Yam D, Eliraz A, Berry EM. Diet and disease--the Israeli paradox: possible dangers of a high omega-6 polyunsaturated fatty acid diet. Isr J Med Sci. 1996 Nov; 32(11): 1134-43

123. Shah PK. Plaque disruption and coronary thrombosis: new insight into pathogenesis and prevention Clin Cardiol 1997; 20(11 Suppl 2):II-38-44.

124. Colpo A, LDL Cholesterol: Bad. Cholesterol or Bad Science? Journal of American Physicians and Surgeons Volume 10 Number 3 Fall 2005

125. Felton CV, Crook D, Davies MJ, et al. Dietary polyunsaturated fatty acids and composition of human aortic plaques. Lancet 1994; 344:1195-1196.

126. Waddington E, Sienuarine K, Puddey I, Croft K Identification and quantitation of unique fatty acid oxidation products in human atherosclerotic plaque using high-performance liquid chromatography. Anal Biochem. 2001 May 15; 292(2):234-44

127. Colpo A. 57

References

128. Eaton SB, Eaton SB 3rd, Sinclair AJ, Cordain L, Mann NJ Dietary intake of long-chain polyunsaturated fatty acids during the Paleolithic Period. World Rev Nutr Diet 1998; 12-23

129. Simopoulos,A.P. 1999 Essential fatty acids in health and chronic disease. AM J Clin Nutr; 70(suppl): 560S-9S

130. Simopoulos AP. The importance of the ratio of omega-6/omega-3 essential fatty acids. Biomed Pharmacother. 2002 Oct; 56(8):365-79

131. McKeown P, Close Your Mouth-Buteyko Clinic handbook for perfect health, Buteyko Books, 2004, 9-13

132. Gerster H., Can adults adequately convert alpha-linolenic acid (18:3n-3) to eicosapentaenoic acid (20:5n-3) and docosahexaenoic acid (22:6n-3)? Int J Vitam Nutr Res. 1998; 68(3):159-73

133. Levine, Barbara S. Most Frequently Asked Questions About DHA. Nutrition Today 1997 November/December, vol. 32, pp. 248-49

134. Gamma-Linolenic Acid By Mary G. Enig, PhD, viewed at http://www.westonaprice.org/knowyourfats/gamma-linolenic.html

135. Enig M. Know Your Fats: The Complete Primer for Understanding the Nutrition of Fats, Oils and Cholesterol, Bethesda Press, 200, 239

136. Sinzinger HF, Prostaglandins in the Cardiovascular System, Birkhauser Boston, 1992, pages 151-156

137. Cambridge International Institute for Medical Science, The Scientific Calculation of the Optimum Omega6/3 Ratio, Page 24

138. Chapkin RS, Metabolism of essential fatty acids by human epidermal enzyme preparations: evidence of chain elongation, Journal of Lipid Research, Volume 27, pages 945-954, 1986.

139. Andersson A. et al. Fatty acid profile of skeletal muscle phospholipids in trained and untrained young men, American Journal of Endocrinological Metabolism, 279: E744-E751, 2000

140. Shah PK. Plaque disruption and coronary thrombosis: new insight into pathogenesis and prevention Clin Cardiol 1997; 20(11 Suppl 2) :II-38-44.

409

141. IBID

142. Figures based upon Enig M. Know Your Fats, Appendix C: food Composition Tables, page 283

143.   Colpo A. 104,105

Chapter 26

144. Stone M. 124

Golomb BA,Criqui MH, White H,Dimsdale JE. The UCSD Statin Study: A randomized controlled trial assessing the impact of statins on noncardiac endpoints" Control Clin Trials., 2004 Apr; 25(2):178-202

Golomb BA,Criqui MH, White H,Dimsdale JE., Conceptual Foundations of the UCSD Statin Study: A Randomized Control Trial Assessing the Impact of Statins on Cognition, Behavior, and Biochemistry") Arch Intern Med. 2004 Jan 26; 164(2):153-62.

145. Golomb BA, McGraw J. "Lack of Physician Response Toward Perceived Statin Adverse Events" paper presented at the American Heart Association, 45th Annual Conference on Cardiovascular Disease Epidemiology and Prevention in association with the Council on Nutrition, Physical Activity and Metabolism April 29–May 2, 2005, Washington D.C.

146.   Kauffman J. Myth 7 - 176

147.   NIH ClinicalTrials.gov identifier NCT00044213

148. Fallon S. and. Enig M. Dangers of Statin Drugs: What You Haven't Been Told About Popular Cholesterol-Lowering Medicines, Viewed at http://www.westonaprice.org/moderndiseases/statin.html

149. Kapoor R, Huang YS. Gamma linolenic acid: an antiinflammatory omega-6 fatty acid. Curr Pharm Biotechnol. 2006 Dec; 7(6):531-4.

150. Leng GC, Lee AJ, Fowkes FG, Jepson RG, Lowe GD, Skinner ER, Mowat BF, Randomized controlled trial of gamma-linolenic acid and eicosapentaenoic acid in peripheral arterial disease.Clin Nutr. 1998 Dec; 17(6):265-71

151. Kruger MC, Horrobin DF. Calcium metabolism, osteoporosis and essential fatty acids: a review. Prog Lipid Res .1997; 36:131-151

152. Horrobin DF. The role of essential fatty acids and prostaglandins in the premenstrual syndrome. J Reprod Med. 1983; 28(7):465-468.

153. Grundy SM et al, Diagnosis and Management of the Metabolic Syndrome An American Heart Association/National Heart, Lung, and Blood Institute Scientific Statement, Circulation. 2005; 112:2735-2752

154. Nutrition Science News, July 1999, Kilmer McCully, M.D. Connects Homocysteine and Heart Disease

155. Lahera V et al. Endothelial dysfunction, oxidative stress and inflammation in atherosclerosis: beneficial effects of statins. Curr Med Chem. 2007; 14(2):243-8

156. Yoshida M et al, HMG-CoA reductase inhibitor modulates monocyte endothelial interaction under physiological flow condition in vitro: involvement of Rho GTPase-dependent mechanism, Arterioscler Thromb Vasc Biol. 2001; 21: 1165–1171

157. Chopra V et al, Beyond Lipid Lowering: The Anti-Hypertensive Role of Statins., Cardiovasc Drugs Ther. 2007 Apr 28

158. Ray KK, Lipid-independent Pleiotropic Effects of Statins in the Management of Acute Coronary Syndromes., Curr Treat Options Cardiovasc Med. 2007 Feb; 9(1):46-51

159. Monetti M et al, Rosuvastatin displays anti-atherothrombotic and anti-inflammatory properties in apoE-deficient mice. Pharmacol Res. 2007 May; 55(5):441-9

160. Krum H et al, Double-blind, randomized, placebo-controlled study of high-dose HMG CoA reductase inhibitor therapy on ventricular remodeling, pro-inflammatory cytokines and neurohormonal parameters in patients with chronic systolic heart failure, J Card Fail. 2007 Feb;13(1):1-7

161. Habib A et al, Modulation of COX-2 expression by statins in human monocytic cells Faseb J. 2007 Feb 22;

162. Shirakawa I et al. Atorvastatin attenuates transplant-associated coronary arteriosclerosis in a murine model of cardiac

transplantation., Biomed Pharmacother. 2007 Feb-Apr; 61(2-3):154-9

163. Alegret M, Silvestre JS. Pleiotropic effects of statins and related pharmacological experimental approaches. Methods Find Exp Clin Pharmacol. 2006 Nov; 28(9):627

164. Bruegel M, Teupser D,Haffner I,Mueller M, Thiery J. Statins reduce macrophage inflammatory protein-1alpha expression in human activated monocytes. Clin Exp Pharmacol Physiol. 2006 Dec; 33(12):1144-9.

165. Saijonmaa O, Nyman T, Fyhrquist F. Atorvastatin inhibits angiotensin-converting enzyme induction in differentiating human macrophages.. Am J Physiol Heart Circ Physiol. 2007 Apr; 292(4):H1917-21

166. Ray KK, Cannon CP, Ganz P Beyond lipid lowering: What have we learned about the benefits of statins from the acute coronary syndromes trials. Am J Cardiol. 2006 Dec 4;98(11A):18P-25P

167. Xing XQ, Gan Y, Wu SJ, Chen P, Zhou R, Xiang XD. Statins may ameliorate pulmonary hypertension via RhoA/Rho-kinase signaling pathway. Med Hypotheses. 2007;68(5):1108-13

168. Tahara N, Kai H, Ishibashi M, Nakaura H, Kaida H, Baba K, Hayabuchi N, Imaizumi T. Simvastatin attenuates plaque inflammation: evaluation by fluorodeoxyglucose positron emission tomography. Am Coll Cardiol. 2006 Nov 7;48(9):1825-31.

169. Kurumazuka D et al.Gender difference of atorvastatin's vasoprotective effect in balloon-injured rat carotid arteries. Eur J Pharmacol. 2006 Dec 28;553(1-3):263-8

170. Nagassaki S, Sertorio JT, Metzger IF, Bem AF, Rocha JB, Tanus-Santos JE. eNOS gene T-786C polymorphism modulates atorvastatin-induced increase in blood nitriteFree Radic Biol Med. 2006 Oct 1;41(7):1044-9

171. Souza-Costa DC, Sandrim VC, Lopes LF, Gerlach RF, Rego EM, Tanus-Santos JE. Anti-inflammatory effects of atorvastatin: Modulation by the T-786C polymorphism in the endothelial nitric oxide synthase gene. Atherosclerosis. 2006 Aug 26

References

172. Aprahamian T, Bonegio R, Rizzo J, Perlman H, Lefer DJ, Rifkin IR, Walsh K. Simvastatin treatment ameliorates autoimmune disease associated with accelerated atherosclerosis in a murine lupus model., J Immunol. 2006 Sep 1;177(5):3028-34

173. Rizzo M, Rini GB. Statins, fracture risk, and bone remodeling: What is true? Am J Med Sci. 2006 Aug ;332(2):55-60

174. Ito MK, Talbert RL, Tsimikas S. Statin-associated pleiotropy: possible beneficial effects beyond cholesterol reduction. Pharmacotherapy. 2006 Jul; 26(7 Pt 2):85S-97S

175. Hayward RA, Hofer TP, Vijan S. Narrative review: lack of evidence for recommended low-density lipoprotein treatment targets: a solvable problem. Ann Intern Med. 2006 Oct 3;145(7):520-30.

176. Hayward RA, Hofer TP, Vijan S. Narrative Review: Lack of Evidence for Recommended Low-Density Lipoprotein Treatment Targets: A Solvable Problem., Annals of Internal Medicine, Oct 3, 2006; 145 (7): 520-530

177. Statins and Lipid-Lowering Therapy: How Far Will the Benefits Go? Medscape Cardiology, 01/26/2004

178. Keys A., Atherosclerosis: A problem in newer public health. Journal of Mount Sinai Hospital 20, 118-139, 1953

179. Ravnskov U., 16-19

180. Rosamond w et al. Heart Disease and Stroke Statistics—2007 Update: A Report from the American Heart Association Statistics Committee and Stroke Statistics Subcommittee, Circulation 115 (5) e69-e171.

181. Zareba G. Torcetrapib and atorvastatin: a novel combination therapy for dyslipidemia., Drugs Today (Barc). 2006 Feb; 42(2):95-102.

182. USA TODAY Loss of heart drug is 'shocker' Robert Davis and Julie Schmit Dec. 3, 2006 http://www.usatoday.com/news/health/2006-12-03-pfizer-heart-drug_x.htm

183. Pfizer ends development of key cholesterol drug Pharmaceutical giant likely to slash staff, accelerate merger deals MSNBC

News Services Dec. 4, 2006
http://www.msnbc.msn.com/id/16027217/

184. Nytimes End of Drug Trial Is a Big Loss for Pfizer December 4, 2006

185. USA TODAY Loss of heart drug is 'shocker' Robert Davis and Julie Schmit Dec. 3, 2006
http://www.usatoday.com/news/health/2006-12-03-pfizer-heart-drug_x.htm

186. Kastelein JJ, van Leuven SI, Burgess L, Evans GW, Kuivenhoven JA, Barter PJ, Revkin JH, Grobbee DE, Riley WA, Shear CL, Duggan WT, Bots ML; RADIANCE 1 Investigators. Effect of torcetrapib on carotid atherosclerosis in familial hypercholesterolemia. N Engl J Med. 2007 Apr 19;356(16):1620-30

187. Nissen SE, Tardif JC, Nicholls SJ, Revkin JH, Shear CL, Duggan WT,Ruzyllo W, Bachinsky WB,Lasala GP, Tuzcu EM; ILLUSTRATE Investigators. Effect of torcetrapib on the progression of coronary atherosclerosis. N Engl J Med. 2007 Mar 29;356(13):1304-16.

188. Kauffmann JM. 166

189. Late thrombosis in drug-eluting coronary stents after discontinuation of antiplatelet therapy. The Lancet, 2004 Oct 23-29;364(9444):1519-21. E. McFadden, E. Stabile, E. Regar, E. Cheneau, A. Ong, T. Kinnaird, W. Suddath, N. Weissman, R. Torguson, K. Kent

190. Boston Scientific Acknowledges Risks Tied to Stent, Wall street journal, Sylvia Pagan Westphal and Ron Winslow,September 7, 2006; Page A3

191. Camenzind E. Safety of drug-eluting stents: A meta-analysis of first generation drug-eluting stent programs.

Nordmann A. Safety of drug-eluting stents: Insights from a meta-analysis – see also:

Nordmann AJ, Briel M, Bucher HC Mortality in randomized controlled trials comparing drug-eluting vs. bare metal stents in coronary artery disease: a meta-analysis.. Eur Heart J. 2006 Dec; 27(23):2784-814

192. Boden WE, et al. Optimal medical therapy with or without PCI for stable coronary disease, N Engl J Med. 2007 Apr 12;356(15):1503-16

193. "Stent Thrombosis After Implantation of Drug Eluting Stent and Bare Metal Coronary Stents in Western Denmark", Dr. Michael Maeng, presented at the March 2007 American College of Cardiology Convention

194. Camenzind EN. Treatment of in-stent restenosis--back to the future? Engl J Med. 2006 Nov 16;355(20):2149-51

195. Lange H, et al, Folate therapy and in-stent restenosis after coronary stenting. N Engl J Med. 2004 Jun 24;350(26):2673-81.

196. Nishida T, Shimokawa H, Oi K, Tatewaki H, Uwatoku T, Abe K, Matsumoto Y, Kajihara N, Eto M, Matsuda T, Yasui H, Takeshita A, Sunagawa K. Extracorporeal cardiac shock wave therapy markedly ameliorates ischemia-induced myocardial dysfunction in pigs in vivo Circulation. 2004 ;110:3055-3061

197. Gutersohn A, Caspari G, Erbel R, Short and Long Term clinical improvement in patients with refractory angina using cardiac shock wave therapy., Presented at the International Academy of Cardiology, 12th world Congress on Heart Disease, Vancouver, B.C. Canada July 16-19,2005

198. Fukumoto Y, Shimokawa H,et al, Extracorporeal cardiac shock wave therapy ameliorates myocardial ischemia in patients with severe coronary artery disease. Coron Artery Dis. 2006 Feb; 17(1):63-70.

199. New York Times, Lessons of Heart Disease, Learned and Ignored, April 8, 2007

200. Caspi O, Lesman A, Basevitch Y, Gepstein A, Arbel G, Habib IH, Gepstein L, Levenberg S. Tissue engineering of vascularized cardiac muscle from human embryonic stem cells., Circ Res. 2007 Feb 2;100(2):263-72.

Chapter 27

201. Flavius Josephus Contra Apionem, I, (Against Apion book 1)

202. Bishop of Bristol Robert Gray, The Connection Between the Sacred Writings and the Literature of Jewish and Heathen Authors Sec Ed, 1819 page 69

203. Schenck SE, The Live Food Factor: A comprehensive guide to the ultimate diet for body, mind spirit & planet, 1st Impression Publishing, 2006, 177

    The Connection Between the Sacred Writings and the Literature of Jewish and Heathen Authors: By Bishop of Bristol Robert Gray, page 70

204. Schenck SE, 177

205. Food Science for All and a New Sunlight Theory of Nutrition – Lectures to Teachers of Domestic Economy, M. Bircher-Benner, Fourth Lecture, page 51, Republished 1960 by Health Research

206. Hans Fischer, The Nobel Prize in Chemistry 1930, Nobel Lecture, On haemin and the relationships between haemin and chlorophyll, December 11,1930

207. Hughes JH, Latner AL. Chlorophyll and haemoglobin regeneration after haemorrhage. J Physiol. 1936 May 4;86(4):388-395

208. Meyerowitz S. Power Juices, Super Drinks: Quick, Delicious Recipes to Prevent & Reverse Disease Kensington, 2000, page 92

209. Fox C, Ramsoomair D, Carter C., Magnesium: its proven and potential clinical significance. South Med J. 2001 Dec;94(12):1195-201

210. Shechter M, Bairey Merz CN, Stuehlinger HG, Slany J, Pachinger O, Rabinowitz B., Effects of oral magnesium therapy on exercise tolerance, exercise-induced chest pain, and quality of life in patients with coronary artery disease. Am J Cardiol. 2003 Mar 1;91(5):517-21

211. Wigmore A. The Wheatgrass Book: How to Grow and Use Wheatgrass to Maximize Your Health and Vitality, Avery 1985, 10,11,18,21,29,36,44, 46,34,47, 48, 59, 61, 83

212. Wigmore A., 21,34,36,47,48,59,61

Meyerwitz S. Wheatgrass Nature's Finest Medicine: The Complete Guide to Using Grasses to Revitalize Your Health Book Publishing Company, 1999, 63,69

213. Rudolph T. Chlorophyll Nature's Green Magic, Nutritional Research, 1957

214. Jensen B. Dr. Jensen's Juicing Therapy,: Nature's Way to Better Health and a Longer Life. McGraw-Hill, 2000, 56

215. Meyerwitz S. 132

216. Wigmore A. 105-106

Fallon S. 615

217. Boutenko V. Green for Life, Raw Family Publishing, 2005, 12, 16, 17, 41, 49, 50

218. Derek E. Wildman, et al. "Implications of Natural Selection in Shaping 99.4% Nonsynonomous DNA Identity Between Humans and Chimpanzees: Enlarging Genus Homo." Proceedings of the National Academy of Sciences. May 19,2003 (#2172)

219. Pilbeam D. Genetic and morphological records of the Hominoidea and hominid origins: a synthesis. Mol Phylogenet Evol. 1996 Feb;5(1):155-68

220. Harding R, Teleki G. Omnivorous Primates: Gathering and Hunting in Human Evolution, Columbia Univ. Press, 1981, 303-343

221. Scientific American, July 2001, Sigma Chi Chimpy, Forget The Ladies--For Chimps, Hunting Is About Fraternity By Meredith F. Small

222. American heart Disease website: http://www.americanheart.org/presenter.jhtml?identifier=4574

Chapter 28

223. As of this writing, on display at the University of Pennsylvania Museum of Archaeology and Anthropology

224. Health and Nutritional Properties of Probiotics in Food including Powder Milk with Live Lactic Food and Agriculture Organization of the United Nations World Health Organization, October 2001

225. Mann,G.V.1977.Hypocholesterolemic effect of milk. Lancet 10:556

Howard, A.N., and J. Marks. 1977. Hypocholesterolemic effect of milk. Lancet 30:255.

Mann, G. V. 1977. A factor in yogurt which lowers cholesterol in man. Atherosclerosis 26:335.

226. Based on the research of Dr. Kurt Oster, summarized in Homogenized Milk May Cause Your Heart Attack - The XO Factor by Kurt A Oster. There is dispute among researchers today regarding the validity of this premise.

227. Gilbère G. Nature's Prescription Milk, Freedom Press, 2002, 27

228. Belanger J Raising Dairy Goats: Breeds, Care, Dairying. Storey Publishing, 2000, 122

229. Gilbère G. 28

230. US Food And Drug Administration Center for Veterinary Medicine, May/June 2000 FDA Veterinarian Newsletter

231. Douglass WC. 62

232. Sally Fallon and Mary G. Enig, PhD. The Ploy of Soy, Price-Pottinger Nutrition Foundation, San Diego, CA

233. Gilbère G. 26

234. IBID

235. Rodriguez EM, Sanz AM, Diaz RC, 1999 Chemometric Studies of Several Minerals in Milks, Journal of Agriculture and Food Chemistry, 47: 1520-4

236. Jernigan D&S. 273

237. Gilbère G. 27

238. Fomon SJ. Infant Nutrition Sec ed, W B Saunders Co. 1974, 206

239. Maugh, T.H. Milk may be the carrier of Crohn's. The Advocate, ES, December 5, 2000.

Maugh TH II. Milk may be the carrier of Crohn's. Los Angeles Times 2000 Sep 18:S1.

240. Stockton S. The Terrain Is Everything, Power of One Publishing, 2000, 207-208

241. Fallon S. 87

References

242. The Milwaukee Journal Sentinel, Apr 17, 2007, Whey's price going way up; Increase should be benefit for state, by Rick Barrett

243. Vasey C. The Whey Prescription The Healing Miracle in Milk, Healing Arts Press, 2006, Chap 1 The history of Whey

244. Fallon S. 89

245. Fallon S. 92

246. Townsend Letter for Doctors and Patients, July, 2003, Consuming whole foods in their raw, uncooked state: a personal interview with raw food nutrition expert, David Wolfe - Medicinal Properties in Whole Foods – Interview, Gina L. Nick

247. Kroeger H. 64

Chapter 29

248. Plain Language About Shiftwork, Rosa R, Colligan M, U.S. Department of Health and Human Services, Public Health Service, Centers for Disease Control and Prevention, National Institute for Occupational Safety and Health, July 1997

249. Daytime cardiac autonomic activity during one week of continuous night shift., Fletcher A, Dorrian J, Roach G, Dawson D., J Hum Ergol (Tokyo). 2001 Dec; 30(1-2):223-8.

250. Nedley N. Proof Positive: How to Reliably Combat Disease and Achieve Optimal Health Through Nutrition and Lifestyle, Nedley Publishing 1999, Chapter 9

251. Manchester LC, Tan DX, Reiter RJ, Park W, Monist K,Qi W., High levels of melatonin in the seeds of edible plants: possible function in germ tissue protection., Life Sci. 2000 Nov 10;67(25):3023-9

252. Reiter RJ, Manchester LC, Tan DX. Melatonin in walnuts: influence on levels of melatonin and total antioxidant capacity of blood. Nutrition. 2005 Sep; 21(9):920-4

253. Colpo A. 164

254. Lee CO, Complementary and alternative medicines patients are talking about: melatonin.,Clin J Oncol Nurs. 2006 Feb;10(1):105-7

255. Nedley N. 68

256. Chen CY, Milbury PE, Lapsley K, Blumberg JB. Flavonoids from almond skins are bioavailable and act synergistically with vitamins C and E to enhance hamster and human LDL resistance to oxidation. J Nutr. 2005 Jun; 135(6):1366-73

257. Hanna Kroeger H. 64

258. Schmid 100

259. Colpo A. 126

260. Kritchevsky D., Cholesterol vehicle in experimental atherosclerosis. A brief review with special reference to peanut oil. Arch Pathol Lab Med. 1988 Oct; 112(10):1041-4

261. Fallon S. 563 513

Chapter 30

262. Stone M. 184

263. Grisanti R. How to Really Lose Weight After 40, third edition, ebook, Busatti Corporation, 2006 Chapter(s) 12

264. Meyer, et al. Interval vs. continuous exercise training after coronary bypass surgery: A comparison of training-induced acute reactions with respect to the effectiveness of the exercise methods. Clin Cardiol. Dec, 1990 :851-61.

265. Inbar O, Skinner JS, Bar-Or O. The Wingate Anaerobic Test, Human Kinetics, 1996, 1

266. Lunde, et al Skeletal muscle fatigue in normal subjects and heart failure patients. Is there a common mechanism? Acta Physiol Scand. 1998.

267. Lee IM, Sesso HD, Oguma Y, Paffenbarger RS Jr. Relative intensity of physical activity and risk of coronary heart disease. Circulation. 2003 Mar 4;107(8):1110-6.

268. MacDougall et al. Muscle performance and enzymatic adaptations to sprint interval training. J Appl Physiol. June, 1998

269. Burgomaster, et al. Six sessions of sprint interval training increases muscle oxidative potential and cycle endurance capacity in humans. J Appl Physiol. Feb, 2005

References

270. Rugnmo, et al. High intensity aerobic interval exercise is superior to moderate intensity exercise for increasing aerobic capacity in patients with coronary artery disease. Eur J Cardiovasc Prev Rehabil. June, 2004.

271. Parra J,Cadefau JA, Rodas G,Amigo N,Cusso R. The distribution of rest periods affects performance and adaptations of energy metabolism induced by high-intensity training in human muscle. Acta Physiol Scand. 2000 Jun; 169(2):157-65.

272. IBID

273. Robergs R.A, Landwehr R. The surprising history of the "HRmax=220-age" Equation. Journal of Exercise Physiology Official Journal of The American Society of Exercise Physiologists (ASEP) Volume 5 Number 2 May 2002

274. Kauffmann JM. 155 -160

275. Indoor Air Quality (IAQ), U.S. EPA and the U.S. Consumer Product Safety Commission, Office of Radiation and Indoor Air (6609J) EPA Document # 402-K-93-007, April 1995

276. New York Times December 24, 1972. Charles Atlas, 79, dies; Body-Building Pioneer

277. Helgerud J, Høydal K, Wang E, Karlsen T, Berg P, Bjerkaas M, Simonsen T, Helgesen C, Hjorth N, Bach R, Hoff J.,Aerobic high-intensity intervals improve VO2max more than moderate training. Med Sci Sports Exerc. 2007 Apr; 39(4):665-71

Chapter 31

278. Heil M, Eitenmuller I, Schmitz-Rixen T, Schaper W. J. Arteriogenesis versus angiogenesis: similarities and differences. Cell Mol Med. 2006 Jan-Mar; 10(1):45-55.

279. Tex Heart Inst J. 2004; 31(1): 47–60

280. Keith Brewer K. The High pH Therapy for Cancer Tests on Mice and Humans. Pharmacology Biochemistry & Behavior, v. 21, Suppl., 1, pp 1-5

281. Safian RD, Mark S. Freed MS, Cindy Grines C, The Manual of Interventional Cardiology, Physician's Press, 2001, 292

282 Safian RD, Mark S. Freed MS, Cindy Grines C, The Manual of Interventional Cardiology, Physician's Press, 2001, 287

283. Chronic Total Occlusions, Ron Waksman (Editor), Shigeru Saito (Editor), Blackwell Publishing, page 8

284. Flowcardia Inc, the manufacturer of the Crosser® CTO Recanalization Catheter http://www.flowcardia.com/patient_cto.htm – viewed Mar 1, 2010 .

285 Chronic Total Occlusions, Ron Waksman (Editor), Shigeru Saito (Editor), Blackwell Publishing, page 104, Re-entry Technique – Pioneer Catheter, Nicolaus Reifart,

286. King SB, et al. A randomized trial comparing coronary angioplasty with coronary bypass surgery. Emory Angioplasty versus Surgery Trial (EAST). N Engl J Med 1994;331(16):1011-1050

287. Dr. Clyde Yancy, president of the American Heart Association, reported by Cristian Salazar and Maryilynn Marchione, Associated Press Writers Feb 12,2010.

288. Dr. Raj Makkar, director of interventional cardiology and the cardiac catheterization laboratory at Cedars-Sinai Medical Center in Los Angeles, reported in New York Times Feb 11 ,2010

Chapter 33

289. Ravnskov U. 207

290. Colpo A. 62-64

Chapter 34

291. Time Magazine Letters to the Editor Monday, May. 12, 1980

292. University of Maryland Medical Center web site http://www.umm.edu/altmed/articles/turmeric-000277.htm viewed Feb 19, 2010

293. Verma SK, Bordia A, Jain P, Srivastava KC, Antioxidant property of ginger in patients with coronary artery disease, South Asian J Prevent. Cardiol.,Volume 8 Number 4, October - December 2004

294. Yance D, Valentie A, Herbal Medicine, Healing & Cancer, McGraw-Hill , 1999, 218

References

295 Colpo A. The Great Cholesterol Con sec edition- ebook page 289

296. Enig M. 105,106

297. Enig M. 128, 129, 250

298. Enig M. 197

299. Manku MS, Morse-Fisher N, Horrobin DF. Changes in human plasma essential fatty acid levels as a result of administration of linoleic acid and gamma-linolenic acid. Eur J Clin Nutr. 1988 Jan; 42(1):55-60

300. Barre DE, Holub BJ., Chapkin R.S. The effect of borage oil supplementation on platelet aggregation, thromboxane B_2, prostaglandin E_1 and E_2 formation. Nutr. Res. 1993; 13:739-751

301. Keen CL, Holt RR, Oteiza PI, Fraga CG, Schmitz HH, Cocoa antioxidants and cardiovascular health, Am J Clin Nutr. 2005 Jan;81(1 Suppl):298S-303S

    Vita JA, Polyphenols and cardiovascular disease: effects on endothelial and platelet function, Am J Clin Nutr. 2005 Jan;81(1 Suppl):292S-297S

302. Gerster H, The use of n-3 PUFAs (fish oil) in enteral nutrition. Int J Vitam Nutr Res. 1995; 65(1):3-20.

303. Fallon S. 113

304. Fallon S. 25

305. Vasey C, The Acid-Alkaline Diet for Optimum Health: Restore Your Health by Creating Balance in Your Diet, Healing Arts Press 2004, 53

306. Schmid R. 100

307. Vasey C, 55

308. Colpo A. (first ed) 62-64

309. Groschel K, Ernemann U, Schulz JB, Nagele T, Terborg, Kastrup A. Stain therapy at carotid angioplasty and stent placement: effect on procedure-related stroke, myocardial infarction, and death. Radiology. 2006 Jul; 240(1):145-51

310. Langsjoen PH. The clinical use of HMG CoA-reductase inhibitors (statins) and the associated depletion of the essential co-factor coenzymeQ_{10}; a review of pertinent human and animal data.

http://www.fda.gov/ohrms/dockets/dailys/02/May02/052902/02 p-0244-cp00001-02-Exhibit_A-vol1.pdf

311. Moosmann B, Behl C. Selenoprotein synthesis and side-effects of statins., Lancet. 2004 Mar 13;363`(9412):892-4

312. Matthias Heil, Wolfgang Schaper. Influence of Mechanical, Cellular, and Molecular Factors on Collateral Artery Growth (Arteriogenesis),Circulation Research. 2004 ;95:449.

313. Heil M, Eitenmuller I, Schmitz-Rixen T,Schaper W. J. Arteriogenesis versus angiogenesis: similarities and differences. Cell Mol Med. 2006 Jan-Mar; 10(1):45-55.

314. Schaper W; Scholz D. Factors Regulating Arteriogenesis. Arteriosclerosis, Thrombosis, and Vascular Biology. 2003;23:1143

315. Schaper W, Buschmann I., Arteriogenesis,the good and bad of it, European Heart Journal (1999)20,1297–1299

316. Heil M, Eitenmuller I, Schmitz-Rixen T,Schaper W. Arteriogenesis versus angiogenesis: similarities and differences. J Cell Mol Med. 2006 Jan-Mar; 10(1):45-55.

317. Heil M, Schaper W. Influence of Mechanical, Cellular, and Molecular Factors on Collateral Artery Growth (Arteriogenesis), Circulation Research. 2004; 95:449

318. Summarized from: Buschmann I, Schaper W, Arteriogenesis Versus Angiogenesis: Two Mechanisms of Vessel Growth News Physiol Sci. 1999 Jun; 14:121-125.

319. Weis M, Heeschen C, Glassford AJ, Cooke JP. Statins have biphasic effects on angiogenesis. Circulation. 2002 Feb 12;105(6):739-45

    Skaletz-Rorowski A,Walsh K. Statin therapy and angiogenesis. Curr Opin Lipidol. 2003 Dec; 14(6):599-603

    Urbich C,, Dernbach E, Andreas M. Zeiher AM, Dimmeler S. Double-Edged Role of Statins in Angiogenesis Signaling, Circ. Res. 2002; 90;737-744

320. Available online http://www.nci.nih.gov/cancertopics/understandingcancer/angio genesis/allpages and http://www.cancer.gov/cancertopics/understandingcancer/angio

genesis
(accessed March 25, 2007)

see also Tumor angiogenesis and accessibility: role of vascular endothelial growth factor., Jain RK., : Semin Oncol. 2002 Dec; 29(6 Suppl 16):3-9

321. Folkman J. Tumor angiogenesis: therapeutic implications. N Engl J Med. 1971 Nov 18;285(21):1182-6.

322. Ferrara N. Role of vascular endothelial growth factor in physiologic and pathologic angiogenesis: therapeutic implications. Semin Oncol. 2002 Dec; 29(6 Suppl 16):10-4

323. Newman TB, Hulley SB. Carcinogenicity of lipid-lowering drugs. JAMA 1996; 275: 55-60

324. Duncan RE, El-Sohemy A, Archer MC. Statins and Cancer Development, Cancer Epidemiology Biomarkers & Prevention Vol. 14, 1897-1898, August 2005

325. Fallon S, Enig M. The Dangers of Statin Drugs- What you haven't been told about cholesterol-lowering medicines. Viewed at http://www.westonaprice.org/moderndiseases/statin.html

326. Arbiser JL, Klauber N, Rohan R, et al. Curcumin is an in vivo inhibitor of angiogenesis. Mol Med. 1998;4(6):376-383.

327. Alber HF, et al. Effect of atorvastatin on peripheral endothelial function and systemic inflammatory markers in patients with stable coronary artery disease. Wien Med Wochenschr. 2007 Feb; 157(3-4):73-78

O'Driscoll G, Green D, Taylor RR. Simvastatin, an HMG-coenzyme A reductase inhibitor, improves endothelial function within 1 month. Circulation. 1997 Mar 4;95(5):1126-31.

328. Taneva E, Borucki K, Wiens L, Makarova R,Schmidt-Lucke C, Luley C, Westphal S. Early effects on endothelial function of atorvastatin 40 mg twice daily and its withdrawal, Am J Cardiol. 2006 Apr 1;97(7):1002-6.

329. Matsunaga T, Warltier DC, Weihrauch DW, Moniz M, Tessmer J, Chilian WM. Ischemia-Induced Coronary Collateral Growth Is Dependent on Vascular Endothelial Growth Factor and Nitric Oxide, Circulation. 2000; 102:3098

330. Ii M, Losordo DW. Statins and the endothelium. Vascul Pharmacol. 2007 Jan; 46(1):1-9.

331. Stefanie Dimmeler, et al. HMG-CoA reductase inhibitors (statins) increase endothelial progenitor cells via the PI 3-kinase/Akt pathway J Clin Invest. 2001 August 1; 108(3): 391–397.

Llevadot J et al, HMG-CoA reductase inhibitor mobilizes bone marrow–derived endothelial progenitor cells J Clin Invest. 2001 August 1; 108(3): 399–405

Vasa M, Fichtlscherer S, Adler K, Aicher A, Martin H,. Zeiher AM, Dimmeler S. Increase in Circulating Endothelial Progenitor Cells by Statin Therapy in Patients With Stable Coronary Artery Disease *Circulation.* 2001; 103:2885

332. Pourati, Isaac et al. Statin Use Is Associated with Enhanced Collateralization of Severely Diseased Coronary Arteries. American Heart Journal, November 2003, Volume 146, Number 5, Pages 876-881.

333. Dincer I, Ongun A, Turhan S, Ozdol C, Kumbasar D, Erol C. Association between the dosage and duration of statin treatment with coronary collateral development. Coron Artery Dis. 2006 Sep;17(6):561-5

334. Forte A, Cipollaro M, Cascino A, Galderisi U. Pathophysiology of stem cells in restenosis. Histol Histopathol. 2007 May; 22(5):547-57

335. Wahl P, Bloch W, Schmidt A. Exercise has a Positive Effect on Endothelial Progenitor Cells, which Could be Necessary for Vascular Adaptation Processes Int J Sports Med: DOI: 10.1055/s-2006-924364

336. Heil M, Schaper W. Insights into pathways of arteriogenesis. Curr Pharm Biotechnol. 2007 Feb;8(1):35-42

337. Schaper W. Scholz D. Factors Regulating Arteriogenesis, Arteriosclerosis, Thrombosis, and Vascular Biology. 2003 ;23:1143.

338. Colpo A. 166, 167

339. Prior BM, Lloyd PG, Ren J, Li Z, Yang HT, Laughlin MH, Terjung RL Arteriogenesis: role of nitric oxide., Endothelium. 2003; 10(4-5):207-16.

340. CNN News - Sharon heart operation set for Thursday Sunday, January 1, 2006

References

341. Law MR, Wald NJ, Rudnicka AR, Quantifying effect of statins on low density lipoprotein cholesterol, ischaemic heart disease, and stroke: systematic review and meta-analysis.BMJ. 2003 Jun 28;326(7404):1423

342. Heil M, Schaper W, Influence of Mechanical, Cellular, and Molecular Factors on Collateral Artery Growth (Arteriogenesis) Circulation Research. 2004; 95:449.

343. IBID

    Tuttle JE et al. VZ Shear level influences resistance artery remodeling:wall dimensions,cell density,and eNOS expression. *Am J Physiol Heart Circ Physiol* 281:H1380–H1389,2001

344. Laufs U, et al. Running exercise of different duration and intensity: effect on endothelial progenitor cells in healthy subjects. Eur J Cardiovasc Prev Rehabil. 2005 Aug; 12(4):407-14

345. Hill JM,Zalos G,Halcox JP, Schenke WH, Waclawiw MA, Quyyumi AA, Finkel T. Circulating endothelial progenitor cells, vascular function, and cardiovascular risk..N Engl J Med. 2003 Feb 13;348(7):593-600

    Werner N. Circulating endothelial progenitor cells and cardiovascular outcomes. N Engl J Med. 2005 Sep 8;353(10):999-1007

346. Parra J,Cadefau JA, Rodas G,Amigo N,Cusso R. The distribution of rest periods affects performance and adaptations of energy metabolism induced by high-intensity training in human muscle. Acta Physiol Scand. 2000 Jun; 169(2):157-65.

    Grisanti R. How to REALLY Lose Weight After 40 Sec edition – ebook, 2005, chapter 12

347. Colpo A. 103

348. Batmanghelidj,F, Your Body's Many Cries for Water, Global Health   Solutions, 2004, 160-162

    Stone M. 132-135, 138

Chapter 35

349. UN General Assembly- in December 1948 and came into effect in January 1951

350. Nytimes December 4, 2006 End of Drug Trial Is a Big Loss for Pfizer

351. American Heart Association, 2007 update at-a-glance- Our guide to current statistics and the supplement to our "Heart and Stroke Facts" Update: Chapter 2 e73

352. Centers for Disease Control and Prevention, National Center for Health Statistics, Leading Causes of Death, 1900-1998, 67

353. Id at 44

354. C.G. Grulee et al, Breast and Artificial Feeding, Journal of the American Medical Association Sept 1934, 103(10):735

355. Douglass WC. 157

356. Id at 155, 158

357. Id at 152

Chapter 36

358. Fuster V et al. 7

Chapter 37

359 Golomb BA, Kane T, Dimsdale JE. Severe irritability associated with statin cholesterol-lowering drugs. QJM. 2004 Apr;97(4):229-35

About the author

Mike Stone grew up in Baltimore, Maryland and graduated from the University of Maryland with a bachelor's degree in Business and Public Administration. He immigrated to Israel in 1975.

In the early 80's Mike made a career change with a practical engineering degree in computer programming. After a long stint as senior systems analyst and programmer at Israel Military Industries, he made the transition to the emerging Internet field, and for eight years served as the site webmaster of a major governmental website.

Married for over 20 years, Mike and Esty live on the outskirts of Jerusalem with their four kids, Lambchop (family dog), Nivi (the cat), and a whole bunch of Nivi's relatives and friends who pop over at snack time...............